WHAT DO THESE PEOPLE HAVE IN COMMON?

- A 40-year old reporter loses his ability to write, falls when he attempts to walk, and becomes so confused that his wife suspects early-onset Alzheimer's …

- A beautiful, normal eight-month-old baby gradually loses her speech, stops responding to her parents and eventually can't even sit up by herself …

- A 20-year-old woman becomes severely depressed and attempts to kill herself …

- A ballet dancer undergoes cosmetic surgery and ends up nearly unable to walk …

- A 69-year-old woman develops balance problems, falls and fractures her hip …

- A 38-year-old woman condemned to life in a wheelchair after gastric bypass surgery …

- An 86-year-old man becomes delusional and kills his wife …

- A 54-year-old woman experiences paranoid delusions and violent outbursts, coupled with symptoms her doctor diagnoses as multiple sclerosis …

- A 4-year-old boy is diagnosed with autism …

- A 73-year-old whose doctors attribute his repeated falls to old age or possible "mini-strokes" …

- A young woman unable to conceive …

- A grandfather transforms, in less than a year, from a healthy jogger to a depressed, confused man diagnosed with senile dementia.

Here's what these patients don't have in common: a correct diagnosis. Instead they have a plethora of incorrect, often hopeless diagnoses: developmental disability, autism, multiple sclerosis, psychosis, senile dementia, transient ischemic attacks, depression or diabetic neuropathy. But, in reality, they all suffer from the same medical condition …

VITAMIN B$_{12}$ DEFICIENCY

"Vitamin B_{12} deficiency is an epidemic causing more health damage than the polio epidemic and it can now be prevented through simple screening and treatment."

—**Sally M. Pacholok, R.N., B.S.N.**

"Sally Pacholok, R.N., B.S.N., and Jeffrey Stuart, D.O., authors of the *Could It Be B₁₂?*, are to be congratulated for calling attention to this common disorder that affects a significant proportion of the population, particularly among the elderly. I enjoyed reading this book and was impressed by the thoroughness of their documentation. The citations to the medical literature and the detailed information in the appendices support the main conclusions of the book. The authors are correct that deficiency of vitamin B_{12} is often under diagnosed and under treated by the medical profession.

America must understand that finding the underlying cause of disease, like B_{12} deficiency, threatens the power structure of the medical establishment. Diagnosing B_{12} deficiency and treating patients with B_{12} calls into question the practice of giving drugs that suppress symptoms of disease without addressing the underlying cause. Part of the motivation is competition for subjects with vitamin B_{12} deficiency, who would be lost as prospective patients if they were treated with inexpensive and effective vitamin therapy. The news media are not interested in effective vitamin therapy, partly because of the financial support of the pharmaceutical industry to the media through lucrative advertisements.

I recommend this book to professionals and patients alike who are interested in finding the underlying cause and cure of many common diseases and conditions related to deficiency of vitamin B_{12}."

—**Kilmer S. McCully, M.D.**, author of *The Homocysteine Revolution* and *The Heart Revolution* and winner of the 1998 Functional Medicine Linus Pauling Award

COULD IT BE B$_{12}$?
An Epidemic of Misdiagnoses

Second Edition

Sally M. Pacholok, R.N., B.S.N.
Jeffrey J. Stuart, D.O.

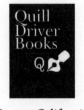

Fresno, California

Could It Be B$_{12}$? Second Edition
Copyright © 2011 by Sally M. Pacholok and Jeffrey J. Stuart.
All rights reserved.

Published by Quill Driver Books,
an imprint of Linden Publishing
2006 South Mary, Fresno, California 93721
559-233-6633 / 800-345-4447
QuillDriverBooks.com

Quill Driver Books and Colophon are trademarks of
Linden Publishing, Inc.

ISBN 978-1-884995-69-9

3579864

Printed in the United States of America
on acid-free paper.

Library of Congress Cataloging-in-Publication Data
Pacholok, Sally M., 1963-
  Could it be B12? : an epidemic of misdiagnoses / Sally M. Pacholok, Jeffrey J. Stuart,. -- 2nd ed.
      p. cm.
  Includes bibliographical references and index.
  ISBN 978-1-884995-69-9 (pbk. : alk. paper)
  1. Vitamin B12 deficiency--Popular works. I. Stuart, Jeffrey J., 1965- II. Title.
  RC627.V55P33 2011
  615'.328--dc22

                              2010050579

Acknowledgments

We would especially like to thank the many dedicated scientists, researchers, and clinicians who have contributed a vast amount of medical literature over the last century regarding cobalamin (vitamin B_{12}) deficiency.

We are very grateful to Stephen Blake Mettee, Kent Sorsky, and Jaguar Bennett from Quill Driver Books, who recognized the importance of making the public aware of this crucial health issue and enabled us to make this book a reality. Special thanks also to Alison Blake for her hard work and good humor in the face of innumerable changes and additions of new research in both editions of the book.

We are indebted as well to the late Dr. Bernard Rimland for his invaluable support and encouragement. Spiritual thanks go to Tracy M. Weick, whose friendship and warmth over the past 30 years are beyond what even a sister could envision. Eternal thanks to Susan Peacock from England, who brought Dr. Joseph Chandy and us together to work on this special assignment in life. Private thanks to Alice Vandemergle, Teddy Harasymiw, Anna Dutko, Anna Pijanowska, Sue Harvey, Grace Izzi, Richard Nimbach, D.O., Karen Balaska-O'Donnell, R.N., Patricia Quaine McDonnell, R.N., and Larry Slabosz.

This book is dedicated to all those who are presently suffering, have suffered, are injured, disabled, institutionalized, or have died because of the continued ignorance and misdiagnosis of vitamin B_{12} deficiency.

In memory of and for my parents
Andrew William Pacholok and Anna June Nykiforuk-Pacholok
Without your deep love, support, and early teachings of responsibility, ethics, and humanity, this book would never be a reality.

For our world-wide B_{12} advocates and "B_{12} Buddies"
The Groover Family, Joseph Chandy, M.D., Hugo Minney, Ph.D., Martyn Hooper, Joshua Luckasavitch, Pat Kornic, Linda and Ken Woolcock, Margaret Venske, Helen Kosy, Eric Norman, Ph.D., Glenn Medina, Kelly Genzlinger, Robin Gould, Susan Stuart, Peggy Demmin, John Leone, Norbert Biebuyck, Rick Solecki, John Dommisse, M.D., Kathy Reichenbach, R.N., B.S.N., Barb Darga, R.N., Wasyl Schumylowych, M.S., R.D., David Carr, M.D., Charles Liu, R. Ph., M.B.A., Richard Reidy, D.O., Joseph Flynn, D.O., Brian Liska, D.O., Elissa Leonard, Kimberley Epton, Charles A. Bentley, Jr., J.D. Michael Mattingly, D.O., and Michael Kitto, D.O.

In memory of B_{12} Advocates and B_{12} Buddies:
Dale and Charlene Back
Joannes Dutko, D.D.S.
W. Michael Forgette, D.D.S.
John Hotchkiss, M.D.
Connie Lamb, R.N.
Milton and Jean Lute
Jim Mundy
Bernard Rimland, Ph.D.
Mary Stuart

Sometimes it takes a group of individuals afflicted with a disease to make positive change, create awareness, and become advocates for others who are suffering.

"When justice is done, it brings joy..." Proverbs 21:15

Please note: The names of patients mentioned in this book have been changed to respect patient confidentiality.

Contents

Foreword

Recently, at a European conference where both Sally Pacholok and I were speakers, I conveyed to the delegates how much I value this book by stating that wherever I travel, two books always accompany me.

One is the Holy Bible. The other is Sally's book, *Could It Be B₁₂?*

Could It Be B₁₂? speaks only the truth, and in doing so it "gives life back" to those with B_{12} deficiency who were well on their way to losing their lives altogether.

The authors, Sally M Pacholok, R.N., and Jeffrey J Stuart, D.O., have committed themselves to this noble cause. They have made this book an invaluable resource for medical students, practicing physicians, and other healthcare professionals. And while it is written in a scientific and highly professional manner, Sally and Jeffrey have succeeded in making the book clear and simple enough to be useful to B_{12} deficiency patients, their families, and friends.

It is unfortunate that despite all the up-to-date evidence that is now available, the medical profession as a whole are taught to believe that B_{12} deficiency only affects the hemopoeitic system—in other words, that it is simply a blood disorder causing anemia and producing megaloblastic (pernicious) red blood cells in the marrow.

What Sally and Jeffrey have accomplished in this remarkable book is to establish the opposite. B_{12} deficiency is a multi-system, polyglandular, multi-point metabolic poisonous (homocysteine) disease/syndrome.

Sally's interest in this problem began in 1985, when she herself was misdiagnosed time after time, in spite of typical megaloblastosis and a strong family history clearly indicative of B_{12} deficiency. This prompted Sally, an emergency room nurse, and her husband, Jeffrey, an emergency medicine physician, to conduct their own research, as well as to gather, analyze, and collate numerous supporting papers published by reputable universities and well-known researchers.

Since I read *Could It Be B$_{12}$?* in 2005, five quotations from the book keep coming back to me. I wondered why. Then l realized that l am also enduring the same burden as Sally and Jeffrey, since I stumbled on my first case of B$_{12}$ deficiency in 1981. Since that time, I have been diagnosing, treating, and continually monitoring over 1,000 B$_{12}$-deficient patients—in other words, 18% of my practice population, as opposed to the 0.01% nationally diagnosed.

The five striking quotes from the book:

"Noted physicians had fought the battle to bring the B$_{12}$ deficiency epidemic to light and had lost. What chance did l have of making a difference?"

"An epidemic is raging, invisible to the public and virtually undetected by medical professionals."

"But l could not come to terms with the continuing parade of lives ruined by failure to detect and treat a simple-to-identify, simple-to-treat, simple-to-cure disorder."

"This is one of the most preventable and most curable of all medical scourges, but only if we choose to act."

"Together, we can stop this epidemic in its tracks."

I ask myself why the crucial evidence-based knowledge outlined in this book is not accepted, and why the diagnosis and treatment of B$_{12}$ deficiency is not part of mainstream practice throughout all the continents.

Is there a deliberate conspiracy to suppress and discredit this knowledge and the people who have been battling to bring this to the world's attention? Who is currently profiting from blocking this simple, innocuous treatment of a vitamin deficiency? This treatment can save patients from a miserable existence which eventually leads to a slow, painful, and premature death. Caring for these patients during their often prolonged course of illness costs governments billions of dollars, and relatives and friends time, money, and pain.

And yet, these are the alarming facts:

- The attention paid to B$_{12}$ deficiency by medical and government bodies is steadily decreasing, not increasing.

- Awareness of this condition is almost non-existent among the current generation of physicians and neurologists.

- Information about this deficiency disease is downplayed and even presented in a confusing manner in the most recent editions of reputable medical textbooks.

Even when clinicians know that they should be treating in accordance with good medical practice (investigate, diagnose, treat, and save lives), they are afraid to commence treatment because they lack up-to-date national guidelines. This results in worldwide misdiagnosis, mistreatment, untold misery, and tragic deaths.

It is a huge challenge to change entrenched medical ideas, even when these ideas lead to the death or disability of patients. It is an even bigger challenge when pharmaceutical companies make billions of dollars annually by promoting symptom-modifying drugs that merely mask symptoms of B_{12} deficiency and fight against those who seek a cure[*].

But Sally and Jeffrey, please do not get disheartened. We in the UK, and many others across the world, admire and love you and are most grateful to you both for your valuable contribution.

"Who so ever shall endure till the end shall reap the reward in due season."

Joseph Chandy (Kayalackakom), M.D.
UK National Health Service Medical Practitioner
2010 Glory of India Award winner for medical services to the community

---

[*] Alliance for Natural Health v. Sibelius court case, F.Supp.2d, 2010 WL 2110071 (D.D.C. May 27, 2010)

Preface to the Second Edition

More than half a decade has passed since we published the original version of our book. The response from the public has been overwhelming. We've touched more lives than we ever expected, and in this new edition, we relate the stories of people—young and old—whose B_{12} deficiency diagnoses saved their health and even their lives. We will also update you on the latest research, new case studies in the medical literature, and the best tests and treatments.

Sadly, the response from many in the medical community has been apathy or even outright hostility.

We have been actively educating the public and health care professionals about vitamin B_{12} deficiency and its frequent misdiagnosis for more than ten years. In 2005, we wrote the first edition of *Could It Be B_{12}?* Four years later, we declared 2009 as the Year of B_{12} Awareness, trying to get health care professionals and governmental agencies to support our efforts and recognize the fourth week in September as B_{12} Awareness Week annually. Our efforts are making slow progress, but we are not yet winning the war on misdiagnosed vitamin B_{12} deficiency.

Not only is most of the health care community still apathetic about this disorder, but so are the government, the media, and the insurance industry—despite the fact that untreated B_{12} deficiency can cause serious health problems, injury, disability, and even premature death.

There is a pattern of ignorance and accepted neglect regarding vitamin B_{12} deficiency that must change. Unfortunately, the only avenue may be the courtroom. Million-dollar malpractice settlements are now being awarded to injured B_{12}-deficient victims. But prevention is a far better solution for everyone.

Much is said about preventative medicine, but is it all so much hot air? Diagnosing B_{12} deficiency is simple and inexpensive, and treating it costs only a few dollars per month. Failure to treat this disorder at an early stage allows conditions to develop that often cause lifelong disability, re-sulting in enormous treatment costs or even death. After the release of the first edition of the book, we have reached out to the medical community, health care community, hospitals, and the government (including three Surgeons General, Congressional representatives from both parties, direc-tors of insurance companies, and Medicare officials). Yet overwhelm-ingly we encounter apathy. Hardly anyone cares and very few want to get involved, or are proactive in changing this system failure.

Yet there are small signs of change. In June 2009, for example, the Centers for Disease Control and Prevention—one of the most prestigious bodies in the field of medicine—issued a report stating that one out of every 31 people over age 50 is B$_{12}$ deficient. The number is much smaller than our findings, but the CDC's report is a step in the right direction.

There have been highs and lows since the first edition of *Could it Be B$_{12}$?* came out. The public response, in the form of letters and testimoni-als, has been astonishing. We *are* making a difference. A 10-month old baby was diagnosed in March 2006 with severe B$_{12}$ deficiency because the baby's grandmother read our book and gave it to her daughter-in-law to read. The family had the baby tested, and the results revealed he was severely B$_{12}$ deficient—a problem undetected by his pediatrician. You'll read this mother's triumphant story in Chapter 12.

Another bittersweet victory is that of the Groover family, whose night-mare we also detail in Chapter 12. Their child was severely injured by B$_{12}$ deficiency in 2001, and as a result, the Groovers have joined us in our B$_{12}$ Awareness campaign and are vocal B$_{12}$ advocates.

The Groovers wrote to their Governor, Bob Riley of Alabama, de-scribing their son's needless misdiagnosis and life-long brain injury. In response, Governor Riley assigned State Health Officer Donald E. Wil-liamson, M.D., to investigate what is being done in Alabama regarding vitamin B$_{12}$ deficiency and what the state might do in the future to alert their citizens and health care practitioners to this epidemic.

In August of 2009, Dr. Williamson directed his staff to develop and disseminate a B$_{12}$ Deficiency/B$_{12}$ Awareness press release to newspapers, public health clinics, the Women, Infants and Children (WIC) program, and the Health Provider Standards section of the Alabama Department of Public Health, which regulates standards for nursing homes. He also sent the release to the Alabama chapter of the American Academy of

Pediatrics, the Alabama Academy of Family Physicians, and the Alabama Hospital Association.

Governor Riley and Dr. Williamson are the first governmental leaders in the United States to address the problem of misdiagnosed B_{12} deficiency. This is exactly what politicians and people in power should be doing, but few are. We hope that Governor Riley and Dr. Williamson will be role models for other leaders to follow.

In 2009, Martyn Hooper, Executive Chairman of the Pernicious Anaemia Society (PAS) of the United Kingdom, joined forces with us and created U.K. B_{12} Awareness Week in the last week of October. Together with the PAS, we gathered in the House of Commons in London on October 28, 2009, to discuss this issue with Members of Parliament. On May 28, 2010, as a result of the ongoing work of the PAS, the Medical Director of the National Health Service (NHS) in Wales, Dr. Stephen Hunter, became involved and requested a review of vitamin B_{12} deficiency and its diagnosis and treatment by the National Institute for Health and Clinical Excellence (NICE) in the U.K. Dr. Hunter studied the PAS website forum group, which contains hundreds of testimonials from patients who were misdiagnosed and are receiving improper treatment. We were pleased to learn that the first edition of our book helped to galvanize Dr. Hunter's resolve to get B_{12} deficiency reviewed by NICE. This is a major victory for those who suffer from B_{12} deficiency. We hope that NICE will approve the review and create new protocols that will impact patients worldwide.

On another positive note, in 2009 we became acquainted with Dr. Joseph Chandy, a general practitioner working with four doctors in the U.K. with a registered list of 5,700 patients. Little did we know that a seasoned clinician some 3,500 miles away and an ocean apart had been silently fighting the same battle as Sally had for so many years—and had shared the same motivation, passion, dedication, and persecution. Patients and fate would bring us together. Dr. Chandy has been treating patients with neuropsychiatric symptoms with or without macrocytosis, using B_{12} replacement, since 1981. In contrast to the national estimate that pernicious anemia only affects 0.01% of the population, Dr. Chandy finds that 18% of his patient population exhibit symptoms consistent with B_{12} deficiency and, perhaps more importantly, benefit from B_{12} therapy. On two occasions, each for more than 18 months at a time (in 2002 and 2007), B_{12} treatment was withdrawn from his patients at government insistence, causing untold and sometimes irreversible damage and suffering.

Dr. Chandy and his assistant, Hugo Minney, Ph.D. (himself a B$_{12}$ deficiency sufferer), are making tremendous changes in the U.K., fighting for their patients by writing letters to Parliament, assisting the PAS, writing academic papers for publication, and assembling evidence for submission to regulatory bodies in the U.K. Hugo authors the B$_{12}$ Deficiency Patient Support Group web site (www.B12d.org), which gives valuable first line advice to thousands of people worldwide.

On a low note, we ended 2009 with two tragic e-mails. The first was from a mother from the Midwest, telling us how her six-month-old baby began showing signs of developmental delay. Her daughter's pediatrician was aware of this but just continued to watch her closely. At 13½ months of age, the child was finally diagnosed with severe B$_{12}$ deficiency and began treatment in November 2008. Two years later, the child has improved somewhat, but it appears that she was diagnosed and treated too late and will suffer a permanent brain injury. The second e-mail was from a cardiothoracic surgeon who went to Harvard Medical School. He wrote in December telling us of his misdiagnosed and mistreated B$_{12}$ deficiency, which occurred in 2009 and has caused him neurologic injury.

Clearly, we are still not winning the war on B$_{12}$ deficiency—and we need your help. Who will be next in this insidious chain of ignorance, secrecy, and misdiagnosis? Who needs to be injured for this disorder to finally be recognized and diagnosed early? Will it take a president, a pope, a politician, a movie star, a TV personality, a newscaster, or a sports hero? What and who will it take for the world to take notice?

We need to address not just the medical community, but also insurance providers, legislators, and trial lawyers. As medical professionals, it goes against our grain to say this—but often only after prodding by the legal profession does any meaningful change occur in medicine. It takes a landmark case, and often several landmark cases, to get the attention of most physicians. Based on our decades of experience, as well as the experience of others, we are convinced this may be the only avenue for meaningful change. And change must happen, because millions of lives and billions of dollars are at stake.

At this moment, the Centers for Medicare and Medicaid Services (CMS) is taking action to improve the quality of care in hospitals and reduce the number of "never events"—preventable medical errors that result in serious consequences for the patient. The evidence you will read in this book clearly shows that undiagnosed and untreated B$_{12}$ deficiency, similar to "never events," is a condition that should never happen. Every day patients are walking in and out of health care institutions with undiagnosed B_{12} deficiency. Yet the ignorance, apathy, and severe knowledge deficit of the medical community allow this poor practice to occur hundreds of thousands of times each year.

Health care professionals and the public must band together to end this global epidemic once and for all. Along with Dr. Chandy, we envision the year 2012 as the year B_{12} Awareness becomes public policy and updated protocols for early diagnosis and treatment are created. We invite all health care professionals, along with the public, to join us in this mission.

In the United Kingdom, we are beginning to see the fruits of our labor. On September 25, 2010, Dr. Chandy received the highly prestigious Glory of India Award, honoring his lifetime of service in primary care and his work on vitamin B_{12} deficiency. Prime Minister David Cameron invited Dr. Chandy to a reception in Downing Street. Members of Parliament Priti Patel and Grahame Morris have written to Secretary of State Andrew Lansley requesting that the UK government investigate how B_{12} deficiency impacts patients, the National Health System, and employers. This is a major victory, and we are hopeful that their investigation will lead to the introduction of a screening program, updated protocols, and on-going research into the diagnosis and treatment of B_{12} deficiency.

In this second edition of *Could it Be* B_{12}?, we include more tragic stories and heartening successes from our own patient population, from readers who have contacted us, and from published case studies in medical journals. We also include a chapter with updated cost-effectiveness statistics that spell out even more clearly the billions of dollars that can be saved by addressing this invisible health crisis. It is our sincere hope that our second edition awakens many more health care professionals and consumers to this overlooked and devastating problem. To keep track of our progress and upcoming B12 Awareness events, please visit our website at **www.B12Awareness.org**.

Sally M. Pacholok, R.N., B.S.N.
Jeffrey J. Stuart, D.O.

Introduction

In 1983, I was the picture of health. I looked fit, I felt great, and I had no idea that a silent crippler lurked inside me, stealthily damaging my brain, nerves, blood vessels, and nearly every organ in my body.

Because of my medical training, however, I noticed small signs that something wasn't right, and I knew enough to be worried even when my doctors dismissed those signs as "nothing to worry about." I pursued the few clues that my potentially deadly disease left, eventually obtaining a diagnosis of pernicious anemia (an autoimmune form of vitamin B_{12} deficiency), and as a result I'll never suffer the terrible symptoms that this disorder can cause.

Millions of other victims of B_{12} deficiency—many of them also victims of doctors who mistakenly ruled out B_{12} deficiency with complete blood counts (CBC), or never considered the diagnosis at all—aren't as lucky. Some are infants and toddlers, left developmentally disabled for life. Some are young adults, mistakenly diagnosed as having multiple sclerosis or told, erroneously, that they are "incurably" infertile. Others are middle-aged men and women, tormented by balance problems, numb hands or feet, or mysterious shooting leg pains so agonizing that they can barely walk. Some are diagnosed with early-onset dementia or pre-Parkinson's disease in their thirties, forties, or fifties. Some are people so depressed that they try to kill themselves. Some appear to be full-blown schizophrenics. And still others are seniors living out their days in nursing homes because their doctors think they have Alzheimer's disease.

It's too late to completely reverse the symptoms of many of these people—but it's not too late to protect yourself, or the people you love, against a similarly tragic fate. In fact, it's extraordinarily simple to prevent or completely reverse the symptoms of B_{12} deficiency if the deficiency is discovered in time. But this condition isn't like other vitamin deficiencies, and simply taking a standard multivitamin pill won't protect you; instead, you need an accurate diagnosis and medical treatment. And getting a diagnosis isn't always easy, as I know from experience.

I had no idea that an invisible disease was attacking my body when I went for a pre-employment physical examination back in 1983, when I was just nineteen. The first clue came when the examining physician reviewed my blood tests and commented on my abnormally large red blood cells. (In retrospect, I may owe my life to the fact that this test came back positive. Many people suffer neurological damage decades before their blood tests become abnormal, and by then it's too late.)

"What kind of diet do you eat?" the doctor asked when he saw my results. When I said that I didn't like vegetables, he told me to eat more of them, dismissing my blood abnormality as merely a sign of a diet low in folic acid.

One month later, another doctor commented again on my large red blood cells, but concluded that my lab results were "insignificant." Like the first doctor, this physician sent me on my way, unaware that he'd just missed diagnosing a disease that could destroy my brain, cripple my body, or even kill me.

Two years later, in nursing school, I bought a manual describing laboratory tests and their meanings. In the section on "macrocytosis"—the medical term for unusually large red blood cells—the manual outlined two different problems, folic acid deficiency and B_{12} deficiency, which could cause this abnormality. Since I loved B_{12}-rich meat and didn't like folate-rich vegetables, I could see why my first doctor picked low folic acid as a likely culprit in my case. But I wondered why he'd never considered B_{12} deficiency as well, since most cases of B_{12} deficiency stem from malabsorption problems rather than diet.

Thinking to myself, "It can't hurt to be sure," I persuaded a doctor I worked with to order a serum folate and serum B_{12} level for me. That night, when I mentioned the tests to my parents, my father surprised me by saying that back in the 1960s my grandfather had been diagnosed with pernicious anemia—the most well-known, although not the most common, cause of B_{12} deficiency. My grandfather's first set of doctors thought he had leukemia and told my dad there was nothing more they could do. It wasn't until my father insisted he be transferred to Henry Ford Hospital in Detroit for a second opinion that he was correctly diagnosed and treated (although it took this second group of doctors nearly four weeks to do so!). So I wasn't completely caught off-guard a few days later when my own B_{12} test came back low. I started receiving B_{12} shots, grateful that I'd obtained a diagnosis before I suffered any symptoms.

But that wasn't the end of my story. Two years later, when I needed surgery, I mentioned my B_{12} deficiency and ongoing treatment to my surgeon. Skeptical because she thought I was "awfully young" to have this problem, she sent me to a hematologist, who dismissed the idea that I had a B_{12} problem, in spite of my earlier diagnosis and abnormal test results showing macrocytosis, low B_{12}, and abnormal Schilling's test. (In fact, the hematologist's chart notes, which I read surreptitiously at a later visit—a nurse's instinct!—suggested that I was merely a hysterical female, imagining problems that didn't exist.) I insisted he run tests anyway.

The hematologist had changed his mind by the time his office called me a week later, asking me to come in "right away." By then, the tests he'd ordered had revealed that I indeed had juvenile pernicious anemia. In fact, he exclaimed exuberantly, I was the youngest patient he'd ever seen with pernicious anemia in his twenty years of practice. I felt like a rare freak of nature. This time around, the doctor was friendly and informative and, I sensed, secretly relieved that I'd insisted he verify my earlier diagnosis. He certainly wouldn't have detected my problem on his own, even with all of the information I'd given him on my first visit, because that surreptitious glance at my chart showed that his suspected diagnoses *didn't even include* B_{12} deficiency.

In short, although I'd virtually handed this doctor my diagnosis, he nearly missed it. If I'd come to him without the benefit of my nursing training and my assertive and inquisitive personality, or without already knowing that I had a history of B_{12} deficiency, his failure could have injured or killed me—because, if I had passively accepted his initial opinion, I would have stopped receiving the B_{12} shots that saved my body from the ravages of pernicious anemia. And yet, in a way, I'm thankful to him.

Why? Because his disbelief led me to ponder an important question: How many other people suffer or die because their doctors don't consider the simple diagnosis of B_{12} deficiency? I was lucky because I had enlarged red blood cells—the easiest-to-spot sign of the problem—and a family history of pernicious anemia. Yet despite these red flags, this doctor, as well as others, missed the correct diagnosis. Studies from the 1980s reveal that, unlike me, more than a third of people with B_{12} deficiency never develop either enlarged red blood cells *or* anemia, meaning that their disease is invisible to routine blood tests. In addition, most have no known family history of B$_{12}$ deficiency. I wondered: Were doctors misdiagnosing such patients on a regular basis?

My curiosity developed, over time, into more than two decades of research on the scope of B$_{12}$ deficiency. I became an expert, reading every textbook and journal article I could get my hands on, and making connections with both clinical doctors specializing in B$_{12}$ deficiency and scientists involved in B$_{12}$ research. My husband Jeffrey, an emergency medicine physician, also conducted research to determine the percentage of B$_{12}$-deficient patients seen in his emergency department. What we learned about the prevalence of B$_{12}$ deficiency, the havoc it wreaks on the entire body, and the number of undiagnosed cases is alarming.

B$_{12}$ deficiency is very common—not just in seniors and middle-aged people, but even in teens, children, and infants. As many as 20 percent of people over sixty (and, according to one new study, 40 percent of seniors with severe mental or physical problems) are suffering, most of them unknowingly, from its ravages. Thousands of young children, teens, and young adults have borderline B$_{12}$ levels, below what's considered necessary to keep their brains functioning optimally. And millions of people labeled as having Alzheimer's, multiple sclerosis, early-stage Parkinson's disease, autism, learning disability, depression, bipolar disorder, vision loss, schizophrenia, diabetic neuropathy, and other severe and often incurable disorders could actually be victims of the easily diagnosable, treatable, and (in its early stages) completely curable problem of B$_{12}$ deficiency.

Initially I was tremendously excited by the extensive research proving that B$_{12}$ deficiency plays a role in so many seemingly hopeless problems. That's because this is a problem that's simple to fix. It's an inexpensive problem as well, with treatment costing only a few dollars a month or ten cents a day—pocket change, compared to the expense of other medical conditions. Thus, diagnosing and treating patients with B$_{12}$ deficiency could both reduce the pain and suffering of these patients and cut medical care costs—a win-win situation, in my opinion.

My excitement was short-lived, however, because most of the doctors I worked with didn't care about an epidemic of undiagnosed B$_{12}$ deficiency. They didn't care that the serum-B$_{12}$ test and other B$_{12}$ markers available to diagnose the problem weren't being used, or that the current lower-end range of "normal" for this test was inaccurate and misleading. They didn't care about the growing number of journal articles warning about the high costs, both to patients and to society, of doctors' rampant failure to identify this problem. Indeed, they accused me of "playing doctor," and they balked at ordering B_{12} tests for patients with clear signs and symptoms of the disorder. In September of 2000, I was forced by my employer to sign a document stating that I would not talk to patients or their families about B_{12} deficiency and I would "stop soliciting physicians to test patients." I was told, in no uncertain terms, to drop the subject, sign the document, or lose my job.

Their attitude didn't stem simply from the fact that I am a nurse, rather than a physician (although that didn't help). My husband encountered a similar level of apathy, even when he showed his colleagues study data revealing that large numbers of his own facility's patients suffered from undetected B_{12} deficiency. Later I learned that other physicians aware of the problem had encountered the same negative response from their own colleagues.

Faced with an impenetrable wall of apathy and, eventually, outright hostility, I slowly and quietly gave up. What else could I do? Those with the ability to diagnose and fight this disease chose instead to ignore it. Noted physicians had fought the battle to bring the B_{12}-deficiency epidemic to light and had lost. What chance did I have of making a difference?

My silent surrender lasted until the day I was asked to discharge a patient who'd been labeled by the preceding shift as a "frequent flyer," a "drug-seeker," and a patient who "doesn't want to go home." When I examined this woman and reviewed her laboratory results and medical history, I saw painfully obvious indications of B_{12} deficiency, evidence that even a first-year medical student should be able to recognize. I also noted the complete absence of any effort by her doctors to test her accurately for this problem during her numerous previous hospital admissions, or even to recommend such testing to her family physician. This sad and frightened woman had suffered for years from crippling and seemingly mysterious symptoms, *every one of which* could be explained by B_{12} deficiency, and yet no one had correctly evaluated her for the disorder. Instead, they'd simply labeled her as nuts.

She wasn't the first patient I'd seen dismissed by doctors who overlooked the signs and symptoms of B_{12} deficiency. In fact, she was only the latest in a long line of patients written off as hopeless by medical professionals who'd failed to diagnose a life-threatening and very common medical problem. Indeed, I'd seen far worse cases, including patients who were on the verge of death or in a permanent state of dementia as a result of undiagnosed B$_{12}$ deficiency. Each case broke my heart. But this time, as I wrote up the discharge papers for this woman who'd received no real help and no real treatment—only a condescending response from her doctors and nurses, a large hospital bill, and a possible death sentence—my anger hit critical mass.

I knew that my own health and life had hung in the balance years earlier, when doctors told me that my troubling lab test findings were "insignificant." Now, on a regular basis, I was watching other patients being sentenced to death or disability by the doctors they trusted. I knew that many of these patients would wind up back in our hospital some day with strokes, dementia, depression, fall-related trauma (fractures and brain injuries), the need for blood transfusions, and other problems stemming from undiagnosed B$_{12}$ deficiency.

I could no longer stand by and be a silent accomplice to an epidemic of apathy and non-diagnosis that is leaving millions of young and old patients crippled or dead. As a medical professional, I'd long since come to terms with the daily tragedy of lives ruined by diseases that can't be prevented or cured. But I could not come to terms with the continuing parade of lives ruined by the failure to detect and treat a simple-to-identify, simple-to-treat, and simple-to-cure disorder. Neither could my husband, a physician who finds it reprehensible to refuse a patient the couple of tests that could prevent nearly *every case* of disability or death due to B$_{12}$ deficiency.

This book was born out of our frustration and anger over these needless injuries and lost lives. But it was also born out of hope—the hope that we can help many current and potential victims of B$_{12}$ deficiency by putting this information in the hands of sufferers and their families, as well as in the hands of concerned medical professionals, the government, media, and the insurance industry.

If you are a medical consumer, this book will empower you to protect yourself and your family members, by helping you to identify loved ones at risk for B$_{12}$ deficiency, and to obtain a real diagnosis and real treatment before it's too late. And if you are a medical professional, we hope you will examine the compelling body of research reviewed in this book and make B$_{12}$ screening (*not* just inaccurate blood counts) part of your standard practice. The hundreds of studies we cite, published in major and respected medical journals, prove that few diseases are more prevalent, simple to diagnose, and easy to treat than B_{12} deficiency—and few carry such a high, yet entirely preventable, risk of deadly disease or infirmity.

Above all, the message of this book is that the suffering caused by B_{12} deficiency, an "invisible" problem so pervasive that it touches the lives of nearly every family in America, is *unnecessary*. We can stop this cruel disorder in its tracks before it destroys more lives. I dodged the bullet of B_{12} deficiency, and so can its other potential victims—but only if patients and doctors alike open their eyes to the scope of this hidden epidemic.

1

An Invisible Epidemic

A silent crippler stalks millions of Americans—and you may be one of them.

This crippler is a master of masquerade, striking different people in different ways. It afflicts one person with tremors, makes another depressed or psychotic, and causes agonizing leg and arm pains or paralysis in still another. It can mimic Alzheimer's disease, multiple sclerosis, early Parkinson's disease, diabetic neuropathy, or chronic fatigue syndrome. It can make both men and women infertile, or cause developmental disabilities in their children. Other times, it lurks silently, stealthily increasing its victims' risk of deadly diseases, ranging from strokes and heart attacks to cancer.

This medical disorder stems from a vitamin deficiency, but your standard multivitamin pill won't prevent it in many cases, and even some higher-dose oral formulas of this vitamin may not help. It's considered an "old people's disease" by doctors, but it can strike any person at any age, and it sometimes hits children the hardest.

The disorder I've described is vitamin B_{12} deficiency. If you develop this deficiency, it's easy to spot, easy to treat, and easy to cure—but only if your doctor diagnoses you before it's too late. Unfortunately, that frequently doesn't happen.

WHO ARE THE VICTIMS OF B_{12} DEFICIENCY?

The cases we'll describe in the pages of this book involve people of every age and from every walk of life: babies, children, young men and women, middle-aged people, and senior citizens.

Among them are the following:

- A thirty-five-year-old man who starts wetting himself, and who can no longer walk steadily or grip with his hands.

- An eight-month-old baby who loses her speech, stops responding to her parents, and eventually can't even sit up by herself.

- A twenty-year-old woman who becomes severely depressed and who attempts to kill herself.

- A grandfather transformed, in three months, from a healthy jogger into a depressed, confused man, diagnosed with senile dementia.

- A two-year-old child who exhibits severe developmental delay and is diagnosed with autism.

- A young woman unable to conceive a baby.

> **All of these very different patients have one thing in common: Their doctors have failed to properly diagnose them.**

- A fifty-four-year-old woman experiencing paranoid delusions and violent outbursts, coupled with symptoms that her doctor diagnoses as multiple sclerosis.

- An eighty-year-old man who develops balance problems, falls, and fractures his hip.

- A ballet dancer who undergoes cosmetic surgery and ends up nearly unable to walk.

- A middle-aged woman accused by her doctors of being an alcoholic and a "drug seeker" when she complains of intense, chronic back and leg pain.

- A seventy-eight-year-old with foot and leg numbness diagnosed as incurable diabetic neuropathy.

- A senior citizen whose doctors attribute his repeated falls to "mini-strokes."

All of these very different patients have one thing in common: Their doctors have failed to properly diagnose them. They've been labeled with a dozen different disorders, ranging from incurable diseases to hypochondria, but in reality, they all suffer from the same medical condition: vitamin B$_{12}$ deficiency.

This isn't a new or fad disease. In fact, you'll find it listed in the textbooks of any first-year medical student. It's not a rare disease, either: If you're over forty, you're at an elevated risk for dangerous B$_{12}$ deficiency,

How Common Is B_{12} Deficiency?

It's important to note that most of the studies mentioned below *underestimate* the prevalence of deficiency, because, as we'll explain later, many deficient people have "normal" serum B_{12} levels.

Tufts University researchers, analyzing data from the large-scale Framingham Offspring Study, found that *nearly 40 percent of participants between the ages of twenty-six and eighty-three* had plasma B_{12} levels in the "low normal" range—a level at which many people begin experiencing neurological symptoms. Nearly 9 percent had outright deficiency, and 16 percent exhibited near-deficiency. Remarkably, low serum B_{12} was as common in younger participants as in the elderly.[1]

Smaller studies report that 15 to 20 percent of seniors have a vitamin B_{12} deficiency.

A recent study found that 40 percent of hospitalized elderly patients had low or borderline serum B_{12} levels.[2]

Over 80 percent of long-term vegans who do not adequately supplement their diets with B_{12}, and over 50 percent of long-term vegetarians, show evidence suggestive of B_{12} deficiency (see Chapter 6).[3, 4]

In June 2009, the CDC reported that B_{12} deficiency is present in one out of every 31 people over the age 50.[5] What's more, this alarming statistic underreports the true incidence of B_{12} deficiency. That's because the researchers defined B_{12} deficiency as a serum B_{12} level under 200 pg/ml. It's well documented that many people whose serum B_{12} is between 200pg/ml and 350pg/ml have a vitamin B_{12} deficiency.[6, 7, 8]

and if you're over sixty, you have up to a 40 percent chance of having potentially dangerous low B_{12} levels. The lower your serum B_{12} gets, and the longer you have signs and symptoms, the greater your potential for injury and poor outcomes.

WHAT IS B_{12} AND WHY IS IT SO IMPORTANT?

To understand why B_{12} deficiency can hurt or even kill you, and why this deficiency is so common even in seemingly healthy people, it's important to know a little about what vitamins are—and why B_{12} is unique.

Your body needs thirteen different vitamins in order to stay alive and remain healthy. These tiny molecules participate in thousands of chemical reactions that build your tissues and organs, provide you with energy from the food you eat, clean the toxins from your body, protect you against infections, repair damage, and allow your cells to communicate with each other.

Your body can't make vitamins by itself, so it depends on you to provide them by eating the right foods. Some (the fat-soluble vitamins) can be stored; others, including the B vitamins, are water-soluble and need to be "restocked" every day. If you don't take in enough of a particular vitamin, your supplies dwindle, causing a marginal deficiency and, eventually, a deficiency disease such as scurvy (vitamin C deficiency) or beriberi (vitamin B$_1$ deficiency). The bigger the drain on your stores, the more serious the consequences will be—up to and including death.

Of the thirteen vitamins your body needs, one is vitamin B$_{12}$. It acts, in many ways, much like the other dozen vitamins. But in other important ways, vitamin B$_{12}$ is an oddity, and some of the quirks that make it different also make it harder for millions of people to get enough of it.

Among its distinctions, B$_{12}$ is the only vitamin that contains a trace element—cobalt—which explains its scientific name, *cobalamin*. Because B$_{12}$ is produced in the gut of animals, it's also the only vitamin that you can't obtain from plants or sunlight. Plants don't need B$_{12}$, so they don't produce or store it.*

To obtain B$_{12}$ from your diet, you need to eat meat, poultry, fish, eggs, dairy products, or foods fortified with B$_{12}$—or, if you don't eat these foods, you need to take supplements. However, even a diet high in B$_{12}$, augmented with a supplement, isn't sufficient for many people.

In fact, while the Institute of Medicine (IOM) reports that you need only a tiny amount of B$_{12}$ each day (two to four micrograms or about a millionth of an ounce), it's remarkably easy to become deficient in this nutrient. While deficiency often occurs in vegans or vegetarians who fail to take the right supplements, *the majority of B$_{12}$-deficient people eat plentiful amounts of the vitamin*—it's just that their bodies can't absorb or use it.

Why? Because to get from your mouth into your bloodstream, vitamin B$_{12}$ must follow a complex pathway, and a roadblock in any part of that

---

* In fact, as we'll explain later, several plants that some supplement manufacturers claim are high in B$_{12}$, such as spirulina and tempeh, actually contain "pseudo-B$_{12}$" analogues that block the uptake of the real vitamin, making it inactive.

pathway can cause your B_{12} levels to plummet. Here's a highly simplified explanation of this pathway:

1. The vitamin B_{12} in your food is bound to animal proteins, and first must be freed. To split the B_{12} and the protein apart, your body uses an enzyme called *pepsin*, which can be produced in sufficient amounts only if there is enough *hydrochloric acid* available in your stomach.

2. Your stomach also produces *intrinsic factor (IF)*, a protein that makes its way into your intestine to be available for a later step in the B_{12} pathway.

3. Next, other proteins called *R-binders* ferry the B_{12} into your small intestine.

4. In the intestine, *intrinsic factor* latches onto the B_{12} (with the help of enzymes called *pancreatic proteases*) and carries it to the last section of the small intestine, the ileum. The cells that line the ileum contain *receptors* that grab onto the B_{12}-IF complex, pulling it into the bloodstream.

5. In the bloodstream, another protein, *transcobalamin II*, carries vitamin B_{12} to the various cells of the body, and then transports the excess to the liver for storage.

> **The majority of B_{12}-deficient people eat plentiful amounts of the vitamin—it's just that their bodies can't absorb or use it.**

This complicated B_{12} metabolism process, far more complex than that for any other vitamin, can break down at any point. The most famous (but not the most common) breakdown in this process is pernicious anemia (an autoimmune disease), a hereditary disorder that once subjected its sufferers to physical and mental deterioration and eventually a terrible death. The disease occurs when the body fails to produce intrinsic factor, making the B_{12} consumed in the diet useless. In 1926, two doctors, George Richards Minot and William Parry Murphy, discovered that feeding half a pound of liver per day to their patients with pernicious anemia dramatically reversed their symptoms.* The physicians, along with Dr. George Hoyt Whipple (who had earlier found that

---

* Most of the people categorized as having pernicious anemia during this era may have actually suffered from other, more common, forms of B_{12} deficiency.

liver reversed pernicious anemia symptoms in dogs), won the 1934 Nobel Prize in medicine for their life-saving discovery.*

It is unknown whether people in the early twentieth century died from "pernicious anemia," which is an autoimmune phenomenon, or whether other causes of B$_{12}$ deficiency played a role. The bottom line is that even today, untreated B$_{12}$ deficiency, whatever its cause, can be "pernicious" or deadly.

A far more common cause of B$_{12}$ deficiency, especially in people over fifty, is a condition called *atrophic gastritis*, an inflammation and deterioration of the stomach lining. Atrophic gastritis reduces the secretion of the stomach acid that is needed to separate vitamin B$_{12}$ from protein—a problem often made worse by proton-pump inhibitors and antacids or other medications (see Chapter 2). In addition, older people have smaller numbers of the cells that produce intrinsic factor.

It's not just the elderly, however, who are at risk. People of any age who undergo gastric surgery for weight loss (gastric bypass), or have partial or complete stomach resections for other reasons, are also candidates for B$_{12}$ deficiency. This is because they lose the cells that produce hydrochloric acid and intrinsic factor. Intestinal surgery involving partial or complete removal of the ileum will also cause B$_{12}$ deficiency, because receptors needed for the absorption of B$_{12}$ are located in this area.

In addition, gastrointestinal disorders such as Crohn's disease (an inflammatory intestinal disease), enteritis, "blind loop" syndrome, or celiac disease can interfere with the absorption of B$_{12}$, even if it's broken down correctly by the body. So can alcohol and many medications, ranging from gastroesophageal reflux (GERD) drugs to ulcer drugs to diabetes medications. Exposure to nitrous oxide, either during surgery (including dental surgery) or through recreational drug abuse, can inactivate B$_{12}$. Toxins such as mercury interfere with B$_{12}$'s ability to cross the blood–brain barrier and reach the neurons where it's needed. And, a variety of inborn errors of B$_{12}$ metabolism, which we'll discuss in later chapters, can interfere with B$_{12}$ metabolism at any step from beginning to end. This is why people who say, "I can't be deficient—I take a vitamin pill every day" are wrong.

---

* Frieda Robshneit-Robbings, together with Whipple, discovered that a diet containing large amounts of liver cured anemia in dogs. Although she coauthored many papers with Whipple, he alone received the Nobel Prize for their joint work.

People who can't metabolize B_{12} from food often can't make use of it efficiently in pill form either, so many of the supplements on the market won't guarantee that you're safe. The National Institute of Health acknowledges that only about 10 mcg of a 500 mcg oral supplement (which is listed as 8,333% of daily value [DV]) is actually absorbed by healthy people.[9] And, if you're already B_{12}-deficient, the few micrograms of B_{12} you'll get from a standard supplement (6 mcg) will do as little good as trying to fill an empty swimming pool with a teaspoon of water each day. A person with B_{12} deficiency needs thousands, not just tens or hundreds, of micrograms of B_{12} every day—and in some cases, even people taking thousands of micrograms of oral B_{12} may benefit more by being treated with injections.

Some high-dose over-the-counter lozenges (containing more than 1,000 mcg of B_{12}) can be effective over time, but people who are severely deficient and have neurologic symptoms initially need to be treated aggressively with B_{12} injections (see Chapter 11). Since B_{12} symptoms eventually become irreversible, it's important to treat the problem

> **Most doctors frequently fail to diagnose people with B_{12} deficiency, mistakenly ascribing their symptoms to pre-existing conditions.**

quickly and aggressively. Patients can be switched to high-dose B_{12} lozenges afterward, but must be monitored by their physicians to assure that this route is effective.

WHY IS B_{12} DEFICIENCY EPIDEMIC?

Given the dangers of B_{12} deficiency, it would be natural to assume that doctors put the disorder high on their list of suspects when they see patients with weakness, dizziness, nerve pain or numbness, mental illness, falls, dementia, multiple sclerosis-like symptoms, chronic fatigue, infertility, or other medical problems that can stem from B_{12} deficiency. You'd probably guess, too, that they automatically screen children with developmental delays or failure to thrive to determine if B_{12} deficiency is to blame. And you'd assume that they routinely screen patients in the highest-risk age group of sixty and over, and especially patients with unexplained Alzheimer's-like symptoms.

These assumptions, however, are wrong. In reality, most doctors frequently fail to diagnose people with B_{12} deficiency, mistakenly ascribing their symptoms to pre-existing conditions, other diseases, aging, heavy drinking (even when patients deny this), or mental illness—and the results can be catastrophic.

A few years ago, a fifty-four-year-old woman named Rebecca arrived at the hospital in a near-coma after suffering a fall. The description on her chart was "unresponsive," but an equally accurate description would be "victim of an unresponsive medical system."

Why? Because throughout Rebecca's life, her body offered up clue after clue of her B$_{12}$ deficiency, but no one noticed. Her mother died at an early age of stomach cancer, a rare cancer in the Western world, but one that often targets people with pernicious anemia. Three of Rebecca's children died shortly after birth—also a red flag for B$_{12}$ deficiency. Rebecca received numerous blood transfusions over the years for anemia, but her doctors never discovered the cause of that anemia. She'd undergone a complete hysterectomy at a relatively early age, possibly as a result of abnormal cells in the cervix and uterus—also a phenomenon that can occur in B$_{12}$-deficient women. In middle age, she'd begun experiencing excruciating headaches, and she complained of left-side weakness and pains in her arms and legs. She also found it increasingly hard to walk because of her worsening dizziness, and she frequently fell. (The subdural hematoma—bleeding between the brain and the brain's lining—that doctors detected in the emergency room resulted from a fall and from repeated blows to her head over the previous few months, which occurred when she lost her balance trying to get into their truck.) In recent months, according to her daughter, Rebecca's memory and personality had changed. All of these problems—weakness, leg and arm pains, dizziness, loss of balance, mental changes—are classic symptoms that can occur when B$_{12}$ deficiency progressively damages the brain and nervous system.

The proximate cause of Rebecca's near-coma when she arrived in the emergency department was a subdural hematoma resulting from hitting her head in repeated falls. The real cause, however, was the dizziness, weakness, and imbalance that made her fall—problems that stemmed directly from her B$_{12}$ deficiency.

Rebecca was severely anemic and required multiple blood transfusions. Her serum B$_{12}$ level was very low and her red blood cells were very enlarged. (You'll remember that enlarged red blood cells are a classic sign of B$_{12}$

deficiency.) In addition, her platelets were dangerously low, which made it difficult for her blood to clot.

Doctors diagnosed Rebecca with pernicious anemia and a subdural hematoma. Before giving her blood transfusions, they ordered additional tests for B_{12} deficiency. (These tests measure levels of methylmalonic acid and homocysteine, explained later in this book). The test results came back several days later and were also grossly abnormal. Rebecca survived emergency brain surgery, but her hematoma enlarged dangerously afterward, and, as a result of the ensuing damage to her brain, she is now in a vegetative state and will never recover.

Rebecca's descent into a permanent coma at the age of only fifty-four, as a result of chronically misdiagnosed vitamin B_{12} deficiency, is a tragedy and unacceptable. But it's only one in a string of tragedies resulting from her misdiagnosis. Rebecca lost years of her life to debilitating vitamin B_{12} deficiency, and it's a virtual certainty that all three of her babies who died at birth or in infancy were victims of her disorder, because Rebecca's depleted stores couldn't nourish them during pregnancy or breast-feeding. (The babies, too, may have suffered from an inherited—and easily detectable and treatable—form of B_{12} deficiency [see Chapter 6].) Simply by testing for B_{12} deficiency, Rebecca's doctors would have uncovered her problem, and early treatment would have prevented the damage her body suffered for years. Almost undoubtedly, a correct diagnosis also would have saved the lives of Rebecca's babies. But nobody ordered the tests because none of the physicians Rebecca encountered were knowledgeable about vitamin B_{12} deficiency.

As medical professionals, we see cases like Rebecca's on a regular basis. Most of the patients with undiagnosed B_{12} deficiency that we encounter aren't at death's door, but a few are—and the majority have suffered terribly, both physically and emotionally, from symptoms that are destroying their health and quality of life.

How can something as simple as a vitamin deficiency cause so much suffering? One explanation is that doctors receive surprisingly little training (much of which is outdated) in the diagnosis and prevention of B_{12} deficiency.

In general, doctors are trained to recognize only the *blood* abnormalities associated with B_{12} deficiency. In particular, they're trained to look for evidence of *macrocytosis*, or the presence of large, immature red blood cells, a classic sign of B_{12} deficiency anemia. (Anemia, which causes extreme fatigue and weakness, occurs when your red blood cells don't have enough hemoglobin—the substance that ferries oxygen throughout your body. "Macrocytic" or "megaloblastic" anemia, in which the red blood cells are enlarged, stems from too little B$_{12}$ or folic acid.) In addition, many doctors who treat severely anemic patients give these patients blood transfusions *before* ordering sensitive tests to rule out underlying B$_{12}$ deficiency. When doctors order these tests later, the healthy donor blood may mask the abnormalities in the patient's blood or make serum B$_{12}$ levels appear normal. Doctors who look only for classic blood abnormalities (macrocytic anemia) can misdiagnose the *neurological* abnormalities that stem from B$_{12}$ deficiency, including tingling or "pins and needles" sensations in the hands and feet,

> B$_{12}$ deficiency mimics many other diseases, so your doctor can't know if you're low in B$_{12}$ simply by analyzing your symptoms.

memory loss, depression, personality changes, dizziness and loss of balance, or even outright dementia. These nervous system symptoms often precede classic blood abnormalities by many years—and the neurologic damage that underlies them can be permanent by the time tests for the blood abnormalities traditionally associated with B$_{12}$ deficiency begin to come back abnormal.

Many doctors also fail to recognize that high levels of another B vitamin, folic acid (folate), can make the complete blood count (CBC) test results appear normal even when a B$_{12}$ deficiency exists. In 1998, new U.S. government rules mandated the fortification of grains with folic acid, increasing the likelihood of missing B$_{12}$ deficiency due to high folate levels, which normalize the size of blood cells that otherwise would appear enlarged. Enriching foods with folic acid is a good idea because it helps prevent spina bifida and related birth defects linked to low folic acid levels; but ironically, the same enrichment that protects many babies from harm also endangers other babies and adults whose doctors rely solely on a complete blood count to detect B$_{12}$ deficiency. New studies reveal B$_{12}$ is also essential to prevent spina bifida (see Chapter 6).

B$_{12}$ deficiency mimics many other diseases, so your doctor can't know if you're low in B$_{12}$ simply by analyzing your symptoms. Also, your doctor can't determine if you're deficient or not simply by ordering a blood count or smear (a test for anemia, enlarged red blood cells and abnormal white

Types of Tests for B_{12} Deficiency

Serum Vitamin B_{12} Test

Measures the level of vitamin B_{12} in your blood serum. There is much controversy as to what constitutes a normal result for this test (see discussion later in this box). Because of this controversy, this test is often used in conjunction with other markers of B_{12} deficiency (MMA, Hcy, and more recently the holoTC).

However, it appears that these markers demonstrate B_{12} deficiency primarily in patients whose serum B_{12} is in the "gray zone" (a serum B_{12} result between 200 pg/ml and 450 pg/ml). We believe that the "normal" serum B_{12} threshold needs to be raised from 200 pg/ml to at least 450 pg/ml because deficiencies begin to appear in the cerebral spinal fluid (CSF) below 550 pg/ml.[10, 11, 12]

At this time, we believe normal serum B_{12} levels should be greater than 550pg/ml. For brain and nervous system health and prevention of disease in older adults, serum B_{12} levels should be maintained near or above 1,000 pg/ml.

We commonly see patients with clinical signs of B_{12} deficiency who are not being tested. Others who are being tested are not being treated because their serum B_{12} falls in the gray zone. This error results in delayed diagnosis and an increased incidence of injury.

Moreover, of the total serum B_{12}, only about 20% is transcobalamin II—the biologically active form. The other two proteins (I and III) are thought to be inactive, but will be included in the total serum B_{12} result, yielding higher results and giving false assurance that a patient's B_{12} status is fine. This is yet another reason why the serum B_{12} lower end range must be raised. (See more below in the HoloTC test section.)

Methylmalonic Acid (MMA) Test

Measures the amount of MMA in the urine or blood. Elevated levels of MMA indicate B_{12} deficiency (see Chapter 11). According to Dr. Eric Norman of Norman Clinical Lab, Inc., MMA is 40 times more concentrated in the urine than in the blood, and the urinary MMA (uMMA) is the preferred test over the serum MMA. **The urinary MMA can be helpful in ruling out B_{12} deficiency, especially since our current lower limit range for B_{12} deficiency is much too low (typically less than 200pg/ml).** (See above.)

However, after reviewing past and present literature as well as thousands of patients' results over a ten year period, we believe it does not make sense to use the MMA test to identify B$_{12}$ deficiency when the serum B$_{12}$ can do the job in the majority of cases if doctors use an updated threshold (greater than 450pg/ml), along with a clinical exam. We often see symptomatic patients whose serum B$_{12}$ is low or in the "gray zone" and whose MMA is normal—and these patient often respond well to B$_{12}$ treatment. It would be dangerous not to treat these patients because their MMA is normal, or to wait for the MMA to become abnormal and the serum B$_{12}$ to fall further—resulting in poor health or worse yet, permanent neurologic injury.

Moreover, the serum MMA also has limitations and can cause false positives and false negatives. The specificity of these tests is debated.[13, 14, 15] We have seen symptomatic patients denied treatment because their serum B$_{12}$ was in the "gray zone" and their urinary MMA, serum MMA, and/or homocysteine (see next section) was normal, only for these patients to return many months later in worse shape and with tests showing deficiency.

In addition, MMA values can be normal in B$_{12}$-deficient patients receiving antibiotics, which can eradicate the intestinal flora needed to synthesize propionic acid.[16]

HOMOCYSTEINE (HCY) TEST

Measures the level of homocysteine in the plasma. Elevated levels of Hcy can indicate vitamin B$_{12}$, vitamin B$_6$, or folate deficiency. Hcy may also be elevated in a few other medical conditions (see Chapter 11). The Hcy test is not necessary to diagnose B$_{12}$ deficiency, but is a valuable adjunct to the serum B$_{12}$ test, because the higher your Hcy level, the higher your risk of cardiovascular disease (see Chapter 5). Patients with vascular disease should always have their Hcy, serum B$_{12}$, and RBC-folate levels measured to determine if B vitamin deficiencies are causing or contributing to their health problems. As with the MMA tests, we have seen many B$_{12}$-deficient patients with normal Hcy levels who were symptomatic and either had a serum B$_{12}$ level less than 200 pg/ml or were in the gray zone.

HOLOTRANSCOBALAMIN (HOLOTC) TEST

Vitamin B$_{12}$ in serum is bound to two proteins, transcobalamin and haptocorrin. The transcobalamin-cobalamin complex is named *holotranscobalamin* (HoloTC) or "active-B_{12}." Only around 20% of total serum B_{12} is in the active form our bodies use, and the HoloTC test measures this fraction. The test detects active-B_{12} or holotranscobalamin (HoloTC), which may be a helpful way of determining vitamin B_{12} deficiency. The test has been available for decades, but has been termed investigational until recently. Coverage for this test will depend on individual insurance policies. As with the MMA test, this test would most likely not be necessary if we raised the lower limit for the serum B_{12} test and used updated clinical exams. A group of researchers concluded that the HoloTC and the serum B_{12} test had equal diagnostic accuracy in screening for metabolic B_{12} deficiency. They found that both tests used in combination provided a better screen than either assay alone.[17] (See "Reference Ranges for Diagnostic Tests" on page 14 for ranges considered acceptable for these tests.)

As you read through all of these tests, remember this bottom line: If we simply raised the lower limit of serum B_{12}, the expensive and "presumably more sensitive" tests (MMA, Hcy, and holo-TC) would not be needed to diagnose B_{12} deficiency in the majority of people with this problem.

What we see is that when a patient is *severely* B_{12} deficient, typically all lab results agree with one another. The serum B_{12} is low, the MMA is elevated, and the Hcy is elevated. When these three laboratory tests all agree with one another, the patient has been B_{12} deficient for a long time and is being diagnosed in the later stages of B_{12} deficiency (in which damage often is permanent). This is why the current lower-end normal range for the serum B_{12} test must be raised, and why we need to educate clinicians that symptomatic patients with a serum B_{12} between 200pg/ml and 450pg/ml almost certainly have a B_{12} deficiency that must be addressed. We have seen cases of severe clinical B_{12} deficiency where the serum MMA was normal, the B_{12} was very low, and the Hcy was very high (renal function and RBC-folate levels normal). **For our part, we advocate treating all patients who are symptomatic and have serum B_{12} levels under 450pg/ml, regardless of what the MMA, Hcy, and HoloTC results are. In addition, we advocate treating symptomatic patients with normal serum B_{12} but elevated urinary/serum MMA or Hcy, and/or low HoloTC.**

> Also, be aware that when it comes to B$_{12}$ deficiency, many physicians tend to treat the paper laboratory report rather than the patient. Numerous times in our experience, a symptomatic patient's serum B$_{12}$ was between 200 pg/ml and 450 pg/ml and the doctor told the patient, "You do not have a B$_{12}$ deficiency." Given the remarkable safety of B$_{12}$ treatment and the horrific consequences of ignoring a deficiency, it is always best to err on the side of treatment.
>
> While raising the lower limit for B$_{12}$ is the most crucial step in accurate diagnosis, we also want to be clear that there are times when the additional markers for B$_{12}$ deficiency (urinary MMA, Hcy, HoloTC) are needed and may be useful. (You'll find more on this in chapters 3, 11, and 12).

blood cells [neutrophils] seen in some clear-cut cases of B$_{12}$ deficiency). **The major problem—indeed, the most important factor—is that most physicians fail to contemplate B$_{12}$ deficiency, are poorly educated about it, and therefore fail to test for it.**

Also, the serum B$_{12}$ test will uncover many cases of B$_{12}$ deficiency, but it's possible to have a B$_{12}$ deficiency and still have "normal" lab results because of the accepted normal range used in the U.S. and world-wide. Most doctors don't understand that a serum B$_{12}$ result in the gray zone (200 pg/ml-450pg/ml) can most certainly be a B$_{12}$ deficiency, and choose not to treat patients in this range or order additional B$_{12}$ tests (see box page 15). The accepted normal range, created many decades ago, is based on hematologic (blood) changes and not neurologic changes, and thus contributes significantly to late diagnosis.

The urinary MMA test described above costs insurance companies or patients around $150 to $256, which isn't much money, especially when you compare it to thousands of dollars for CT scans, MRIs, and other tests that doctors routinely order. Moreover, the MMA and Hcy tests are covered by insurance, but not all doctors know this. The unfortunate result of this lack of awareness is that many physicians forgo these tests in situations where they are indicated, and also forgo treating patients in the "gray zone" who are symptomatic, thus condemning these patients to ill health and unknowingly setting them up for neurologic injury and poor outcomes in the near future.

REFERENCE RANGES FOR DIAGNOSTIC TESTS

COMMON REFERENCE RANGES FOR THE SERUM B_{12} TEST

Serum B_{12}: 211–911 pg/ml
180–914 pg/ml
200–1,100 pg/ml

EXAMPLE SERUM B_{12} REFERENCE RANGES FROM A HOSPITAL WITH GUIDELINES *STRONGER* THAN THE RANGES ABOVE:

Deficient: < 200 pg/ml
Borderline: 200–270 pg/ml
Normal: 271–870 pg/ml

As you can see, a few institutions are making physicians aware that a serum B_{12} between 200 and 270 pg/ml is problematic, using the term "borderline." This gives a hint to the doctor that the patient's B_{12} needs to be higher.

Serum B_{12} Gray Zone: 200–450 pg/ml (We advocate B_{12} treatment in all symptomatic patients with serum B_{12} below 450 pg/ml).

Urinary MMA: < 3.8 µg MMA/mg creatinine
(3.6 µmole/mmole creatinine)

Serum MMA: 0.04–0.27 µmol/L or 40–270 nmol/L
0.07–0.40 µmol/L or 70–400 nmol/L

Homocysteine (plasma): 4.0–12.0 µmol/L

HoloTC (Active-B_{12}): 35–101 pmol/L (Specialty Laboratories in Santa Monica, California, currently performs this test)

Ironically, this misplaced concern over the expense of B_{12} testing costs the medical system far more than it saves, because B_{12} deficiency is remarkably simple to detect and even easier to treat. Patients treated in the early stages of the disease usually experience complete recovery, with even severe symptoms such as vision loss, agonizing leg pains, paralysis, multiple sclerosis-like symptoms, psychosis, and dementia often receding in months or even weeks. Moreover, unlike many medical problems, B_{12} deficiency is very inexpensive to treat. Treatment for one year involving bi-monthly injections and a series of six initial daily injections costs $36 per year when patients or family members administer the injections (which are similar to the insulin shots diabetics give themselves).

An alternate option, high-dose methyl-B$_{12}$ lozenges (2,000 mcg), costs around $48 to $72 per year depending on the brand used. Compare this to the cost of giving a depressed or demented patient with undiagnosed B$_{12}$ deficiency unnecessary antidepressants or dementia drugs, which can run over $1,000 a year—or to the cost of caring for a B$_{12}$ deficient patient misdiagnosed as having Alzheimer's, multiple sclerosis, or developmental disability, an expense that can run $60,000 a year or more for decades. The cost in human terms, of course, is far greater. There is no price one can place on the pain of individuals whose undiagnosed B$_{12}$ deficiency leads to severe, irreversible physical and mental disability. Here are a few examples:

In 2000, a fifty-year-old Illinois woman, Vicki Lambert, received a $3 million out-of-court settlement from two hospitals and two physician groups. Lambert charged doctors at each of these institutions failed to diagnose her B$_{12}$ deficiency, leaving her permanently crippled. She suffers from chronic painful neuropathy, uses specialized crutches to walk, and has irreversible cognitive deficits. She is unable to work as a nurse because of her disability and has moved to a one-story home because she could no longer go up and down stairs.

"Unless someone were in my shoes, you can't imagine," Lambert told a newspaper reporter. "I remember lying in bed and feeling death would be better because I was so sick."[18]

In a similar 1999 case, a sixty-four-year-old Georgia woman was awarded $3.1 million after a missed diagnosis of B$_{12}$ deficiency. The woman now requires a wheelchair as a result of permanent nerve damage due to her doctors' failure to identify her condition.[19]

In December 2007, the Toronto Sun *reported the case of a 12-year-old boy named J.J. who suffered great neurologic injury due to misdiagnosed vitamin B$_{12}$ deficiency. J.J. was in and out of the Hospital for Sick Children for more than eight months, slowly losing his ability to walk, write, and draw. J.J.'s neurologic status continued to deteriorate to the point where he needed a wheelchair, and none of his doctors could figure out why. He then became jaundiced, and his pediatrician worried that J.J.'s organs were shutting down.*

"I was watching my son dying in front of my eyes and no one would do anything," his mother said. "Later I overheard the doctors saying that when

we brought him in, he was close to death. He stumped everyone, he hit the medical history books because no one has been as bad as him."

J.J. didn't have a bizarre or rare disorder; he simply had vitamin B_{12} deficiency. Yet none of his doctors knew the signs or symptoms, despite J.J.'s classic presentation.[20] (More on J.J. in Chapter 6.)

Two cases of severe B_{12} deficiency were reported in Madison, Wisconsin, in the American Journal of Emergency Medicine *(2007). Both patients were diagnosed in the emergency department (ED) rather than by their primary care doctors or neurologists. Both had prolonged and progressive symptoms and "had had rather extensive outpatient workups without diagnosis." Their previous doctors and specialists never contemplated vitamin B_{12} deficiency as the cause of their progressive neurologic decline. The diagnosis was only suggested when blood abnormalities were found in the ED. These blood changes (severe anemia and macrocytosis) are very late signs of B_{12} deficiency.*

The first woman was fifty years old and presented to the ED complaining of progressive weakness and increasing numbness of her arms, feet and legs. Her serum B_{12} was critically low at 72 pg/ml, despite the fact that she was on a multi-vitamin. Her neurologic signs and symptoms were slightly improved at a one-week follow-up.

The second woman was twenty-five years of age and came to the ED complaining of increasing weakness. She had a six-month history of decline which led to her using a walker for three months. Later, she began to use a wheelchair because she was too unstable to use the walker. Her serum B_{12} was undetectable in lab tests, and she was severely anemic and required four blood transfusions. However, she was not macrocytic. Two months after starting B_{12} treatment, her sensory abnormalities improved, but her motor deficits were unchanged and she continues to use a wheelchair.

Prior to this woman's arrival in the ED, it was reported, her own doctors ordered tests including an MRI of her brain and spine and even an electromyogram (EMG). But they didn't contemplate or investigate vitamin B_{12} deficiency, even though her signs and symptoms were obvious as well as numerous. As a result, this young woman will have a life-long disability and her physicians may have a costly malpractice suit.[21]

How B$_{12}$ deficiency attacks the body

As you can guess from the cases we described at the start of this chapter, it's impossible to paint a simple picture of what B$_{12}$ deficiency looks like. When B$_{12}$ deficiency attacks the body, it takes many guises, depending in part on the age and genetic vulnerabilities of its victims, and the length and severity of the deficiency. Also, because B$_{12}$ deficiency is progressive, signs and symptoms may take years to develop. The following list outlines signs and symptoms that can stem from B$_{12}$ deficiency.

Note: If you have any of the following signs or symptoms, it does not necessarily mean that you have a B$_{12}$ deficiency. These symptoms can stem from many causes. However, it does mean that your doctor needs to rule out B$_{12}$ deficiency as a possible culprit.

Mental changes

- irritability
- apathy
- sleepiness
- suspiciousness (paranoia)
- personality changes
- depression (including postpartum depression)
- memory loss
- dementia, intellectual deterioration
- hallucinations
- violent behavior
- in children, developmental delay and/or autistic behavior

Neurological signs and symptoms

- abnormal sensations (pain, tingling and/or numbness of legs, arms, trunk, or other area)
- diminished sense of touch, pain, and/or temperature
- loss of position sense (awareness of body position)
- weakness (legs, arms, trunk, or other area)

- clumsiness (stiff or awkward movements)
- tremor
- symptoms mimicking Parkinson's disease or multiple sclerosis
- spasticity of muscles
- incontinence (urine and/or stool)
- paralysis
- vision changes (decreased vision or loss of vision)
- damage to the optic nerve (optic neuritis, inflammation, or atrophy of the optic nerve)

Vascular problems

- transient ischemic attacks (TIAs, or "mini-strokes")
- cerebral vascular accident (CVA or "stroke")
- coronary artery disease
- myocardial infarction ("heart attack")
- congestive heart failure
- palpitations
- orthostatic hypotension (low blood pressure when standing, which can cause fainting and falls)
- deep vein thrombosis (blood clot to the leg or arm)
- pulmonary embolism (blood clot to the lung)

Additional signs and symptoms

- shortness of breath
- generalized weakness
- chronic fatigue or tiredness
- loss of appetite/weight loss or anorexia
- epigastric pain (poor digestion, full or bloated feeling after eating small or normal sized meals)
- gastrointestinal problems (diarrhea, constipation)

- osteoporosis

- increased susceptibility to infection

- in newborns and infants, failure to thrive

- tinnitus (ringing or roaring in the ears)

- vitiligo (white patches of skin) or, conversely, hyperpigmentation of skin

- prematurely gray hair

Systems Affected by Vitamin B$_{12}$ Deficiency

Neurologic
Numbness, tingling, and/or burning sensation in arms, legs, or body, balance problems, difficulty ambulating, falling, weakness, tremor, paralysis, confusion, forgetfulness, dementia, depression, mental illness, psychosis, incontinence, impotence, headaches, vision loss.

Hematologic (blood)
Fatigue, weakness, anemia, shortness of breath, enlarged spleen or liver, enlarged red blood cells (macrocytes), hypersegmented neutrophils, ovalocytes.

Immunologic
Poor wound healing, increased susceptibility to infections, increased risk of cancer, poor antibody production after vaccines.

Vascular
Coronary artery disease, myocardial infarction (heart attack), pulmonary embolism (blood clot(s) in lungs), deep-vein thrombosis (DVT) of extremities, mini-stroke, stroke.

Gastrointestinal
Indigestion, abdominal pain, constipation, diarrhea, gastroesophageal reflux disease (GERD), gastric stasis, weight loss (in some people).

Musculoskeletal
Fractures, osteoporosis, suppressed activity of osteoblasts (cells that build new bone).

Genitourinary
Abnormal PAP smears, urinary incontinence, impotence, infertility.

It amazes many people that a single medical problem—B_{12} deficiency—can cause so many medical symptoms. But the reason is simple: B_{12} wears many hats, playing key roles in the health of your nerves, your brain, your blood, and your immune system, as well as in the formation of DNA (the molecular blueprint for making the substances that create and maintain your body). Thus, B_{12} deficiency can impair the functioning of almost any part of your body.

In particular, B_{12} deficiency often strikes the nervous system, causing damage to the soft fatty material called *myelin* that surrounds and protects nerve fibers. This damage (*demyelination*), which can be compared to the fraying of an electrical wire, can cause you to develop mysterious and frightening neurological problems, ranging from numb, tingling, or painful legs and arms, to loss of balance, vision loss, impotence, or incontinence. Because your brain and nervous system control your mental state, the demyelination caused by B_{12} deficiency can also lead to memory loss, "fuzzy" thinking, personality changes, depression, or even psychosis or dementia. In a child, the damage can be even worse, because the young brain is still forming and requires adequate B_{12} to grow normally.

> B_{12} deficiency can impair the functioning of almost any part of your body.

As B_{12} deficiency continues, your immune system also falls prey, because it can no longer produce enough disease-fighting white blood cells. Thus, you become an easier target for viral or bacterial infections. Your gastrointestinal system suffers as well, because your body can't make enough cells to replace your intestinal lining efficiently, so you may experience diarrhea, nausea, or severe appetite loss. And eventually, as your B_{12} deficit grows, you're likely to feel exhausted and weak due to the anemia that occurs when your body can't make enough healthy blood cells to carry oxygen to the cells of your body.

At the same time, B_{12} deficiency causes a breakdown in a crucial metabolic pathway that detoxifies the potentially dangerous amino acid homocysteine. As homocysteine accumulates in your blood, it dramatically increases your risk of coronary artery disease, stroke, and blood clots. If you become pregnant, high homocysteine levels will also make you more vulnerable to preeclampsia, a potentially fatal pregnancy complication.

If you're a woman, the blood abnormalities resulting from B_{12} deficiency may affect the lining of your uterus and cervix, causing cervical dysplasia (abnormal cervical cell appearance) that can be mistaken for a pre-cancerous condition. But B_{12} deficiency doesn't just mimic cancer warning signs; it also puts you at higher risk for certain cancers, whether you're male or female. Pernicious anemia, the classic form of vitamin B_{12} deficiency, is a strong risk factor for stomach cancer, and there is mounting evidence linking deficient levels of B_{12} to breast cancer, as well.

THE BAD NEWS…AND THE GOOD NEWS

So far, what we've told you is frightening. Millions of Americans and millions of other people world-wide suffer from undiagnosed B_{12} deficiency—and you may be one of them. If you are, this disease could be attacking your brain, your nervous systems, your cardiovascular system, and your immune system, putting you at risk for everything from Alzheimer's-like dementia to heart disease and cancer. You're not safe even if you get regular checkups, because your doctor may miss the correct diagnosis until it's too late to reverse your symptoms. And if you're a woman who is B_{12} deficient and you don't find out about your condition in time, even your children may suffer permanent damage to their bodies and brains.

That's the bad news. The good news is that if it's caught early, B_{12} deficiency is one of the simplest disorders in the world to treat. In fact, many formerly B_{12}-deficient people say that getting a diagnosis was the best thing that ever happened to them, because it meant that the "incurable" neuropathy, weakness, infertility, MS-like symptoms, depression, or other problems that afflicted them weren't untreatable after all. In this book, we'll share the stories of once-bedridden people who can walk again… people freed from excruciating leg and back pain… individuals cured of memory loss, depression, schizophrenic symptoms, and even dementia… people freed from the need for repeated blood transfusions for mysterious anemia… people able to conceive healthy babies after B_{12} treatment… and even developmentally disabled or autistic children who made almost miraculous gains after their deficient B_{12} levels were detected and treated. All of these individuals experienced dramatic improvement after undergoing the simplest and safest of treatments: a few shots (or, in some cases, pills) containing megadoses of vitamin B_{12}.

> The good news is that if it's caught early, B_{12} deficiency is one of the simplest disorders in the world to treat.

Who's at Greatest Risk for B$_{12}$ Deficiency?

Anyone, at any age, can become B$_{12}$-deficient. Thus, you need to be tested immediately if you develop any of the symptoms we've described in this chapter. However, certain people are at an elevated risk. They include the following:

- Vegetarians, vegans, and people eating macrobiotic diets
- People aged sixty and over
- People who've undergone any gastric and/or intestinal surgery, including bariatric surgery for weight loss purposes (gastric bypass)
- People who regularly use proton-pump inhibitors, H2 blockers, antacids, metformin and related diabetes drugs, or other medications that can interfere with B$_{12}$ absorption
- People who undergo surgeries or dental procedures involving nitrous oxide, or who abuse this drug recreationally
- People with a history of eating disorders (anorexia or bulimia)
- People with a history of alcoholism
- People with a family history of pernicious anemia
- People diagnosed with anemia (including iron deficiency anemia, sickle cell anemia, and thalassemia)
- People with Crohn's disease, irritable bowel syndrome, gluten enteropathy (celiac disease), or any other disease that causes malabsorption of nutrients
- People with autoimmune disorders (especially thyroid disorders such as Hashimoto's thyroiditis and Graves' disease), type 1 diabetes, vitiligo, lupus, Addison's disease, ulcerative colitis, infertility, acquired agammaglobulinemia, or a family history of these disorders.
- Women with a history of infertility or multiple miscarriages
- Infants born to and/or breast-fed by women who are symptomatic or are at risk for B$_{12}$ deficiency

Their stories are a powerful counterpoint to the horrific stories of patients who have suffered devastating injuries, years of poor health or terrible illnesses, and who have incurred huge medical expenses as well, due to the non-diagnosis or late diagnosis of their B$_{12}$ deficiency.

We want it to be perfectly clear at the outset of this book that B$_{12}$ isn't a "magic bullet." The symptoms we've outlined have many causes, and B$_{12}$ deficiency is only one of them. But patients and doctors need to be aware that B$_{12}$ deficiency often *does* cause these symptoms, and that doctors who fail to rule it out

> **Vitamin B$_{12}$ treatment is quite possibly the safest medical treatment on earth.**

or treat it may be condemning their patients to unnecessary debility or even death. Conversely, the brief amount of time and money required to identify B$_{12}$ deficiency is a small investment to make—and whether you're a doctor or a medical consumer, it may be the most important investment you'll ever make.

Note: Vitamin B$_{12}$ treatment is quite possibly the safest medical treatment on earth. However, one small group of people—those with a rare disorder called Leber's hereditary optic neuropathy—should never take cyanocobalamin, one specific form of B$_{12}$. Information about safe forms of B$_{12}$ treatment for these individuals is contained in Chapter 11.

Chapter 1 Notes

1. Study cited in "B$_{12}$ deficiency may be more widespread than thought," Judy McBride, Agricultural Research Service website, U.S. Department of Agriculture, August 2, 2000. http://www.ars.usda.gov/is/pr/2000/000802.htm.

2. Shahar, A., Feiglin, L., Shahar, D. R., Levy, S., and Seligsohn, U. High prevalence and impact of subnormal serum vitamin B$_{12}$ levels in Israeli elders admitted to a geriatric hospital. *Journal of Nutrition, Health and Aging* (2001) 5:124-7.

3. Crane, M. G., Register, U. D., Lukens, R. H., and Gregory, R. Cobalamin (CBL). Studies on two total vegetarian (vegan) families. *Vegetarian Nutrition: An International Journal* 1998, 2(3):87–92.

4. Bissoli, L., Di Francesco, V., Ballarin, A., Mandragona, R., Trespidi, R., Brocco, G., Caruso, B., Bosello, O., and Zamboni, M. Effect of vegetarian

diet on homocysteine levels. *Annals of Nutrition and Metabolism* 2002, 46(2):73–9.

5. http://www.cdcgov/ncbddd/b12/introlhtml.

6. Stabler, S. P. Screening the older population for cobalamin (vitamin B_{12}) deficiency. *J Am Geriatr Soc.* 1995 Nov;43(11):1290–1297.

7. Pennypacker, L. C., Allen, R. H., Kelly, J. P., et al. High prevalence of cobalamin deficiency in elderly outpatients. *J Am Geriatr Soc.* 1992 Dec; 40(12):1197–1204.

8. Dharmarajan, T. S., Adiga, G. U., Norkus, E. P. Vitamin B_{12} deficiency. Recognizing subtle symptoms in older adults. *Geriatrics* 2003;58:30–8.

9. Dietary Supplement Fact Sheet: vitamin B12. http://ods.od.nih.gov/factsheddts/vitaminb12/.

10. VanTiggelen, C. J. M., et al. Assessment of vitamin-B_{12} status in CSF. *American Journal of Psychiatry* 141, 1:136–7, 1984.

11. Mitsuyama, Y., Kogoh, H. Serum and cerebrospinal fluid vitamin B_{12} levels in demented patients with CH3-B_{12} treatment-preliminary study. *Japanese Journal of Psychiatry and Neurology* 42, 1:65–71, 1988.

12. VanTiggelen, C. J. M., Peperkamp, J. P. C., TerToolen, J. F. W. Vitamin-B_{12} levels of cerebrospinal fluid in patients with organic mental disorder. *Journal of Orthomolecular Psychiatry* 12:305–11, 1983.

13. Solomon, L. R. Cobalamin-responsive disorders in the ambulatory care setting: unreliability of cobalamin, methylmalonic acid, and homocysteine testing. *Blood*, 2005;105:978–985.

14. Green, R. Unreliability of current assays to detect cobalamin deficiency: "nothing gold can stay." *Blood*, 2005;105: 910–911.

15. Solomon, L. R. Disorders of cobalamin (Vitamin B_{12}) metabolism: emerging concepts in pathophysiology, diagnosis and treatment. *Blood*, 2007;21:113–130.

16. Ibid.

17. Miller, J. W., et al. Measurement of total vitamin B_{12} and holotranscobalamin, singly and in combination, in screening for metabolic vitamin B_{12} deficiency. *Clinical Chemistry* (2006) 52:2;278–285.

18. Ordower, G. "Batavia woman makes appeal to Bush," *Daily Herald*, January 6, 2005.

19. www.emarcusdavis.com/practice/practice_hmom.html.

20. *Toronto Sun*, December 17, 2007. Boy paralyzed by "forgotten disease." By Michele Mandel. http://www:torontosun.com/News/Columnist/Mandel_Michele/2007/12/17/pf-4728358

21. Svenson, J. Case Report: Neurologic disease and vitamin B$_{12}$ deficiency. *American Journal of Emergency Medicine* (2007) 25, 987.e3–987.e4.

2

Is It Aging—or Is It B₁₂ Deficiency?

"The lack of knowledge about vitamin B₁₂ deficiency is astounding, especially when you consider the number of elderly individuals that are afflicted now and, with the graying of society, the number that will soon be at risk."
—Robert Schmidt, M.D., board member, American Society on Aging[1]

Emily came into the emergency department during my shift, bruised and shaken after a frightening fall. X-rays revealed a fracture in her right arm, but the tiny, fragile eighty-nine-year-old had more problems than just a broken bone. She seemed confused, made little sense when she talked, and couldn't tell me the date or time. She walked slowly and unsteadily, with a wide-based gait, as though she couldn't tell where her feet were. She looked thin, pale, and malnourished, and she needed to wear Depends because she wet herself.

Emily came to us with a diagnosis of dementia. Luckily for her, the doctor on my shift ordered a serum B₁₂ level; it came back 156pg/ml, revealing deficiency. Her low B₁₂ levels could explain every one of her symptoms— the fall, the confusion and memory loss, her abnormal gait, her pallor and incontinence—yet none of her previous doctors had ever checked her B₁₂ levels. They just thought she was old and had Alzheimer's.

Being old isn't easy. Being an elderly patient is even harder. That's because the medical profession, like the public in general, tends to stereotype seniors. They're "drifty." They forget things. They fall a lot. They have aches and pains everywhere. They get senile.

But in reality, these problems aren't "normal" or "typical." When we see them in a patient who's twenty, thirty, or forty, we usually search until we find a cause. But when a seventy-year-old complains of forgetfulness, depression, or incontinence, medical professionals too often think to themselves, "That's to be expected when you get old." As a result, vast numbers of seniors suffer unnecessarily from problems that go undiagnosed and untreated—frequent falls, difficulty in walking, memory lapses, depression, and crippling aches and pains—simply because we fail to look for their causes.

If we do take note of these problems, all too often, we simply say, "It's just a new symptom of your existing medical conditions." We blame leg pains on diabetes or arthritis, and falls on failing vision or poor reflexes. We dismiss depression as a normal response to losing a spouse or friends, and we say that memory lapses are simply part of the aging process. But when we dismiss aging patients' suffering as "normal," we consign many of these patients to nursing homes, or even to death, when they have treatable problems. And one common problem in people over sixty is vitamin B$_{12}$ deficiency.

Seniors are a high-risk group for severe B$_{12}$ deficiency for several reasons. One is that 30 percent of them develop a condition called *atrophic gastritis*, or inflammation and wasting of the stomach lining. This drastically decreases their levels of stomach acid, which is needed to free B$_{12}$ from animal proteins so that it can be absorbed.

Doctors commonly treat elderly patients' stomach upsets and indigestion with drugs such as Prevacid, Prilosec, Zantac, Pepcid, Aciphex, Nexium, and Protonix, and seniors frequently dose themselves with over-the-counter antacids. Unfortunately, all of these medications reduce stomach acid even more, causing B$_{12}$ levels to drop still further.

> **Seniors are a high-risk group for severe B$_{12}$ deficiency.**

In addition, many seniors eat poorly, and those who live on limited budgets often forgo vitamin supplements and meat (the primary dietary source of B$_{12}$) to save pennies. Older individuals frequently lose interest in food, especially if they live alone and have to prepare it themselves or if they find it difficult to eat due to indigestion or sore mouths. Many have trouble chewing their food—which again makes them avoid meat—because of bad teeth or poorly fitting dentures. And a high percentage of seniors have a history of gastric or intestinal surgeries, or of radiation treatment for cancers of the abdominal or pelvic organs, either of which can dramatically increase the risk of having dangerously low B$_{12}$ levels.

Some older people actually suffer not from an age-related problem in extracting and absorbing B$_{12}$, but from true pernicious anemia (an autoimmune disease; see Chapter 1) that has gone undiagnosed for years. One case we witnessed involved a seventy-seven-year-old woman with symptoms so advanced that she'd been placed under hospice care. Doctors had misdiagnosed her increasing motor problems for many years, eventually labeling them as "multiple sclerosis" when she was seventy-two years old.

When seniors start showing symptoms of B$_{12}$ deficiency, their doctors often mask these symptoms with drugs—Detrol for incontinence; Aricept or Namenda for Alzheimer's-like deterioration; Haldol or Risperdal for psychotic behavior; Prozac, Zoloft, Effexor, or Serzone for depression; Paxil, Xanax, or Ativan for anxiety—without ever determining their cause. This makes patients feel better, but not for long. That's because the damage caused by the deficiency is still eating away at these patients' brains, nervous systems, and cardiovascular systems.

It's ironic that in the name of cost containment (one reason for failing to order B$_{12}$ tests), doctors often prescribe expensive drugs to treat symptoms that could, in cases where these symptoms stem from B$_{12}$ deficiency, be eliminated by high-dose B$_{12}$ lozenges (2,000 mcg) or B$_{12}$ shots costing about around $36 per year. Compare this cost to more than $1,200 a year for Namenda, often prescribed for patients with dementia due to undiagnosed B$_{12}$ deficiency—or to the over $2,000-per-year tab for the drug Neurontin, often used to treat numbness and leg pains that can be caused by deficient stores of B$_{12}$. These drugs are "penny wise and pound foolish" for yet another reason: They often allow B$_{12}$ deficiency symptoms to progress, undiagnosed and untreated, to the point where patients need expensive hospital or nursing home care.

> Between 15 and 40 percent of people over sixty have low serum B$_{12}$ levels.

A PROBLEM OF EPIDEMIC PROPORTIONS

How many seniors suffer or die because B$_{12}$ deficiency impairs their minds and wreaks havoc on their hearts, blood vessels, and nervous and immune systems? The data we've seen indicate that there are millions—enough to have a huge impact on medical care expenses in the United States, and to touch almost every family in some way. As we noted in the last chapter, between 15 and 40 percent of people over sixty have low serum B$_{12}$ levels. This means that at least one in seven people over sixty—and possibly as many as four in ten—are at risk of suffering from

COMMON DRUGS THAT CAN PUT SENIORS AT RISK FOR B$_{12}$ DEFICIENCY

The following drugs impair absorption of B$_{12}$ in various ways. Seniors who take these medications regularly, or take a combination of them, are at increased risk of developing B$_{12}$ deficiency:

Drug	Reason for Use
Proton pump inhibitors (PPIs): Prevacid, Prilosec, Protonix, Nexium, Aciphex, Omeprazole	Heartburn/gastritis GERD (acid reflux) Ulcers Upper GI bleeding H. Pylori infection
H2 blockers: Zantac, Tagamet, Axid, Pepcid	Heartburn/gastritis GERD Ulcers Upper GI bleeding
Antacids: Alternagel, Maalox, MOM, Mylanta, Riopan, Tums	Heartburn/gastritis Acid indigestion Peptic ulcer disease GERD Hiatal hernia
Biguanides: Metformin, Glucophage, Riomet, Fortamet, Glumetza, Obimet, Dianben, Diabex, Diaformin, Glucovance	Diabetes
K-Lor, K-Lyte, Klotrix, K-Dur, Micro-K, Slow-K, potassium chloride	Potassium deficiency—often prescribed for patients with congestive heart failure, kidney failure, or cirrhosis of the liver, and for patients who receive diuretics ("water pills") such as Lasix, Bumex, and hydrochlorothiazide (HCTZ)
Colchicine	Gout
Questran	Elevated cholesterol levels
Neomycin	Infections
Para-aminosalicylic acid	Tuberculosis

Common Drugs that Can Be Misprescribed for the Signs and Symptoms of B$_{12}$ Deficiency

Doctors who prescribe the following drugs to treat B$_{12}$-deficient patients' symptoms, without uncovering the cause of those symptoms, can allow undetected B$_{12}$ deficiency to progress to incurable or even life-threatening stages:

Drug	Commonly used for
Celexa, Effexor, Elavil, Nardil, Pamelor, Paxil, Prozac, Serzone, Sinequon, Tofranil, Wellbutrin, Zoloft	Depression
Ativan, Klonopin, Librium, Paxil, Serax, Tranxene, Valium, Xanax	Anxiety and panic disorder
Viagra, Cialis, Levitra	Erectile dysfunction
Aricept, Cognex, Namenda, Exelon, Reminyl	Dementia
Antivert	Dizziness, imbalance, and vertigo
Detrol, Ditropan, Levbid	Incontinence
Compazine, Geodon, Haldol, Navane, Risperdal, Stelazine, Tegretol, Thorazine	Psychosis
Ambien, Dalmane, Halcion, Restoril	Insomnia
Cylert, Ritalin	Fatigue
Diamox, Inderal, Mysoline, Symmetrel	Tremors
Elavil, Neurontin, Tegretol	Numbness and tingling
Folic acid (folate), Folvite, Apo-Folic (folate is a nutrient often given to alcoholics and patients with poor diets, and also used to lower the risk of colon cancer or to treat high homocysteine levels)	Blood abnormalities (enlarged red blood cells)

nerve, brain, heart, and blood vessel damage caused by an often "silent" deficiency.

In 1996, hematologist Dr. Ralph Carmel estimated that more than 800,000 people in the United States over the age of sixty had undiagnosed and untreated pernicious anemia.[2] This is only the tip of the iceberg when it comes to B$_{12}$ deficiency, because the number of seniors with deficiency due to poor diet or malabsorption problems is believed to be significantly greater than the number of people with pernicious anemia.

Furthermore, the number of new cases of B$_{12}$ deficiency is rising each year as the senior population grows. In 1993, Dr. Eric Norman used the urinary MMA test to re-evaluate 299 independently living seniors aged sixty-five and older whose screenings for B$_{12}$ deficiency had been normal approximately one year earlier. The re-testing showed that more than 2 percent had developed B$_{12}$ deficiency over the year. "Thus," Dr. Norman says, "for the thirty million United States elderly, 600,000 new cases per year are possible."[3] His findings strongly indicate that yearly B$_{12}$ screening is warranted for the elderly population.

Yet only a small percentage of seniors will be sent for even a serum B$_{12}$ test, and almost none will receive the urinary MMA test that can some-times be helpful in diagnosing B$_{12}$ deficiency. Another problem is that most B$_{12}$-deficient seniors will not actually receive treatment because physicians typically do not treat symptomatic patients in the gray zone—a serum B$_{12}$ between 200 pg/ml and 450 pg/ml (see Chapters 1 and 11). As a result, many will wind up wheelchair-bound or bedridden, develop ir-reversible dementia, or even suffer unnecessary strokes or heart disease.

Why is this obvious diagnosis so often missed in older patients? There are a number of reasons, involving time pressures, stereotypes about the elderly, and concerns about money. The following are the excuses we hear most often from our colleagues:

1. *"They're just old."* As we've noted, far too many medical profession-als equate old age with decrepitude. As a result, they don't spend the time and effort it takes to determine whether an elderly person's leg pains, difficulty in walking, falls, confusion, memory loss, neuropa-thy, or other symptoms are "just old age," or stem from treatable B$_{12}$ deficiency.

2. *"We can't screen for everything."* The doctors who say this are unaware of the high rate of B$_{12}$ deficiency in older patients, as compared to

the rates of other problems for which they routinely screen. At one hospital we studied, for instance, 316,000 patients used the laboratory's services in 1999, but doctors screened only 121 patients for B_{12} deficiency. Therefore, doctors ordered B_{12} tests for only one of every 2,612 patients (0.04 percent) using the facility's laboratory services. Yet, as we noted, a minimum of 15 percent of people over the age of sixty, and potentially as many as 40 percent, have deficient or borderline B_{12} levels. (In contrast, this hospital ordered more than 600 serum calcium tests *per week*, even though only about 10 percent of patients had abnormal serum calcium levels.)

3. *"It's someone else's job."* Elderly patients often have a primary care doctor and a host of specialists, and these doctors frequently assume that another physician will check for B_{12} deficiency. The emergency room doctor assumes that it's the primary care doctor's responsibility. The primary care doctor assumes that it's the cardiologist's, gastroenterologist's, endocrinologist's, surgeon's or neurologist's problem. And all too often, nobody follows through.

4. *"His last doctor probably checked it."* Under managed care, seniors often get shuffled from plan to plan and from doctor to doctor. Each new doctor may assume—usually incorrectly—that a previous physician did a B_{12} level.

5. *"A complete blood count (CBC) is good enough."* As we explained in Chapter 1, a CBC *isn't* good enough, by a long shot. Many patients present with neurologic signs and symptoms long before blood changes occur. What's more, when patients are anemic, physicians typically don't consider B_{12} deficiency, but only contemplate iron-deficiency anemia. When patients are macrocytic, they tend to ignore it. If the serum B_{12} is above 200pg/ml or is in the ballpark, most doctors think they've ruled out B_{12} deficiency.

How widespread is ignorance about testing and treating B_{12} deficiency? As we noted earlier, one test that's helpful is the urinary MMA. In the study mentioned above, which we conducted at a hospital that treated tens of thousands of elderly patients and had a total of 316,000 patients of all ages using laboratory services in 1999, doctors ordered the serum MMA test to rule out B_{12} deficiency only twenty-nine times during the entire year. This means that only one out of every 10,897 patients, or 0.01

percent of all patients, had additional tests to help diagnose or rule out B$_{12}$ deficiency that year. *No urinary MMAs were performed.*

6. *"I already have a logical explanation for her symptoms."* Elderly patients often have one or more pre-existing diseases, and it's easy to dismiss new symptoms as part of an existing medical problem.

For instance, I recently talked to a once-active man who began suffering years ago, at the age of sixty-eight, from foot and leg numbness. He's now barely able to walk far enough to do a little grocery shopping, and he's dangerous when he drives, because he can't feel his feet. For a decade, every doctor he saw assumed that his symptoms were side effects of diabetes. But given his age, his poor eating habits, and his history of iron-deficiency anemia* and hospitalization for this severe and unexplained anemia, I knew that his symptoms were also quite likely to be due to B$_{12}$ deficiency. Yet despite the fact that he'd seen fifteen doctors in the past two years alone, he'd never been tested.

Why does it matter? Because if the numbness stems from B$_{12}$ deficiency, it's treatable, at least in its early stages. If it stems from diabetes, it usually isn't. It might not make a difference to the doctor, but it makes all of the difference in the world to a patient who wants to continue to enjoy driving, shopping, and living independently. Moreover, the neuropathy due to B$_{12}$ deficiency is just one step in a process that, left uncorrected, is likely to become a long slide into severe debility, or even death. The man I just described was saved from this fate because he took my advice, got tested, and found out that he is indeed B$_{12}$-deficient. It may be too late to reverse his leg pain and numbness, but it's not too late to save him from the psychosis or dementia that chronically depleted B$_{12}$ levels can cause.

Blaming a patient's problems on a single condition also overlooks the fact that many older patients' problems are multifactorial; in other words, they have more than one cause. Even if a patient's symptoms can be linked to diabetes or Parkinson's disease or another known condition, a B$_{12}$ deficiency may very well be contributing to these symptoms. Identifying one disorder is no justification for ignoring another. (As an old medical saying goes, "If a patient has six nails in his foot, and you remove one, he still has a sore foot.")

---

* B$_{12}$ deficiency can cause severe anemia, requiring blood transfusions. Doctors typically equate severe anemia with internal bleeding and fail to order B$_{12}$ and iron studies before giving transfusions. Testing patients for B$_{12}$ and iron status after blood transfusions are given yields inaccurate results, clouding the clinical picture.

7. *"The insurance company isn't going to pay for this."* This is a common response in a cost-cutting era in which every test comes under scrutiny. We have two answers for doctors who are concerned about the financial aspects of B$_{12}$ testing. One is that when they code for B$_{12}$ tests correctly (see Appendix S), insurers will cover them. The other is, "Would your patient think it's worth around $90 (the cost of a serum B$_{12}$) or $150 (the cost of a urinary MMA*) to prevent a stroke, congestive heart failure, a crippling fall, chronic disability, or dementia?"

We guarantee that patients would say yes. So would doctors and insurers, if they realized that they could save the health care and insurance industries enormous amounts of money by diagnosing B$_{12}$ deficiency before it causes expensive, chronic illnesses. Dr. Eric Norman, the biochemist who developed the urinary MMA test for B$_{12}$ deficiency in 1985, says that widescale identification and treatment of B$_{12}$ deficiency would "help seniors maintain their productivity, dignity, and independence while saving billions of dollars annually in health care costs."[4]

THE LONG DARKNESS: WHEN LOW B$_{12}$ DESTROYS THE MIND

The first time you forget your best friend's name, you laugh and write it off as a "senior moment." But the moments start happening more and more often.

You drive to the grocery store and can't remember where you parked. You forget to pay the electric bill three months in a row. You set out for the doctor's office and wind up miles away, not sure how you got there. As time passes, you find yourself unable to add a simple column of numbers or address a birthday card. Familiar people begin to look like strangers, and the crossword puzzles you once loved become a meaningless blur of words. You forget what day it is, where you live, what your children's names are. You begin wetting yourself, and one winter morning the neighbors find you outside in your underwear. You become angry, frightened, and confused.

Your daughter cries when your doctor says you need to be moved to a long-term care facility. Soon, you find yourself living in a tiny room, being led to cafeteria meals by people you don't know. Eventually, the same people need to dress you, bathe you, and help you go to the bathroom, because you

---

* The cost of the uMMA test from Norman Clinical Laboratory, Inc. is $150.00. At the Mayo Clinic and Specialty Laboratory, the cost of urinary MMA test is $249.00.

can no longer care for yourself. You don't know why you're there. You don't know what's become of your home, your family, and your life. In time, you don't even know who you are.

This is the tragic pattern of dementia, a relentless decline in memory and mental ability. Striking more than five million Americans, dementia turns victims' "golden years" into years of torment, devastates families emotionally and financially, transforms loving spouses and children into exhausted full-time caretakers, and fills America's nursing homes with sad, bewildered patients with no hope of recovery.

If you're dealing with someone suffering from dementia, you know the pain of watching a vibrant individual become a different person—one who becomes agitated, inconsolably sad, paranoid, or even violent or hateful. You know the agony of watching a friend or relative stare at you vacantly, wondering who you are. And you know the guilt of hoping for a loved one to die, because dying is preferable to the slow and inexorable loss of self that dementia causes.

But what you may not know is that *dementia isn't always incurable—even when doctors say it is.* As neurologist Sydney Walker III, M.D., noted, "Many patients do suffer from Alzheimer's and other dementias; but [many others], who are labeled as having dementia, are actually suffering from problems that can be corrected. Studies suggest, in fact, that up to 60 percent of patients tentatively labeled as having 'dementia' actually have treatable and reversible disorders."[5] There are millions of people with true dementias, such as Alzheimer's disease and Pick's dementia (although even Alzheimer's may be linked to B$_{12}$—see later in this chapter), but for each of them it's likely that there's another "demented" patient with a disorder that's treatable and curable. And in many cases, that disorder is B$_{12}$ deficiency.

If you review the statistics we've already cited, this isn't surprising. Remember that:

- Up to 15 percent of seniors, and up to 40 percent of symptomatic people over sixty, have low or borderline B$_{12}$ levels.

- The symptoms of B$_{12}$ deficiency can include confusion, memory loss, personality changes, paranoia, depression, and other behaviors that look just like incurable dementia. Dementia stemming from B$_{12}$ deficiency also mimics other dementias in its progress, which usually is gradual but relentless. Thus, it's all too easy to mistakenly write off B_{12}-deficiency dementia as incurable.

- There is no test that can diagnose Alzheimer's conclusively in a living patient. Thus, the only way to differentiate between Alzheimer's and other causes of dementia is to rule out all other causes, something that's too rarely done. (A recent study in Finland, a country with a highly advanced medical system that is comparable to that of the United States, found that only 20 percent of patients with symptoms of dementia were screened for B_{12} deficiency.[6])

- As we've noted, a serum B_{12} test is too infrequently ordered for elderly patients, and even those who *are* tested rarely receive treatment if their serum B_{12} is in the gray zone. Moreover, what the medical community accepts as "normal" B_{12} status for the elderly may be far too low. Behavioral medicine specialist Dr. Mark Goodman has treated four demented patients whose seemingly normal serum B_{12} levels masked a severe B_{12} deficiency. When he gave these patients B_{12} injections, every one of them improved dramatically.[7] Similar results have been reported by other physicians treating the elderly, and we've witnessed many such cases first-hand.

While most doctors are unaware of the prevalence of B_{12} deficiency in patients with symptoms of dementia, the medical literature clearly shows that the problem is not a rare one. One study, for instance, found that one in seven demented patients seen consecutively by a clinic had subnormal serum B_{12} levels.[8] Identifying such patients early is crucial, because prompt treatment in the early phases of B_{12} deficiency can restore patients to normal or near-normal functioning.

In an article in Discover *magazine, Leslie Bernstein, M.D. told of her shock when she saw "Pop," a formerly active, healthy patient of hers. "If his grandson hadn't been holding him up, he'd have pitched straight forward onto his face," she said. "Saliva dribbled from the corners of his mouth. His eyes were vacant." Over time, Pop had changed from a healthy jogger and loving grandfather into a confused, incontinent man whose doctors diagnosed him as having senile dementia.*

Pop's blood work looked normal, except that his red blood cells were slightly larger than normal. His psychiatrist had concluded that he suffered from "toxic/organic disease without significant depression." Luckily, his *family brought him to see Dr. Bernstein, who almost immediately thought of a more logical explanation for Pop's drastic decline: Due to his age and vegetarian diet, he was probably B$_{12}$-deficient. Dr. Bernstein quickly ordered blood work that showed that Pop had B$_{12}$ levels too low to measure.*

Pop received an injection of B$_{12}$ and by the next morning he could sit up by himself. Within two days, he could control his bowels and bladder, and within a week he could play card games and talk coherently on the phone. He didn't make a full recovery—he continued to have a short attention span and to cry easily—but he didn't need to spend the rest of his life in a nursing home, labeled with "senile dementia."[9]

Unlike Pop, many seniors receive a correct diagnosis for their B$_{12}$-deficiency symptoms only after many years of non-diagnosis. That lost time can translate into lost hope; if Pop's doctors had waited even a few more months to detect the cause of his problem, his dementia probably would have been permanent. There appears to be a critical window of opportunity for treating B$_{12}$ deficiency, and therapy started more than six months after the onset of symptoms may fail to reverse these symptoms.

However, this isn't true in every case, so aggressive treatment is still called for even if symptoms have been present for longer than six months. In one reported case, a patient who'd suffered for nearly a year from "presenile dementia" recovered completely when doctors uncovered and treated his B$_{12}$ deficiency.[10] Also, even at later stages, treatment may lead to slight improvement or at least a leveling-off of symptoms—although the damage to the brain may be permanent, causing life-long cognitive deficits. The degree of recovery may depend on how long the person had B$_{12}$ deficiency, how severe the B$_{12}$ deficiency was, the person's age, and other preexisting diseases.

> There is a critical window of opportunity for treating B$_{12}$ deficiency before permanent cognitive changes or injury result.

Incidentally, while we've put the topic of B$_{12}$-deficiency dementia in our aging chapter, we should note that it can strike even very young people. For instance, doctors reported on a twenty-one-year-old woman who developed bipolar disorder and then full-fledged dementia, both due to deficient B$_{12}$ levels and an accompanying folate deficiency. With treatment, her doctors say, she experienced a "dramatic resolution" of her symptoms.[11]

The medical literature even contains reports of infants and toddlers suffering dementia-like symptoms that were reversed, partially or totally, with B_{12} therapy. (Some children, however, ended up with lower IQs and/or mental retardation.) In these cases, just as with seniors, there is a window of opportunity for effective treatment (see chapters 6 and 12). That's why it's urgent, in either the elderly or the young, to order B_{12} testing for any patient exhibiting signs and symptoms of dementia.

MOUNTING EVIDENCE FOR A B_{12}-ALZHEIMER'S LINK

We differentiate in this chapter between "true" dementias, such as Alzheimer's and Pick's, and the often reversible dementia symptoms produced by B_{12} deficiency. Yet preliminary evidence indicates that deficient B_{12} levels worsen Alzheimer's symptoms, and that B_{12} deficiency may even play some role in causing the disease.

Alzheimer's is the most common type of dementia, affecting up to one-fifth of people over eighty and hundreds of thousands of people in their fifties, sixties, and seventies. The diagnosis is confirmed only after patients' deaths, when autopsies reveal the *plaques* (chemical deposits) and *tangles* (malformed nerve cells) that are hallmarks of the disease. While patients are alive, doctors make a tentative diagnosis by excluding other causes of dementia, and using clues provided by brain scans and tests of mental functioning.

Several years ago, Dr. Robert Clarke and colleagues[12] measured the levels of B_{12}, folate, and homocysteine in 164 patients diagnosed with Alzheimer's, comparing them to a control group of people without Alzheimer's. (You'll remember that high homocysteine levels are a strong indication of B_{12} deficiency.) At the time the researchers reported their findings, 76 of the 164 patients diagnosed with Alzheimer's had died, and autopsies confirmed the diagnosis; the eighty-eight still-living patients were included as "probable" Alzheimer's cases. Clarke and his colleagues found the following conditions:

- Homocysteine levels at the patients' initial visits were significantly higher in the Alzheimer's group than in control group members.

- B_{12} and folate levels were markedly lower in Alzheimer's patients than in control group members.

- Alzheimer's patients with high homocysteine levels showed greater evidence of disease progression, as revealed by atrophy seen on scans, than those with lower levels. A similar but non-significant trend was seen for serum folate and B_{12} levels.

- Homocysteine levels in the Alzheimer's patients didn't change as the disease progressed, which indicates that the differences between patients and control group members weren't caused by the disease itself, but rather predated or coincided with the onset of Alzheimer's.

Clarke suggests that high levels of toxic homocysteine, possibly stemming from B$_{12}$ deficiency, may cause "microinfarcts"—tiny areas of blood vessel damage—that then trigger the formation of the plaques and tangles that eventually clutter the brain of a person with Alzheimer's. He concludes: "Low blood levels of folate and vitamin B$_{12}$, and elevated total homocysteine (tHcy) levels were associated with Alzheimer's disease. The stability of tHcy levels over time and lack of relationship with duration of symptoms argue against these findings being a consequence of disease and warrant further studies to assess the clinical relevance of these associations for AD."*

More evidence implicating low B$_{12}$ as a player in Alzheimer's comes from a United Kingdom study of a family genetically predisposed to the disease. Remarkably, researchers found that four of six family members with confirmed Alzheimer's had low blood levels of B$_{12}$, while only one of twelve without Alzheimer's exhibited B$_{12}$ deficiency.[13] Another study— this one in Sweden—found that seniors with low intakes of vitamin B$_{12}$ and folate are twice as likely to develop Alzheimer's as people with healthy B$_{12}$ levels. The researchers collected blood samples from their subjects *before* the subjects developed the disease, proving that the low vitamin levels weren't merely a side effect of the Alzheimer's.[14] And one more study, conducted recently in Germany, found that Alzheimer's patients with lower-than-normal B$_{12}$ levels exhibited more behavioral and psychological symptoms of dementia than patients with normal B$_{12}$ levels. "Vitamin B$_{12}$," the researchers concluded, "could play a role in the pathogenesis of behavioral changes in Alzheimer's disease."[15]

In 2008, an article in *Neurology* reported that low B$_{12}$ causes brain atrophy (shrinkage) and is linked to cognitive impairment in the elderly.[16] Brain atrophy is associated with confirmed Alzheimer's disease, and so is vitamin B$_{12}$ deficiency. This study's data suggested that subclinical low vitamin B$_{12}$ status—within what is usually considered to be the normal range (what we call the "gray zone")—can affect brain volume even in the early stages of cognitive decline, possibly by disturbing the integrity of

---

*Unfortunately, these researchers did not include serum B$_{12}$ in the gray zone or urinary MMA testing in their study. The key question that future research must address is: How many patients with confirmed Alzheimer's disease have untreated B$_{12}$ deficiency as evidenced by serum B$_{12}$ in the gray zone or elevated urinary MMA?

> **TERMINAL OR TREATABLE?**
>
> George Isajiw, M.D., reports the case of a 92-year-old with perni-
> cious anemia and Alzheimer's dementia who received an inappropriate
> hospice referral because the patient's doctors did not take the time to
> uncover her reversible B_{12} deficiency. Isajiw comments, "This case…
> demonstrates the need to evaluate each patient on a rational, individ-
> ual, clinical basis as opposed to blindly applying so-called 'evidence-
> based medicine' in an extremely diverse population of patients labeled
> with the so-called diagnosis of 'terminal Alzheimer's dementia.'" [17]

brain myelin or by causing inflammation. "Thus," the researchers commented, "early treatment of low vitamin B_{12} status may prevent further
brain volume loss."

This study showed that low B_{12} status at baseline is an important risk
factor for loss of brain volume in older adults. The researchers found that
"plasma vitamin B_{12} status may be an early marker of brain atrophy and
thus a potentially important modifiable risk factor for cognitive decline in
the elderly."

In 2009, another study reviewed the evidence that cognition in older
adults may be adversely affected at concentrations of vitamin B_{12} above
the traditional cutoffs defined as B_{12} deficiency. Using additional B_{12}
markers (holoTC and MMA), it found that cognition is associated with
B_{12} status across the normal range. (This again reinforces the need to raise
the lower range of the serum B_{12} test). In this study, brain atrophy and
white matter brain damage were both associated with low vitamin B_{12}
status.[18]

Since evidence suggests that sub-normal B_{12} levels contribute to Alzheimer's, it's crucial that we educate the health care community and the
public about this apparent association, develop screening protocols, and
initiate early treatment for B_{12} deficiency, as well as keeping serum B_{12}
levels above 1,000 pg/ml in older adults. Researchers should pursue the
evidence aggressively, and hope that it leads to real progress in treating
and/or preventing this insidious disease.

In the meantime, it is crucial for families to serve as advocates for
patients with dementia. In October 2006, for example, we received a letter from a woman in New Jersey whose husband, John, was diagnosed at
the age of fifty-four with cortical basal ganglionic degeneration (CBGD).

This is a progressive dementia with Parkinsonism features, leading to increased cognitive and motor disability, with a mean survival of about eight years.

Julie told us how her life had come "crashing down" on her when her husband, after holding down a steady job for twenty years, could no longer function at work. Over a span of five years he lost twelve jobs.

Julie added, "He started losing his place during presentations to customers, and would stare at his computer and forget what he was doing. I noticed problems on the road with his driving. He would forget to use his turn signals and he had trouble maintaining his lane. He could not do simple math. He is a good carpenter and could not figure out a project."

John's family doctor stated he didn't think it was Alzheimer's and prescribed Cerefolin—a prescription vitamin that contains high-dose methyl-B$_{12}$ (2,000 mcg), high-dose L-methylfolate (5.6 mg) and N-acetylcysteine (600 mg). He ordered blood work and prescribed B$_{12}$, but never ordered a serum B$_{12}$ test to see if B$_{12}$ deficiency was causing John's symptoms, or, if a B$_{12}$ deficiency existed, how severe it was.

Another doctor who evaluated John ordered a serum B$_{12}$ and a brain MRI—but by this point, John had been on daily high-dose B$_{12}$ for three weeks, making the serum B$_{12}$ test results invalid. John also received his first B$_{12}$ injection at this office, after his blood was drawn. Despite the daily high-dose prescription of B$_{12}$ the first doctor gave him, John's serum B$_{12}$ level was in the gray zone and still marginal at 224 pg/ml.

Next, John was referred to a neurologist in Pennsylvania who specialized in cognitive disorders. By this time, John had been on the oral B$_{12}$ (Cerefolin) for eight weeks. After many tests and consultations, John was diagnosed with CBGD. The neurologist told him to quit driving and apply for permanent disability. Other doctors reviewed the lab and scan results and said the same thing: no hope, no cure.

Oddly, it was a laboratory—not John's doctors—who raised a red flag at this point. A note or disclaimer attached to one of John's lab reports said, "Please note: Although the reference range for vitamin B$_{12}$ is 200-1100 pg/ml, it has been reported that between 5 and 10% of patients with values between 200 and 344 pg/ml may experience neuropsychiatric and hematologic abnormalities due to occult B$_{12}$ deficiency; less than 1% of patients with values above 400 pg/ml will have symptoms."

Julie queried the doctors about John's B$_{12}$ level. "The neurologist in Pennsylvania said he would only recognize the deficiency if the homocysteine was high," she told us, "so he ordered a test and it was elevated at 14.5."

What did all of John's doctors fail to realize? His serum B$_{12}$ should have been very high by this point, because he'd been on a prescription high-dose methyl-B$_{12}$ for a little over three weeks before the initial serum B$_{12}$ was ordered. And his homocysteine and MMA levels should have been normal or very low because he was on Cerefolin for 11 weeks before these tests were performed. In other words, his tests were abnormal *despite* treatment—a fact that should have alarmed his doctors.

John's lab report showing low B$_{12}$ bothered Julie and she became fixated on it, while John's doctors ignored or made light of it. Curious, Julie turned to the Internet to search for clues as to why John would be low in B$_{12}$. "This is when I learned about the use of acid inhibitors," she told us. "John was his gastroenterologist's first patient on Prilosec, and he has gone from there to Nexium and has been on these medications for 18 years now with the same doctor, but has never had a B$_{12}$ level drawn."

Eleven weeks after John was placed on Cerefolin and saw the neurologist, Julie went back to the family physician, who was willing to give John a B$_{12}$ injection. "The injection made John feel so focused he could not believe it," Julie says. "When he asked for a second one, two weeks later, the family physician refused. Feeling frustrated, Julie went to another neurologist in New Jersey and begged him to review John's records. After examining John, reviewing his medical records, and hearing John's and Julie's testimony about the results of the one B$_{12}$ injection, this second neurologist agreed to prescribe regular B$_{12}$ injections.

Over a year later, Julie wrote, "During our last visit to the neurologist in New Jersey, John's neuro evaluation was greatly improved. As his wife, I see a remarkable difference in his abilities and his personality. The first neurologist at the University agrees that if John had CBGD by now he would have suffered a decline and that he was most likely incorrect in his diagnosis; yet this doctor still uses the diagnosis of CBGD and doesn't include the diagnosis of vitamin B$_{12}$ deficiency. The second New Jersey neurologist said, 'This is a miracle' and 'You have your wife to thank for this.'"

Why John's doctor contemplated and diagnosed CBGD rather than vitamin B$_{12}$ deficiency, when both may present with Parkinsonism (and

John's history and laboratory evidence supported B$_{12}$ deficiency), is mystifying—yet it eloquently demonstrates the severe knowledge deficit regarding B$_{12}$ deficiency among physicians. In fact, dementia is a very late feature of CBGD[19], the opposite of John's presentation.

Even though John shows improvement on cognitive tests, visual field tests, and behavioral evaluations, his diagnosis and treatment came too late. He still suffers from cognitive difficulties and has a mild to moderate form of dementia which is permanent—the result of delayed treatment for a disorder that is entirely curable if caught in its early stages.

After discovering the first edition of our book, Julie gave several copies to different doctors and to the neurologist who'd agreed to treat John. He reported to her later that he had helped additional patients by treating them with B$_{12}$.

John's story illustrates how doctors often overlook B$_{12}$ deficiency and, as a result, condemn their patients to dementia or even death. Unless we succeed in raising the awareness of the public and the medical community, thousands of people will continue to be at risk. What can you do to protect your own family members? If you are dealing with a loved one who exhibits symptoms of Alzheimer's, or who suffers from mental deterioration and memory loss in general, your task is simple: Have the person tested immediately for B$_{12}$ deficiency. (Again, both a serum B$_{12}$ and a urinary MMA test are in order.) If B$_{12}$ deficiency is causing the symptoms, each day that you wait increases the chances that the damage will become permanent.

But even if your loved one is in the late stages of dementia, insist on obtaining B$_{12}$ tests and then, after testing, perform a trial of high-dose B$_{12}$ lozenges (2,000 mcg–5,000 mcg daily) and/or have the doctor perform a trial of injectable B$_{12}$, as described in Chapter 11. It won't do any harm, and there's a possibility that it could slow down or halt the progression of the dementia or even reverse some symptoms.

And there's another important reason for the tests: If your relative's dementia turns out to stem from B$_{12}$ deficiency, aggressive treatment is in order. Parenteral (injectable) treatment remains indicated for severe neurologic deficits caused by B$_{12}$ deficiency. What's more, if injury has occurred and can be clearly related to B$_{12}$ deficiency, documentation of test results will be needed to pursue a malpractice suit. In addition, other family members may be at risk (since B$_{12}$ deficiency often runs in families) and should be tested themselves.

B$_{12}$ DEFICIENCY: A CAUSE OF FREQUENT FALLS AND FALL-RELATED TRAUMA

Dementia is the saddest consequence of undiagnosed B$_{12}$ deficiency, but it's far from the only one. Another is frequent falling, which strips many seniors of their independence and can cause fatal injuries.

In fact, falling is the most common cause of fatal injuries among people over sixty-five, with nearly ten thousand seniors dying of fall-related injuries each year. Hospitals treat a third of a million hip fractures every year, most of them in elderly patients, and half of these elderly patients never return home or live independently after their injuries.[20]

One reason that B$_{12}$ deficiency is a common cause of falls is that it attacks the nervous system, and particularly the nerves in the lower part of the body. These nerves have an insulating coating

> B$_{12}$ deficiency is a common cause of falls.

known as the myelin sheath, and B$_{12}$ deficiency damages this sheath—in a manner somewhat similar to the fraying of an electrical wire—making it harder for nerve cells to carry messages. As a result, victims often develop weakness, balance problems, leg and back pains, or "glove and stocking" numbness in their hands and feet. Many walk with a slow, foot-slapping gait, because they can't tell when the bottoms of their feet are touching the floor. In addition, B$_{12}$ deficiency can cause visual disturbances, vision loss, dizziness, vertigo, or postural hypotension (a sudden drop in blood pressure upon standing). Together, these problems dramatically increase the risk of falls, and falls in turn can lead to broken bones, hospital stays, and often an end to an independent life.

Arthur came to our emergency department with a nasty gash on his head. He felt weak, he said, and had trouble walking.

It wasn't Arthur's first visit; the seventy-three-year-old's chart showed a history of multiple falls over the past three weeks. After hospitalizing him and running tests to rule out a stroke, the doctors sent Arthur home. He returned five weeks later, again complaining of weakness, and again the doctors discharged him after a short stay.

Nine weeks later, Arthur came in one more time, this time after a fainting episode that led to a serious fall. By this point, his family was considering selling Arthur's home and having him move in with them—an action he dreaded. But this time, an alert doctor ordered a serum B$_{12}$ test, which came

*back very low, and he started Arthur immediately on B$_{12}$ therapy. Thanks
to this doctor's willingness to spend a few extra minutes, Arthur finally
obtained a real diagnosis and real help. With B$_{12}$ therapy, it's likely that his
weakness will clear up completely, and his chronic falls will become a thing
of the past, allowing him to remain independent and keep his home.*

Often, as in Arthur's case, older people's falls stem from problems in
standing and walking. A typical case, involving a sixty-one-year-old,
shows how easy it is to correct these symptoms if they stem from B$_{12}$
deficiency that's detected early enough. This patient first began experiencing numbness and tingling in his toes, which gradually spread throughout
his feet. The tingling turned into pain and weakness, and by the time he
came to the hospital six months later, he could barely walk with assistance
in the daytime and he couldn't walk at all after dark. (This is a common
problem for patients with neurological problems, because when it's dark
they can't use their vision to compensate for the impaired sensory input
from their feet and legs.)

After quickly identifying this patient's B$_{12}$ deficiency, his new doctors started injections of the vitamin. Within two weeks, the man's tone,
strength, and reflexes improved, and within a month he could walk normally again.[21]

In some cases (see Chapter 8), motor problems so severe that they
cause near-paralysis can be reversed within a few months. Such results
are common when doctors catch B$_{12}$ deficiency in its early stages. Often,
people who could barely walk a few feet are able, within a few months of
starting treatment, to resume daily chores, drive, and even exercise again.
Equally important, many are able to live independently, without the
constant fear of becoming victims of crippling falls that could rob them of
their independence.

The benefits to patients are obvious, but there are huge benefits for the
medical system and insurers as well. From a financial standpoint, the
cost of a fall and resulting fracture—emergency department visit, X-rays,
labs, CT scans, casting, admission, possible surgery, physical therapy,
medications, a visiting nurse, and possible placement in an extended care
facility—far exceeds the cost of blood or urine tests to ascertain if vitamin
B$_{12}$ deficiency exists. In 2003, the cost of a hip fracture exceeded $50,000
in six weeks, which included the ambulance ride, ER visit, surgical repair,
hospitalization, physician fees, in-patient rehabilitation, out-patient rehabilitation, and in-home mobility devices.

We find it perplexing that hospitals do not routinely provide B$_{12}$ screening for patients suffering from weakness or repeated falls, particularly in light of the fact that the diagnostic procedures that hospitals *do* order for these patients are so expensive. For example, patients with these symptoms almost always receive a CT scan of the brain, costing approximately $1,000, and each time they return, they receive additional scans. We have no quarrel with ordering expensive CT scans, which can reveal problems other than B$_{12}$ deficiency (although they're useless for diagnosing low B$_{12}$); rather, we have a problem with medical professionals who fail to order equally necessary and far less expensive B$_{12}$ tests.

Arthur, for example, had $3,000 worth of CT scans in five months, and his total hospital bill exceeded $30,000, when less than $100 for a serum B$_{12}$ test on his first visit would have identified his B$_{12}$ deficiency. If he'd suffered a fracture, the three-day hospital stay for his surgery in 1999 would have cost more than $14,000, not including the surgeon's bill or post-hospital rehabilitation. Ten years later, in 2009, the average hospital bill for four days following a hip fracture and surgical repair (no complications) exceeded $30,000.

How common are stories like Arthur's? In 2007, as a community service, we screened 87 residents of an assisted-living center for B$_{12}$ deficiency using the urinary MMA test. Nineteen percent were found to be B$_{12}$-deficient. One man with a history of severe neuropathy, numerous falls, and tremors had a severe B$_{12}$ deficiency as indicated by a sky-high uMMA of 35.0 (normal < 3.8). When we reported these alarming results to the director, the director notified us that the man had fallen again, this time breaking his hip. He died ten days later in a hospital as a result of a blood clot that traveled to his lung, a common complication of a hip fracture. This man was on many medications and had numerous doctors, but none of them considered B$_{12}$ deficiency, even though he had several signs, symptoms, and risk factors.

Of course, not all falls stem from B$_{12}$ deficiency, but statistics suggest that a significant percentage do. Thus, doctors should test for this disorder any time an older patient complains of pain, numbness, weakness, dizziness, difficulty in walking, or falls.

Nurses and directors of health care facilities, too, need to stand up for their patients and advocate for proper screening, diagnosis, and treatment.

All hospitals, ambulatory care centers, clinics, nursing homes, and assisted living communities have fall prevention programs regulated by state and federal guidelines. However, the most common risk assessment models used by these facilities (the Hendrich II Fall Risk Scale and the Morse Fall Scale) do not include assessments for B_{12} deficiency—even though 90 percent of the criteria these models screen for are common signs, symptoms, or risk factors for B_{12} deficiency. By adding B_{12} screening to their fall prevention programs, these facilities could prevent thousands of injuries and deaths every year, and save billions of health care dollars.

THE B_{12}–OSTEOPOROSIS CONNECTION

In 2004, newspapers and national newscasts showcased three new studies showing a strong link between low B_{12} levels and osteoporosis, one of the leading cripplers of seniors. Osteoporosis causes a thinning and weakening of the bones, often leading to debilitating or even fatal fractures.

The first study, which evaluated hip-bone mineral density in eighty-three elderly women, found that those with the lowest levels of B_{12} exhibited much more rapid hip bone loss than those with higher B_{12} levels. Lead author Dr. Katie Stone commented, "We knew that vitamin B_{12} benefited the nervous system, but our findings suggest that it may also benefit bone health."[22]

The two other studies both reported a strong association between high homocysteine levels and bone fractures. (As we've explained, one of the primary causes of high homocysteine is low B_{12}.) One study following nearly 2,000 men and women for two decades found that men with the highest concentrations of homocysteine were nearly four times as likely to break a hip as were those with the lowest concentrations, while the risk for women with the highest homocysteine levels was double that of women with the lowest levels. The researchers reporting this finding noted, "If the homocysteine concentration truly is a causal mechanism for the risk of fracture, the public health implications could be substantial."[23] The other study, involving more than 2,400 Dutch subjects, found that men and women with the highest homocysteine concentrations were twice as likely to break a hip or experience other commonly broken bones as were those with lower homocysteine.[24]

> It's well documented that people with untreated B_{12} deficiency are at high risk for osteoporosis.

While these new studies were treated as ground-breaking, previous research had already established a powerful connection between B$_{12}$ deficiency and osteoporosis. It's well documented that people with untreated pernicious anemia are at high risk for osteoporosis and resulting fractures,[25] which is not surprising because vitamin B$_{12}$ is crucial to the function of osteoblasts (bone-forming cells). In one case study, a patient with severe osteoporosis exhibited a "dramatic response" to treatment with B$_{12}$ and cyclic etidronate (a bone-strengthening drug), with serial bone density measurements demonstrating a 15 percent and 17 percent increase in the lumbar (lower back) and greater trochanter (hip) regions, respectively, and a 79 percent increase in the femoral neck region, over the two-year follow-up period—an effect significantly greater than that which would be expected with etidronate alone. In addition, the patient suffered no new fractures during the course of the study.[26]

More recently, in 2009, researchers reported that patients with pernicious anemia have an elevated risk of hip fracture. The study was based on an evaluation of 9,506 patients with the diagnosis of pernicious anemia who were compared to 38,024 controls.[27]

Given all of these findings, it is our opinion that tests for B$_{12}$ deficiency should be a standard part of the evaluation for any patient with osteoporosis—and in particular for patients who are at high risk of falls, or who have already suffered falls and/or sustained fractures. Moreover, research on the connection between low B$_{12}$ and increased risk for fall-related injuries, fractures, and osteoporosis needs to become a national priority. The evidence indicates that B$_{12}$ deficiency is epidemic among seniors; that low B$_{12}$ and high homocysteine are strong risk factors for osteoporosis; that B$_{12}$ deficiency also leads to falls and injuries by impairing neurological function; and that B$_{12}$ therapy may help stop or reverse bone loss, and can often reverse neurological dysfunction, in B$_{12}$-deficient patients. Translating these research findings into a national effort to combat B$_{12}$ deficiency in seniors could lead to a significant drop in the numbers of crippling or fatal falls suffered by the elderly—and an equally large drop in America's health-care costs.

OTHER B$_{12}$ ILLS THAT MASQUERADE AS AGING

In Chapter 5, we'll further discuss how low B$_{12}$ levels increase levels of homocysteine, and how high levels of this toxic amino acid can harm the heart, circulatory system, and immune system. This can contribute to congestive heart failure, coronary artery disease, transient ischemic attacks (TIAs or "mini-strokes"), cerebral vascular accidents (strokes), heart attacks, pulmonary embolisms (blood clots in the lung), and deep vein thromboses—all problems that plague the elderly, in particular.

But B$_{12}$ deficiency disables its older victims in still more ways. The nervous system impairment stemming from this deficiency can cause tremors, handwriting difficulties, and other symptoms severe enough to resemble the early stages of Parkinson's disease. (See Chapter 3 for more on this.)

And because B$_{12}$ deficiency affects all of the nerves, it can also affect the nerves of the eye and lead to reduced vision or even blindness. In young adults, blindness caused by B$_{12}$ deficiency is so unexpected that it often leads to an accurate diagnosis. But the elderly, and especially diabetics, aren't as lucky: If their failing eyesight stems from B$_{12}$ deficiency, it's likely to be attributed to age, macular degeneration, or diabetic eye damage. New research, while preliminary, also links B$_{12}$ deficiency to one form of cataracts.[28]

Again, these disorders have many causes, and B$_{12}$ deficiency is just one of them. But even if only one in seven seniors suffers from problems linked to deficient B$_{12}$ levels—and that's likely to be a substantial underestimate—identifying and treating these individuals can save billions of dollars, and, more important, can improve or even save millions of lives. The moral for medical professionals is clear: We owe it to our patients to diagnose B$_{12}$ deficiency and save our patients from preventable debility or death.

CHAPTER 2 NOTES:

1. Schmidt, cited in "Americans lack critical knowledge about potentially debilitating condition," *Doctor's Guide*, November 19, 1997 http://www.docguide.com.

2. Carmel, R. Prevalence of undiagnosed pernicious anemia in the elderly. *Archives of Internal Medicine* 1996, 156(10):1097–1100.

3. Norman, E. J. and Morrison, J. A. Incidence estimate of cobalamin deficiency in independently living elderly subjects using the urinary methylmalonic acid assay. *Blood*, 1993, 82(10 Suppl 1):1850.

4. Norman, Eric. Vitamin B$_{12}$ deficiency. *Journal of Family Practice* (1993), 36:597.

5. Walker III, Sydney. *Dose of Sanity*. New York: John Wiley & Sons, 1996, p. 192.

6. Lopponen, M., Raiha, I., Isoaho, R., Vahlberg, T., and Kivela, S. L. Diagnosing cognitive impairment and dementia in primary health care—a more active approach is needed. *Age and Ageing*, 32(6):606–12.

7. Interview with Mark Goodman in *Clinical Pearls News* (1997), 7(10):132–134.

8. Teunisse, S., Bollen, A. E., Van Gool, W. A., Walstra, G. J. M. Dementia and subnormal levels of vitamin B₁₂: effects of replacement therapy on dementia. *Journal of Neurology* (1996), 243(7):522–529.

9. Bernstein, Leslie. Vital signs: Dementia without a cause. *Discover* (February 2000), 21(2):31–2.

10. Cited by Hector, Melvin, and Burton, John, What are the psychiatric manifestations of vitamin B₁₂ deficiency? *Journal of the American Geriatrics Society* (1988), 36:1105–1112.

11. Reid, S. D. Pseudodementia in a twenty-one-year-old with bipolar disorder and vitamin B₁₂ and folate deficiency. *West Indian Medical Journal* (2000), 49(4):347–8.

12. Clarke, R., Smith, A. D., Jobst, K. A., Refsum, H., Sutton, L., and Ueland, P. M. Folate, vitamin B₁₂ and serum total homocysteine levels in confirmed Alzheimer's disease. *Archives of Neurology* (1998), 55:1449–55.

13. McCaddon, A., and Kelly, C. L. Familial Alzheimer's disease and vitamin B₁₂ deficiency. *Age and Ageing* (1994), 23(4):334–7.

14. Wang, H. X., Wahlin, A., Basun, H., Fastbom, J., Winblad, B., and Fratiglioni, L. Vitamin B₁₂ and folate in relation to the development of Alzheimer's disease. *Neurology* 2001, 56:1188–94.

15. Meins, W., Muller-Thomsen, T., and Meier-Baumgartnerm, H. P. Subnormal serum vitamin B₁₂ and behavioural and psychological symptoms in Alzheimer's disease. *International Journal of Geriatric Psychiatry* (2000), 15(5):415–8.

16. Vogiatzoglou, A. et al. Vitamin B₁₂ status and rate of brain volume loss in community-dwelling elderly. *Neurology* 2008;71:826–832.

17. Isajiw, G. To peg or not to peg: A case of a hospice referral for vitamin B₁₂ deficiency. *The Linacre Quarterly* 76(2) (May 2009): 212–217.

18. Smith, A. D., Refsum, H. Vitamin B₁₂ and cognition in the elderly *Am J Clin Nutr* 2009;89(suppl):707S–11S.

19. Mitra, K., Gangopadhaya, P. K., Das, S. K. Parkinsonism plus syndrome—A review. *Neurol India*, 2003;51:183–8.

20. Statistics are from "Falls and hip fractures among older adults," Centers for Disease Control and Prevention, November 2000, http://www.cdc.gov.

21. Karantanas, A. H., Markonis, A., and Bisbiyiannis, G. Subacute combined degeneration of the spinal cord with involvement of the anterior columns: A new MRI finding. *Neuroradiology* (2000), 42:115–117.

22. Stone, K. L., Bauer, D. C., Sellmeyer, D., and Cummings, S. R. Low serum vitamin B$_{12}$ levels are associated with increased hip bone loss in older women: A prospective study. *Journal of Clinical Endocrinology & Metabolism* 2004, 89(3): 1217–21.

23. McLean, R. R., et al. Homocysteine as a predictive factor for hip fracture in older persons. *New England Journal of Medicine* 2004, 350:2042–2049.

24. van Meurs, J. B. J., et al. Homocysteine levels and the risk of osteoporotic fracture. *New England Journal of Medicine* 2004, 350:2033–41.

25. Goerss, J. B., et al. Risk of fractures in patients with pernicious anemia. J Bone Miner Res 1992 May; 7(5):573–9. Espallargues, M., et al. Identifying bone-mass related risk factors for fracture to guide bone densitometry measurements: A systematic review of the literature. *Osteoporosis Int.* 2001;12(10):811–22.

26. Mellton, M. E., and Kochman, M. L. Reversal of severe osteoporosis with vitamin B$_{12}$ and etidronate therapy in a patient with pernicious anemia. *Metabolism* 1995, 43(4):468–9.

27. Merriman, N.A, et al. Hip fracture risk in patients with a diagnosis of pernicious anemia. *Gastroenterology*, 2010 Apr;138(4):1330–7.

28. Kuzniarz, M., Mitchell, P., Cumming, R. G., and Flood, V. M. Use of vitamin supplements and cataract: The Blue Mountains Eye Study. *American Journal of Ophthalmology* (2001), 132:19–26.

3

Deadly Mimic: When B_{12} Deficiency Masquerades as Multiple Sclerosis or Other Neurological Disorders

"...Eighty to 90 percent of untreated patients [suffering from a deficiency of vita-min B_{12}] will develop disorders of the nervous system."
—E. Steve Roach, M.D., and William T. McLean, M.D.[1]

B_{12} deficiency strikes large numbers of seniors, but if you think that it's solely an "old person's disease," think again. A deficiency of B_{12} can destroy your nervous system at any age, and we've seen children, teens, young adults, and middle-aged people crippled or killed by this prevent-able disease.

Neurologic symptoms of B_{12} deficiency in young adults (or in children; see Chapter 6) often baffle doctors, particularly when the complete blood count (CBC) is normal and symptoms are subtle. The result, frequently, is a dangerous delay in obtaining treatment. But even if you show obvious signs and symptoms of B_{12} deficiency, there's no guarantee that you'll get a quick diagnosis.

> **A B_{12} deficiency can destroy your nervous system at any age.**

After he'd spent years suffering from odd and frightening symptoms that a neurologist finally diagnosed, Washington Post *writer Thomas Heath described "how close my bewildering illness had come to killing me."*[2]

Barely into his forties, and seemingly in excellent health, Heath began experiencing memory lapses and numbness in his hands and lower legs. His thinking deteriorated to the point that his wife suspected early-onset Alzheimer's. He started losing his balance, and stopped running because he kept falling. Later, he began losing control of his bowels and bladder.

When a physical showed that Heath had low folic acid levels, one doctor put him on folate supplements—which can mask B$_{12}$ deficiency. Another physician attributed his painful tongue, a classic sign of B$_{12}$ deficiency, to a fungus infection. When walking became difficult, Heath went to an ortho-pedic doctor who gave him steroids. A psychiatrist spent several hours trying to coax him into taking antidepressant medications.

Finally, after more than three years of non-diagnosis, Heath went to a neurologist. By then, he was a wreck. "When he asked me to close my eyes and walk a straight line, I almost fell over," Heath says. "I couldn't tell where my legs were without my sight." The doctor, eventually suspecting B$_{12}$ defi-ciency, sent Heath to a hematologist who quickly said two words that saved Heath's life: "pernicious anemia."

Heath immediately started B$_{12}$ injections, and his hands are now com-pletely functional. He can jog again, but only slowly. (He ran marathons be-fore he became ill.) He enjoys books and movies now, but says, "I still seem to have more trouble than usual remembering names, words and appoint-ments." Despite his continuing debility, Heath says he's fortunate: "Although my body, my life, and my marriage were slowly unraveling because of this insidious disease, they have been repaired."

Heath's diagnosis came far later than it should have, but he is luckier than others who never get diagnosed, and who suffer or even die without ever knowing that their problems were curable. Physician Robert Schil-ling cites the tragic case of a thirty-five-year-old man doomed to spend the rest of his life on a Stryker frame (a rotating bed for patients who cannot move) because "no one had thought of vitamin B$_{12}$ deficiency until it was too late."[3] And Heath is lucky that he suffered from "classic" pernicious anemia, rather than other forms of B$_{12}$ deficiency that doctors (including neurologists) often misdiagnose.

Such misdiagnoses occur for several reasons. One is that the symptoms of B$_{12}$ deficiency are easy to mistake for symptoms of other neurologic diseases, such as amyotrophic lateral sclerosis (ALS, also known as Lou Gehrig's disease) or multiple sclerosis (see next section). Another is that, as we've noted, doctors typically look for blood abnormalities when they check for B$_{12}$ deficiency—but *neurological damage can precede blood anomalies by many years*. Still another reason for missed diagnoses is that even doctors somewhat knowledgeable about B$_{12}$ deficiency think of it as a rare disease, or a disease of old age. Those doctors, however, are wrong, because B$_{12}$ deficiency is common, has many causes, and strikes people of all ages.

Because B$_{12}$ deficiency mimics so many other disorders, doctors can't rule out a deficiency simply by examining patients. With the right tests, however, an informed and conscientious doctor can make the right call in a matter of days—and that diagnosis can lead to a dramatic cure. In one case, for instance, mystified doctors sent a twenty-eight-year-old woman to physician Helmut Wilhelm after she developed unexplained vision loss. In addition to checking the woman for other common causes of sudden

---

**IF YOU SUFFER FROM THESE SYMPTOMS…
COULD IT BE B$_{12}$ DEFICIENCY?**

The neurological symptoms of B$_{12}$ deficiency that occur in young and middle-aged people are very similar to those in older people. They include the following:

- Numbness, tingling, or burning sensations of the hands, feet, extremities, or truncal area, often misdiagnosed as diabetic neuropathy or chronic inflammatory demyelinating polyneuropathy (CIDP)
- Tremor, often misdiagnosed as essential tremor or pre-Parkinson's disease
- Muscle weakness, paresthesias, and paralysis, sometimes attributed to Guillain-Barré syndrome
- Pain, fatigue, and debility, often labeled as "chronic fatigue syndrome"
- "Shaky leg" syndrome (leg trembling)
- Confusion and mental fogginess, often misdiagnosed as early-onset dementia
- Unsteadiness, dizziness, and paresthesias, often misdiagnosed as multiple sclerosis
- Weakness of extremities, clumsiness, muscle cramps, twitching, or foot drop, often misdiagnosed as amyotrophic lateral sclerosis (ALS)
- Psychiatric symptoms, such as depression or psychosis (covered in greater length in the next chapter)
- Visual disturbances, vision loss, or blindness

---

blindness, Wilhelm discovered that her serum B$_{12}$ levels were only one-third of the normal limit. He started vitamin B$_{12}$ injections immediately, leading to "an almost complete recovery."[4]

In contrast, a doctor ignorant about the effects of B$_{12}$ deficiency can destroy a patient's life. The late John Hotchkiss, Jr., M.D., a crusader for the accurate diagnosis of B$_{12}$-deficient patients, once offered an example. When Hotchkiss (an ear-nose-throat specialist) practiced in a medical group, one of his partners—a Harvard graduate—objected strenuously to Hotchkiss's insistence on ruling out B$_{12}$ deficiency in patients with neurological disorders or other suspicious signs and symptoms. The doctor grew hostile on more than one occasion when Hotchkiss suggested evaluating a patient's B$_{12}$ levels, and he refused to be swayed by the medical literature Hotchkiss sent him.

"Some years later," Hotchkiss said, "he sent a patient to me for 'dizziness' evaluation." Hotchkiss discovered that the woman was not dizzy, but instead suffered from poor coordination stemming from neurological dysfunction. He wasn't surprised: the woman's history included a gastrectomy twelve years earlier, a surgery that inevitably results in severe B$_{12}$ deficiency if patients don't receive compensatory B$_{12}$ injections.

> **A doctor ignorant about the effects of B$_{12}$ deficiency can destroy a patient's life.**

The woman had been followed by Hotchkiss's colleague ever since the surgery, Hotchkiss said, "but he had done no follow-up studies concerning her B$_{12}$ status." As a result, she suffered from a condition known as "combined systems disease," or "subacute combined degeneration," a complication of chronic B$_{12}$ deficiency in which damage to the spinal cord tracts causes irreversible crippling.

"The doctor not only failed to monitor her and prevent this from happening, a grave dereliction, but he failed to recognize the condition when it occurred," Hotchkiss said. "When we met in the hall some weeks later, he said, 'You got me.'"[5]

Dr. Hotchkiss's story is further evidence that even specialists can miss a simple diagnosis of B$_{12}$ deficiency. It also demonstrates that even the most prestigious doctors, trained at the best schools, aren't immune from this failing. In addition, it's an illustration of why early treatment is crucial. This patient, of course, never should have developed symptoms to begin with, but once she did, a quick diagnosis would have saved her health.

Erica, a personal friend of ours, developed a mild tremor and arm weakness in middle age. When two neurologists failed to diagnose her problem, her son, a physician himself, stepped in and ordered tests that identified a B$_{12}$ deficiency. He immediately began treatment and, ten years later, her tremor is reduced by more than 75 percent and her arm no longer feels weak. The damage done by her B$_{12}$ deficiency was at least partially reversible, and even more important, it will never progress to the point where she will suffer dementia, paralysis, or other crippling symptoms.

If you suffer from neurological symptoms, the only way to rule out B$_{12}$ deficiency is by insisting that a doctor—whether it's your family practitioner, neurologist, psychiatrist, or other specialist—order a serum B$_{12}$, a urinary MMA, a holo TC, and a homocysteine test to help determine your B$_{12}$ status. We recommend a therapeutic trial of B$_{12}$ if even only one of the tests above is abnormal (which would include the serum B$_{12}$ falling in the gray zone). The alternative—never knowing if your symptoms could stem from a diagnosable, treatable, and often fully curable disorder—is simply unacceptable.

Vitamin B$_{12}$ deficiency needs to be ruled out in Parkinson's-type symptoms as well as in patients already diagnosed with Parkinson's disease. Because Parkinson's disease and B$_{12}$ deficiency share some of the same signs and symptoms, and there is no diagnostic test that can confirm Parkinson's disease, it only makes sense to investigate and rule out B$_{12}$ deficiency. This simple step can often save a life.

In one article in the medical literature, for instance, doctors reported the case of a fifty-five-year-old man who suddenly developed Parkinson's-like symptoms, including a slow gait, slow-paced movements, mild hand tremors, and low-volume speech. His doctors reported that he had a reduced blink rate, cogwheel rigidity of all limbs, resting tremors of both hands, and an expressionless face—all of which occur in Parkinson's patients.

After an extensive workup, the man's doctors discovered that he had a severe B$_{12}$ deficiency. His neurologist diagnosed him with acute onset parkinsonism with mild myeloneuropathy secondary to vitamin B$_{12}$ deficiency. He began receiving intramuscular vitamin B$_{12}$ injections and showed dramatic improvement. The neurologist reported that at a five-year follow-up, the man had no neurological deficits and was completely independent.[6]

Because vitamin B$_{12}$ deficiency affects the brain and nervous system in a variety of ways, neurological symptoms can vary widely. For instance, one recent case reported in a neurology journal involved a twenty-six-year-old man with recurrent partial complex seizures.[7] A year before the seizures began, the man had withdrawn socially. He had also started acting abnormally, and he'd developed memory problems. "Prior to admission," his doctor said, "he had neglected self-care, had become severely withdrawn and was disoriented." He was being treated with risperidone (Risperadol) and carbamazepine (Tegretol).

The patient was found to be severely B$_{12}$ deficient (his B$_{12}$ level was 26 pg/ml) and began treatment with vitamin B$_{12}$ injections. He quickly improved, became independent by the end of the third month, and was able to stop his medications after six months. At a twenty-four-month follow-up, his doctor reported that he remained seizure-free and was doing well.

Similar case reports of misdiagnosis or late diagnosis continue to be reported on a regular basis. These are not isolated cases. An array of medical journal articles can be found describing patients who suffered severe neurologic manifestations for months or years because B$_{12}$ deficiency was not included in the differential diagnosis by primary care physicians, internists, neurologists, and other specialists.[8-13]

We often receive firsthand reports of this negligence as well. Recently, for instance, a forty-six-year-old college professor named David wrote to us describing his frustration with his own doctors' lack of knowledge about B$_{12}$ deficiency. In 2006, David went to his family doctor complaining of mild depression and insomnia. "He offered to prescribe an antidepressant and sleep medication but I declined, in favor of trying natural remedies," David said. "I asked if there was a blood test to check for a chemical imbalance or vitamin deficiency. I didn't know anything about B$_{12}$ then." The doctor sent David for lab work, and about a week later his assistant called to report that everything tested normal. But his B$_{12}$ level *wasn't* normal; at 216 pg/ml, it was low and in the gray zone. The laboratory report noted this fact, stating that the results could reflect a hidden B$_{12}$ deficiency.

A year later, by this time suffering from severe depression and severe insomnia, David went to see his doctor again. "He offered an antidepressant and Ambien and this time I accepted it because my condition was so severe," David said. "At the appointment I asked if I should have blood tests but he said 'no need' because I had tests a year earlier and repeated tests would reveal the same thing."

A month after this appointment, after taking the prescribed antidepressant Cymbalta, David spent eight days in a psychiatric hospital because his depression and insomnia were so crippling he couldn't function at work or at home. "I was only sleeping three hours per night," he said. "Of course, the mental hospital did not screen my B$_{12}$ level. They only checked for the use of illegal drugs." Within the next eighteen months, David developed new symptoms: irritability, apathy, memory problems, weakness, fatigue, and paresthesias.

In February of 2009, David began to experience a strange muscle weakness in his legs, particularly in the left hamstring. His fatigue progressed to the point where he spent most of his day in bed. His doctor ordered lab work, including a CBC and basic metabolic panel, and reported that everything tested as normal. After seeing David twice and ordering a wide range of blood tests on two different occasions (none of which included B$_{12}$ tests), the doctor decided to refer David to a neurologist. David said, "He told my wife he suspected multiple sclerosis and was concerned that I might permanently lose the use of my legs."

The neurologist concluded that David had some type of virus that needed to run its course. He told David there was no treatment, the symptoms would take six weeks to six months to pass, and he would reevaluate David in five months. To make this diagnosis, the doctor had ordered more blood tests, an electromyography (EMG), and a nerve conduction velocity (NCV) study, but no tests for B$_{12}$ deficiency. Four weeks later, as David's symptoms grew worse, the neurologist reexamined him and sent him for more blood tests. The neurologist then referred him to another neurologist who specialized in neuromuscular conditions because he acknowledged that something was seriously wrong with David but could not accurately diagnose him.

The second neurologist suspected Guillain Barré syndrome because of David's symptoms, but repeat tests for this disorder were negative. He ordered more blood work, including a myasthenia gravis panel and an MRI of David's brain, neck and spine. "I had a follow-up appointment with the doctor on May 14, 2009, in which he was very concerned," David said. "He had the results of the MRIs, which were normal. He had all the blood test results except B$_{12}$ and B$_6$, which he thought would be normal. So he suspected ALS and was going to refer me to a specialist in San Francisco."

Fortunately, the next day the doctor received the B$_{12}$ and B$_6$ reports and discovered that David's B$_{12}$ level was severely low at 131 pg/ml. "What a huge one-day turnaround, from ALS to B$_{12}$ deficiency!" David said. David began receiving B$_{12}$ shots, which he self-administered daily for a year. He made little progress on the cyanocobalamin he received initially for the first five weeks, but his symptoms rapidly began resolving when his doctor switched to injectable methylcobalamin after David read the first edition of this book and requested this form of treatment (more on this in Chapter 11). "Three months later I had full recovery," he told us.

David reviewed the journals he'd kept during his experience and noted that he had experienced more than ten signs and symptoms of B$_{12}$ deficiency, and scored 13 on the Cobalamin Deficiency Risk Score (see Appendix M). His symptoms included muscle weakness, cramps, spasms, muscle twitches (upper and lower body), muscle atrophy, difficulty walking, balance problems, abnormal gait, tingling in his feet, a buzzing sensation in his lower legs, fatigue, poor memory, difficulty concentrating, apathy, irritability, and depression.

David was extremely lucky, because after three months of daily methyl-B$_{12}$ injections he reported a miraculous full recovery. However, his experience continues to affect his life today. In 2008, he applied for life insurance but was declined because of his history of depression and his stay in the psychiatric hospital. In 2009, after his true chronic B$_{12}$ deficiency was uncovered and treated, he applied again for life insurance but was declined this time as well.

IS IT MULTIPLE SCLEROSIS OR B$_{12}$ DEFICIENCY?

Kathy* *was just twenty-one when she fractured her leg. It healed, but afterward, it felt numb and Kathy found it harder and harder to walk. Then her fingers began tingling, and she started dropping objects frequently. Soon her right foot began dragging when she walked.*

A doctor checked Kathy's serum B$_{12}$ level, which was reported as "normal," but was in the gray zone at 275 pg/ml—actually indicating a deficiency. She was also anemic and her red blood cells were enlarged, two more signs of B$_{12}$ deficiency. Her bone marrow test appeared normal. Reviewing these findings, Kathy's doctor told her the bad news: She had multiple sclerosis (MS), a tragic diagnosis for a young woman. Barely out of her teens,

---

* Our pseudonym for the patient cited in this journal report.

Kathy faced a life burdened by a crippling disease that might eventually leave her paralyzed.

Six years later, however, Kathy found out her doctor was wrong. When Kathy turned twenty-seven, she was admitted to a hospital for increasing weakness and abnormal gait. During her stay, a new bone marrow test showed abnormalities consistent with B$_{12}$ deficiency. A repeat B$_{12}$ test performed at this time was reported as "normal," but actually wasn't normal at all. (The result was 180 pg/ml, which clearly indicates a deficiency, but this lab's reference range was 160 pg/ml—1,018 pg/ml.) Her iron deficiency anemia was growing worse and her red blood cells were still enlarged.

A new doctor reviewed Kathy's history from birth, spotting her early delays in walking and reading, and her poor coordination—as well as her mother's two unsuccessful pregnancies (one ending in a miscarriage, and the other in a stillbirth), and her father's history of hyperthyroidism and early death from heart disease. In his mind, Kathy's current symptoms and past history added up not to multiple sclerosis but to a familial form of B$_{12}$ deficiency. Further tests indeed showed that she suffered from a hereditary defect of B$_{12}$ metabolism, called cobalamin G, a diagnosis her previous doctors had missed for twenty-seven years.

Kathy's doctor started her on weekly B$_{12}$ shots, and gave her another medication (oral betaine) to normalize the high homocysteine levels caused by her inborn error of B$_{12}$ metabolism. Her weakness lessened, and after time she began walking more easily. But according to the physician who reported her case in the New England Journal of Medicine, *she continued to suffer from permanent neurologic damage—a legacy of more than a quarter-century of misdiagnosis.[14] Kathy's case is yet another example of why the accepted "normal" range for serum B$_{12}$ must be changed, and why doctors need to treat patients in the gray zone.*

Your coffee pot and your vacuum cleaner run on electricity, carried through wires. A thin layer of insulation covers these wires, preventing the current from escaping to the outside and disrupting the flow of electricity.

Similarly, the neurons in your brain and spinal cord send electrical messages. They too are insulated, by a protective fatty coating called *myelin*. If this myelin breaks down or becomes swollen, the electrical impulses sent by neurons can go haywire. One common cause of this short-circuiting is multiple sclerosis (MS), a disease that most often strikes young or middle-aged people, most of them women and most of them Caucasian.

We don't know what causes multiple sclerosis. We know that it's an autoimmune disease, possibly triggered by exposure to a virus, in which the body mistakenly attacks its own cells. We know that genes play a role, because having a first-degree relative with MS increases the risk of developing the disease several-fold. And we know that geography is involved: People born above the 40th parallel in the northern hemisphere, or below the 40th parallel in the southern hemisphere, have a higher risk of developing MS than people near the equator, unless they move before puberty.

We know, too, that multiple sclerosis and B$_{12}$ deficiency are different disorders. But the conditions are linked in three crucial ways:

- The symptoms of B$_{12}$ deficiency mimic the symptoms of multiple sclerosis, often leading to misdiagnosis—a mistake with grave consequences, because B$_{12}$ deficiency is completely reversible in its early stages, while MS is incurable.

- MS and chronic untreated B$_{12}$ deficiency both damage myelin, causing lesions or disease in the brain and spinal cord, and both disorders are classified as demyelinating diseases.

- Scientists report intriguing evidence tentatively implicating low B$_{12}$ levels in the development or exacerbation of multiple sclerosis—meaning that even when MS is diagnosed correctly, B$_{12}$ deficiency could possibly be contributing to the disease.

Later, we'll outline the speculative evidence implicating deficient B$_{12}$ levels as a factor in true cases of multiple sclerosis. First, however, let's look at why some of the 400,000 Americans diagnosed with MS may, instead, be suffering from a B$_{12}$ deficiency that can be diagnosed and cured.

> The symptoms of B$_{12}$ deficiency mimic the symptoms of multiple sclerosis, often leading to misdiagnosis.

Diagnosing multiple sclerosis is a challenge because no test can prove or rule out the presence of the disease, and because many other disorders mimic its signs and symptoms. It's estimated, in fact, that as many as 10 percent of people diagnosed with multiple sclerosis *don't actually have the disease.*[15]

Of this group, which translates into as many as 35,000 Americans (with 200 more new cases diagnosed each week), a significant number are likely to have B$_{12}$ deficiency. The resemblance between MS and B$_{12}$ deficiency is striking, with common symptoms including the following:

- gait problems
- numbness
- "pins and needles" sensations
- depression, paranoia, or psychosis
- memory loss, dementia, and other cognitive changes
- weight loss
- tremors
- fatigue
- coordination problems
- incontinence
- pain
- visual disturbances or vision loss

As we noted, there's a simple reason for this resemblance. Multiple sclerosis stems from myelin damage—and B$_{12}$ deficiency, left untreated long enough, also damages myelin, causing the same "short-circuiting" of nerve impulses.

But here's the big difference: When myelin destruction stems from B$_{12}$ deficiency, we can cure the patient's symptoms—all of them—if we catch the problem in time. Thus, it stands to reason that doctors should always rule out B$_{12}$ deficiency in patients with MS. Yet current standards of care do *not* dictate that doctors order the tests needed to do this, and many, as a result, never do. Nor do they give a therapeutic trial of daily or bi-weekly high-dose injectable methyl- or hydroxo-B$_{12}$.

Accurate diagnosis requires ordering a battery of tests that can conclusively prove, or definitively rule out, B$_{12}$ deficiency (see list at the end of this chapter). Even a "definitive" diagnosis of MS based on abnormal MRI findings does not eliminate the need for testing. As physician Robert Schilling notes, "Even though magnetic resonance imaging has been a significant advance in the diagnosis of multiple sclerosis, the findings are not 100 percent specific and cannot be relied on to differentiate MS from cobalamin [B$_{12}$] deficiency or another condition."[16]

Unfortunately, most doctors "rule out" B$_{12}$ deficiency in patients with suspected MS simply by ordering a CBC test, which can be grossly inaccurate. Other doctors who *do* include a serum B$_{12}$ test typically don't acknowledge deficiency or offer treatment when the serum B$_{12}$ is in the gray zone. In addition, physicians don't routinely use other B$_{12}$ markers (MMA, Hcy, or holo-TC) to assist in diagnosis. (Remember that the serum B$_{12}$ test can show "normal" or even high B$_{12}$ levels in markedly deficient patients for a variety of reasons.)

The results can be catastrophic, and for people like the seventy-seven-year-old woman we first mentioned in Chapter 2, they're likely to be fatal. Doctors told this woman when she was in her late fifties that she had MS, even though the disease typically strikes people below the age of fifty. One doctor gave her monthly B$_{12}$ shots for years—during which time her symptoms stabilized—but a new doctor discontinued them around the time of her seventy-second birthday. She deteriorated drastically over the next five years, finally arriving in the emergency room suffering from dementia and respiratory failure. Tests revealed clear evidence of B$_{12}$ deficiency (low serum B$_{12}$, elevated MMA, anemia, and hypersegmented neutrophils), but by then it was too late to save her. When we saw her, she was comatose and rolled into a fetal position. She had large bedsores and a severe blood infection (sepsis). She will spend the remainder of her life in an institution under hospice care.

Sadly, this woman's case is not an isolated anomaly. Robert Schilling and William Williams wrote in 1995, "Many experienced hematologists have seen patients with severe, permanent neurologic damage because the B$_{12}$ deficiency was mistaken for another disorder, such as *multiple sclerosis* [italics added], diabetic neuropathy, amyotrophic lateral sclerosis, or even Guillain-Barré syndrome." One of Schilling's own cases involved a woman diagnosed with MS eight months earlier by another doctor. The tests ordered by Schilling revealed conclusively that the woman suffered from a B$_{12}$ deficiency and did not have multiple sclerosis.[17]

Similarly, Dr. Eric Norman reported in 2000 that of six young women his research team diagnosed with B$_{12}$ deficiency, three were initially suspected of having MS. These three women's original doctors were puzzled and diagnosis was delayed because of the similarities between MS and B$_{12}$ deficiency, and because their patients were young. Norman comments, "This population deserves further evaluations since it has not been considered prone to cobalamin [B$_{12}$] deficiency." Correct treatment of these six patients resulted in a nearly complete recovery for two women, and partial recovery in one other case. The extent of improvement in two other women could not be measured since treatment had just begun when the report was published, and the last woman had not yet developed significant neurologic symptoms.[18]

How many similar cases of B$_{12}$ deficiency are misdiagnosed as MS? We don't know, but cases reported in the medical literature make it clear that the problem isn't an isolated one.

In the American Journal of Psychiatry,[19] *Gary Payinda and colleagues reported the case of a woman who probably owes them her life—and certainly owes them her sanity.*

At fifty-two years of age, Mrs. A suddenly developed paralysis in her legs. Her doctor referred her to a neurologist, who diagnosed her with multiple sclerosis. Over the next two months, Mrs. A was placed on numerous medications, but her leg weakness progressed and the drugs did not help. She required a cane, then used a walker, and eventually needed a wheelchair to get around. As time went by, Mrs. A became agitated and angry. She grew paranoid, and she called the police to report that her family was trying to poison her. She also became violent, throwing furniture and even trying to jump from a moving car.

Mrs. A's family, stunned and frightened by her worsening behavior, finally took her to an emergency psychiatric center. She appeared disheveled, was delirious and disoriented, and paranoid, and could not stand without assistance. The psychiatric facility obtained a B$_{12}$ level, which came back extremely low at 9 pg/ml.

The doctors diagnosed Mrs. A. with subacute combined spinal cord degeneration and psychosis due to a severe vitamin B$_{12}$ deficiency. Additional tests revealed that she suffered from pernicious anemia; earlier physicians missed the diagnosis in part because her folic acid supplements had masked her blood abnormalities.

Two days after starting B$_{12}$ injections, Mrs. A started regaining the strength in her legs. Within eight weeks, her symptoms of mental illness vanished. Unfortunately, she may never fully regain her health and mobility, because of the delay in diagnosing her correctly. The cause of that delay: her *original neurologist failed to diagnose her correctly, instead misdiagnosing her with MS and apparently never considering B$_{12}$ deficiency.*

Patients like Mrs. A suffer terribly, and unnecessarily, because many physicians lack even the most basic knowledge about B$_{12}$-deficiency symptoms. Moreover, this ignorance isn't limited to inexperienced doctors. Recently, we found a noted neurologist offering the following advice to fellow doctors on differentiating between MS and B$_{12}$ deficiency:

"Multiple sclerosis often has the pattern of relapse then [remission] with multiple episodes. B$_{12}$ deficiency progressively worsens.... Multiple sclerosis can have other systems affected—for example, visual, coordination, tremor—and often years apart from the current problem. These are not features of B$_{12}$ deficiency.... In most cases history and exam can tell these two apart, but sometimes one can mimic the other. If so, part of the workup could include a B$_{12}$ level and if suspicion is high, one can check homocysteine and methylmalonic acid levels, metabolites which are more sensitive for B$_{12}$ deficiency—these tests should give an answer if any question of B$_{12}$ deficiency exists."[20]

What's wrong with this advice, offered by a physician at a leading American hospital? Almost everything. Here's why:

- B$_{12}$ deficiency can easily mimic the remission-and-relapse pattern of MS. A patient getting blood transfusions, or receiving tube or IV feedings, can receive enough B$_{12}$ to temporarily replenish B$_{12}$ levels, making the serum B$_{12}$ fictitiously elevated on a lab report. A B$_{12}$-deficient vegetarian who starts eating more animal products or meat again can appear to go into "remission." Steroids administered to patients during an "attack" can increase B$_{12}$ absorption in undiagnosed autoimmune pernicious anemia patients, again mimicking remission.* A patient who starts taking high-dose vitamins may receive enough B$_{12}$ to cause improvement. Doctors who give occasional B$_{12}$ injections, "just in case you need it," can make patients' symptoms vanish temporarily, only to return when the shots' effects wear off. Conversely, stress, pregnancy, infection, administration of immunizations with mercury (see Chapter 12), eating disorders, exposure to

---

* G. R. Lee states in *Wintrobe's Clinical Hematology* (1999, 10th Edition, pp. 941–958), "The fact that some patients with pernicious anemia respond to the administration of adrenal corticosteroids also suggests a possible autoimmune mechanism in the development of the disease. The reported responses include hematologic improvement, increased vitamin B$_{12}$ absorption, histologic improvement in gastric mucosa, appearance of acid and intrinsic factor in gastric juice and decrease in serum titers of intrinsic factor antibody."

nitrous oxide, or a switch to a vegetarian diet can cause a "relapse." Thus, arbitrarily ruling out B$_{12}$ deficiency in a patient with a relapsing and remitting pattern of MS symptoms can be deadly.

- A history, exam, and complete blood count are *never* sufficient to rule out B$_{12}$ deficiency in a patient with suspected MS, because B$_{12}$ deficiency can mimic the signs and symptoms of even classic MS. Remember, both MS and B$_{12}$ deficiency are classified as demyelinating diseases.

- Vision problems (up to and including blindness), tremor, and poor coordination can indeed be symptoms of B$_{12}$ deficiency, and the pattern and timing of symptoms can vary from patient to patient—just as in multiple sclerosis.

- Suggesting that the workup for a patient with multiple sclerosis "*could include* a B$_{12}$ level [italics added]," as though the test is optional, is dangerously misguided. The serum B$_{12}$, urinary MMA, Hcy, and Holo TC are all absolute necessities in every suspected case of MS—particularly because most physicians do not practice treating patients in the gray zone. (See Chapter 11.)

> A history, exam, and complete blood count are *never* sufficient to rule out B$_{12}$ deficiency in a patient with suspected MS.

- The recommendation that only patients whose MS diagnosis is obviously "suspicious" should receive MMA and homocysteine tests is, again, potentially deadly. As we've explained, the standard serum B$_{12}$ test is often inaccurate because of the poor parameters set by many labs. Moreover, tests for anemia and enlarged red blood cells can be misleading because—and this is a critical piece of information that most doctors lack—**the steroids commonly used to treat multiple sclerosis can normalize the anemia and enlarged cells characteristic of B$_{12}$, while allowing the neurologic damage to continue unchecked.** (This is similar to the effects of folic acid supplementation, which we discussed earlier.) In addition, some co-existing conditions (iron deficiency, sickle cell anemia, and thalassemia) can mask enlarged red blood cells.

Thus, in our opinion, a doctor must rule out B$_{12}$ deficiency in all patients suspected of having MS, or actually diagnosed with MS. Failing to order these tests (as well as failing to treat patients in the gray zone) puts patients at risk for permanent injury or even death, and in our opinion constitutes negligence.

As medical professionals, we've seen the results of this negligence first-hand. One case involved Linda, a thirty-six-year-old patient diagnosed with MS. Linda turned up in the emergency room three years after her

---

THE COST OF MISDIAGNOSIS

Four hundred thousand Americans currently are diagnosed with multiple sclerosis. If only 4.2 percent of them actually suffer from B$_{12}$ deficiency—the lowest estimate we can find in the medical literature, and undoubtedly a gross underestimate because of the criteria used[21] —that adds up to 16,800 people.

Using this lowest-possible estimate, let's look at the cost of treating these individuals:

- If these 16,800 people take Betaseron, at $33,165 per year, the cost is: $557 million yearly.

- If these 16,800 people eventually require nursing home care, the cost is: $1.3 billion yearly.

- If these 16,800 people receive a correct diagnosis, the cost of their treatment (initial series of shots, and then weekly self hydroxoco-balamin injections) drops to less than $605,000 yearly—which is over $556 million in savings yearly.

- And, if these 16,800 people did not require nursing home care, the savings would be over 1.299 billion dollars! (See Chapter 13.)

Goodkin et al. found that 32 (19.4%) of 165 patients with multiple sclerosis or idiopathic myelopathy had serum B$_{12}$ levels below 301 pg/ml. They mistakenly concluded that only 4.2% had B$_{12}$ deficiency because they also had elevated MMA or Hcy levels. We now know that MMA and Hcy values are not gold standards and can mislead the clinician (see Chapter 11), and that symptomatic patients in the gray zone need to be treated. Therefore, if we used the 19.4% value rather than the 4.2% statistic, this would equate to 77,600 patients who have a B$_{12}$ deficiency and may respond to B$_{12}$ therapy. If these 77,600 patients were on Betaseron, this equates to $2.57 billion dollars per year!

WE ARE AS SICK AS OUR SECRETS

A film producer passionate about our cause contacted us in late 2009 after she read the first edition of *Could It Be B12?* She is currently producing a documentary about B$_{12}$ deficiency and its underdiagnosis, and has interviewed many patients and physicians to tell the story of this misunderstood and mistreated epidemic. Speaking of one hematologist she interviewed, she says, "I couldn't use the story he told about a medical student diagnosing a patient that the whole neurology department missed, because that raises the question, 'Did someone do something wrong?'"

It most certainly does raise that question! How can we effectively address this treatable disorder if those with the power to help make needed change don't speak out, but hide in fear?

---

initial diagnosis (and several months after delivering a baby), when her symptoms began growing worse. She complained of foggy vision and weakness in her legs, and she'd fallen and injured her left knee.

The tests the ER doctor ordered for Linda revealed a very low B$_{12}$ level. It's likely that Linda's B$_{12}$ stores became dangerously depleted during her pregnancy, triggering the exacerbation of her symptoms. But when the ER doctor notified Linda's neurologist that her B$_{12}$ level was very low and could be causing some or all of her symptoms, the neurologist replied brusquely, "No, this patient has documented MS."

> Copaxone, an MS drug, costs $36,000 per year, while B$_{12}$ therapy costs under $40 per year.

In an age of managed-care cost cutting, many physicians consider comprehensive testing for B$_{12}$ deficiency "too expensive," although in reality the cost of *not* performing these tests is vastly higher. Copaxone, a drug for MS that must be injected daily, costs $36,903 per year; Betaseron and Avonex are nearly as expensive, at $33,165 and $33,299 per year, respectively. In addition, many people with MS require extensive and expensive therapy, and some require long-term care. If even a small percentage of cases diagnosed as MS involve B$_{12}$ deficiency, correct diagnosis could save families, and the American medical system, millions of dollars annually.

When it comes to B$_{12}$ screening, however, physicians and managed care providers are often penny-wise and pound-foolish. Thus, if you've been diagnosed with multiple sclerosis, or if a doctor suggests that your symptoms point to MS, it's up to you to be assertive and insist on thorough testing. Don't assume that your doctor will check you for B$_{12}$ deficiency, and don't assume—even if your doctor says you'll be tested—that he or she will order the right tests. Instead, obtain your test results, check them against the list at the end of this chapter, and keep pushing until every test on the list is performed. Don't take the risk of being diagnosed with an incurable disease, when you may have one that's completely curable in its early stages.

A DOCTOR'S STORY

Even physicians have been misdiagnosed with other neurological disorders when the real diagnosis was vitamin B$_{12}$ deficiency. In 2004, David Carr, M.D., a local pediatrician in Orlando, Florida, began having paresthesias and balance problems which he himself thought may be MS. In 2005, he became very ill.

Carr was misdiagnosed with olivopontocerebellar atrophy (OPCA) or multisystem atrophy at age fifty-five. He lost fifty pounds, lost his vision, and gradually deteriorated to the point where he could not eat or walk. His sister, who trains guide dogs, says, "On his 'death bed' at Shands Hospital in Gainesville, Florida, the doctor discovered that it was pernicious anemia, vitamin B$_{12}$ deficiency." Dr. Carr was told by his doctors that he would probably gain his sight back, but he may never walk again. Fortunately, with the help of physical therapy, forearm crutches, and a specially trained balance dog, Dr. Carr did regain the ability to walk, but he still suffers from neurologic disability caused by chronic untreated B$_{12}$ deficiency.[22]

Dr. Carr relays that the so-called "best neurologist in Florida" misdiagnosed him and told him he was dying and to go into hospice care. Multisystem atrophy is a rare neurological disorder characterized by a combination of parkinsonism, cerebellar and pyramidal signs, and autonomic dysfunction. His friend, a psychologist, carried him to the hospital where a geriatric psychiatrist correctly determined that he was severely B$_{12}$ deficient (serum B$_{12}$ 54 pg/ml). In 2010 (five years later), Dr. Carr still suffers from the result of late diagnosed B$_{12}$ deficiency and needs forearm crutches to ambulate.

Similarly, we advocate comprehensive B$_{12}$ testing in all patients diagnosed with Guillain-Barré, chronic immune demyelinating polyneuropathy (CIDP), seizure disorders, ALS, CBGD, and Parkinson's type disorders.

George, a fifty-two-year-old male, came into the ER with an injured right foot. Wheelchair-bound due to symptoms of MS, George could get up to shave and go to the bathroom, and that's what he'd been doing when he fell and broke his foot. His legs were very weak, and he walked with a spastic gait when he moved from his wheelchair to a regular chair. He complained of chronic mid-back pain and told the ER staff that in addition to his MS (diagnosed eighteen months earlier), he suffered from depression, bipolar disorder, spinal stenosis, an irritable bowel, and neuralgia.

George's history raised red flags, leading the ER doctor to look for additional evidence of B$_{12}$ deficiency. George's blood tests showed enlarged red blood cells, and his MMA came back elevated. The latter clearly indicated B$_{12}$ deficiency, particularly after the doctor ruled out other likely causes of high serum MMA, such as impaired kidney function. Interestingly, George had high serum B$_{12}$ levels, possibly because other doctors—mistaking his symptoms for effects of alcoholism—occasionally gave him intravenous fluids containing vitamins.

The ER doctor called George's primary care doctor one week later, after receiving all of George's results, and explained that the findings indicated that B$_{12}$ deficiency was causing or exacerbating George's symptoms. George's doctor was grateful for the information, saying, "I owe you one."

Speculation: Does true MS involve a B$_{12}$ abnormality?

MS and B$_{12}$ deficiency are two different diseases, and doctors diagnose the great majority of cases of MS correctly. Yet intriguing (although highly speculative) clues are now leading scientists to explore the possibility that even classic multiple sclerosis may involve a defect in B$_{12}$ metabolism.

Interestingly, there are many similarities between MS and pernicious anemia, the autoimmune form of B$_{12}$ deficiency we described in Chapter 1. The two diseases strike both young adults[*] and middle-aged persons,

---

[*] Although it is not well known or extensively documented, autoimmune pernicious anemia can strike people in their twenties, thirties, and forties. Because physicians believe that pernicious anemia typically strikes in the fifth or sixth decade of life, they rarely evaluate young adults for this disease, instead assuming that the neurological symptoms of B$_{12}$ deficiency or pernicious anemia are caused by multiple sclerosis.

IS IT MULTIPLE SCLEROSIS OR B$_{12}$ DEFICIENCY—OR BOTH?

If you're experiencing symptoms that resemble multiple sclerosis, or if you have already been diagnosed with MS, your doctor needs to order the following tests in order to rule out B$_{12}$ deficiency. Defects in B$_{12}$ utilization stemming from inborn errors of B$_{12}$ metabolism or transport are difficult to detect without tests more sensitive than a serum B$_{12}$ test. If your doctor questions the need for any of these tests, refer him or her to Chapter 11:

1. Serum B$_{12}$ (*results falling in the gray zone also need treatment or therapeutic trial*)

2. Urine methylmalonic acid (MMA)

    a. Lab must use gas chromatography/mass spectrometry (GC/MS) technique

3. Plasma homocysteine (Hcy)

4. Holo-TC

If any of these tests come back positive or the serum B$_{12}$ is in the gray zone, your doctor should start you on hydroxocobalamin or methylcobalamin injections. A therapeutic trial is daily or every-other-day subcutaneous methyl-B$_{12}$ injections for three months (see Chapter 11).

Note: If possible, your doctor should order these tests before beginning any treatment with steroids, Copaxone, Betaseron, or Avonex (Rebif). It is unknown if treatment with these drugs can alter the results of MMA, Hcy, or Holo-TC tests. Also, testing should be done before you try any over-the-counter or prescription B$_{12}$, which will skew B$_{12}$ test results.

and both involve immune system abnormalities. Both are more common in cold northern areas than in tropical southern areas, and both affect Caucasians more often than African Americans. Both diseases strike females more often than males, and in the same ratio (1.3 to 1). There are more links, too, between multiple sclerosis and B$_{12}$ deficiency:

- Enlarged red blood cells, a classic sign of B$_{12}$ deficiency, often occur in MS patients. This abnormal finding is seen even in the earliest stages of MS, and thus isn't likely to be merely a side effect of the disease.

> ## Abnormal Vitamin B$_{12}$ Transport or Partial Defect of Transcobalamin II?
>
> Complete transcobalamin II (TC II) deficiency is detected in infancy and causes severe neurological manifestations, anemia, failure to thrive, and death from the inability to transfer cobalamin (B$_{12}$). It is typically detected in the first 6 to 20 weeks of life. But what happens if a person has a partial rather than a complete defect? The TC II or B$_{12}$ deficiency may not manifest until late childhood or early adulthood. The serum B$_{12}$ may be normal because most of the vitamin in plasma is bound to TC I or TC III. It is the body's inability to transport B$_{12}$ to the cells that causes the severe neurologic disease (subacute combined degeneration of the spinal cord) which can be confused with MS and other neuromuscular disorders. Similar to Dr. Kilmer McCully (see Chapter 5) hypothesizing that a partial genetic defect of homocysteine could cause early vascular disease in adults, we hypothesize that some patients diagnosed with MS or other neuromuscular disorders may have a partial TC II defect that manifests itself in early adulthood. This hypothesis deserves research—for many lives could be saved if there is a safe and effective treatment.

- Researchers often report marginal serum B$_{12}$, or B$_{12}$ results in the gray zone in MS patients.

- B$_{12}$ injections do not improve motor function in most people with true MS. However, one study of MS patients found that visual and brain stem auditory evoked potentials—measurements of the nervous system's response to stimuli—improved more frequently during B$_{12}$ treatment than before treatment.[23] (Unfortunately, it's impossible to know if the motor symptoms of the patients in this study might also have improved if B$_{12}$ treatment had been started earlier, before their myelin damage became permanent. We also don't know if aggressive daily treatment with methyl-B$_{12}$ injections could have reduced their motor symptoms.)

- The medical literature contains reports of patients exhibiting symptoms of multiple sclerosis due to a deficiency of R binder, a protein that plays an essential role in B$_{12}$ metabolism.

All of these facts hint that MS and B$_{12}$ deficiency may somehow be intertwined. Unfortunately, only a minority of patients with true MS improve appreciably when they receive injections of vitamin B$_{12}$—although this disappointing result could possibly be influenced by the form, dose, and frequency of B$_{12}$ they are given (see Chapter 11).

To clarify the possible B$_{12}$–MS link, scientists are now focusing on the following two questions:

1. *Does B$_{12}$ deficiency contribute to the development of MS?* Research shows that people who develop multiple sclerosis before the age of eighteen have lower B$_{12}$ levels than those who develop MS in adulthood. Because B$_{12}$ levels are unrelated to the length of the illness, researchers say, "these findings suggest a specific association between the timing of onset of the first neurological symptoms of MS and vitamin B$_{12}$ metabolism."[24] They speculate that B$_{12}$ deficiency—which suppresses the immune system's ability to fight off viruses and bacteria—could leave some people more vulnerable to MS by impairing their defenses against the infections that are widely suspected of playing a role in the genesis of MS.

2. *Does B$_{12}$ deficiency make it harder for the body to repair the myelin damage that occurs in MS?* Vitamin B$_{12}$ plays a crucial role in myelin formation, and research suggests that the body may require normal or even higher-than-normal levels of

> **All of these facts hint that MS and B$_{12}$ deficiency may somehow be intertwined.**

B$_{12}$ in order to reverse the myelin damage caused by MS.[25] If so, MS patients with low levels of B$_{12}$ may be less likely to go into remission.

All of these findings are very preliminary, and we don't yet know if B$_{12}$ deficiency puts people at increased risk for MS, or whether it inhibits their ability to go into remission once they have the disease. However, researchers should focus on finding answers to these questions. Few diseases strike the young and healthy with as much cruelty as MS, and if it turns out that B$_{12}$ can play some role in protecting against the disease, or in improving its course when it occurs, this knowledge could be invaluable to thousands of MS patients.

In the meantime, we urge that any MS patient, with or without signs of B$_{12}$ deficiency, should first be tested and then start a long-term trial of

NOTE FOR PHYSICIANS:
WHAT IS THE END RESULT OF UNTREATED VITAMIN B₁₂
DEFICIENCY OR LATE DIAGNOSIS?

Subacute combined degeneration (SCD) is the term doctors use to describe the damage to the spinal cord caused by chronic vitamin B₁₂ deficiency. It typically involves the posterior and lateral columns of the spinal cord (hence the name *combined system disease*). In medical terminology, this is also abbreviated as SCDSC—*subacute combined degeneration of the spinal cord*. The term SCD is customarily reserved specifically for the spinal cord lesion caused by vitamin B₁₂ deficiency.

In addition to the spinal cord, vitamin B₁₂ deficiency attacks and injures the peripheral nerves, brain, and optic nerves. Prolonged B₁₂ deficiency eventually leads to SCD, but in many cases, psychiatric, cognitive, and visual disturbances appear first. Mood disturbances and mental changes, ranging from mild forgetfulness to severe dementia or psychosis, often occur.

Common early symptoms of SCD include numbness and tingling (paresthesias), difficulty walking, and balance problems. Paresthesias typically occur in the limbs but may involve the trunk, causing a wrapping sensation or constriction in the abdomen or chest.

Abnormal reflexes are often found and spasticity of muscles may develop. Patients report a reduced sense of touch, pain, and temperature. Loss of vibration sense, changes in tendon reflexes, clonus, and extensor plantar responses may occur. Sensory disturbances precede motor disturbances. Progression of the deficiency leads to limb weakness and ataxia. Prolonged untreated B₁₂ deficiency may progress to paraplegia with variable degrees of spasticity and contracture. The spinothalamic tracts may be involved, which manifests as a loss of superficial sensation below a certain level on the trunk.

Mental signs of vitamin B₁₂ deficiency are common and should always raise a red flag. In some cases, beginning dementia may be the first symptom. Damage to the optic nerve, decreased visual acuity, peripheral vision loss, and signs of nerve inflammation may be found during eye and retinal exams. Visual impairment due to optic neuropathy may occasionally be the earliest or sole manifestation of B₁₂ deficiency. The fact that visual evoked potentials may be abnormal in vitamin B$_{12}$-deficient patients without clinical signs of visual impairment reveals that evaluation of the visual pathways may be an important adjunct to the neurologic examination. Some patients may also experience autonomic dysfunction, including urinary sphincteric symptoms and impotence.

B$_{12}$ deficiency causes myelin breakdown, axonal degeneration, macrophage infiltration, and astrocytic gliosis. The process of destruction takes the form of a diffuse though uneven degeneration of white matter of the spinal cord as well as the brain. Swelling of myelin sheaths is an early finding, followed by larger tissue destruction. Both the myelin sheaths and axis cylinders are attacked. Injury begins in the posterior columns of the lower cervical and upper thoracic segment of the cord and fans out from this region up and down the cord as well as into the lateral and anterior columns. Because the lesions are scattered irregularly through the white matter and are not limited to the fibers within the posterior and lateral columns, the term *combined system disease* (often used loosely to describe the myelopathy caused by B$_{12}$ deficiency) is less appropriate than the term SCD.[27]

injectable daily methyl-B$_{12}$. We recommend a methyl-B$_{12}$ trial even if the tests are negative for a deficiency, because we don't yet fully understand the connection between MS and B$_{12}$ metabolism.

We are aware that this is not standard practice for most physicians who treat MS. However, vitamin B$_{12}$ is nontoxic, even in high doses, so it's risk-free, except for patients with rare allergic reactions or a very rare condition called Leber's disease. (People with this disease have an adverse reaction when *cyanocobalamin* is used—see Chapter 11.) Moreover, a small but significant percentage of MS patients report that treatment makes them significantly better. In some cases the improvement is dramatic, and occasionally it occurs even after years of disability. Thus, to our way of thinking, it makes sense—given the lack of a "down side"—for every MS patient to give B$_{12}$ a chance. Doctors will not only be saving lives, but will also be saving enormous amounts of money for their patients and society.

Note: Patients who are being treated for neurologic injury caused by B$_{12}$ deficiency or are using high-dose B$_{12}$ as therapy for MS or other neurologic disorders should not be using cyanocobalamin. Methyl-B$_{12}$

alone or combined with adenosyl-B$_{12}$ should be used instead (see Chapter 11).

In 2009, doctors published a case study in the Journal of the Louisiana State Medical Society[26] *describing an eighteen-year-old woman who presented with significant neurological manifestations but only mild blood abnormalities and a normal serum B$_{12}$ level.*

The woman arrived at the ER complaining that she was unable to walk. For about a month, she'd suffered from severe leg weakness, which was preceded by numbness and tingling and balance problems. Her symptoms progressed to the point where she required a walker to get around her house. As a result, she was unable to attend school. She also had blurred vision, constipation, and problems with urinary retention.

The woman wasn't a vegetarian, and she ate meat and meat products. At the time the ER doctor saw her, she was emotionally "flat," exhibited monotonous speech, and was thin. The motor strength in her legs was markedly diminished, and her leg muscles were atrophied. She had poor sensation in both legs below her thighs, as well as impaired sensation in both feet.

Tests showed that the woman had anemia with macrocytosis, but her serum B$_{12}$ was 415 pg/ml. An MRI of the spine revealed evidence of demyelination in the anterior portion of her spinal cord, extending from the bottom of her neck (C7) through her mid-back (T4). Physical exam revealed abnormal nerve responses from this area. Her blood MMA and homocysteine levels were both severely elevated at 13 μmol/L and 167 μmol/L respectively. Additionally, she was positive for anti-intrinsic factor, a finding consistent with pernicious anemia.

Her doctors began B$_{12}$ treatment and report that after the first injection she "became more alert; her speech improved; and her clonus began to diminish." They add, "By the time she was transferred to our rehabilitation facility several days later, she was taking short steps with assistance and had regained much of her normal cognitive functioning."

This case study shows why patients who present with signs and symptoms of B$_{12}$ deficiency need to have additional B$_{12}$ markers (MMA and Hcy) included in their work-ups. In this case, the patient's serum B$_{12}$ was on the high side of the gray zone, which would have led nearly all physicians to rule out B$_{12}$ deficiency because of her "normal" results. However, her anemia, macrocytosis, and severe neurologic deficits all pointed to B$_{12}$ deficiency—and her grossly elevated MMA and Hcy revealed a severe deficiency and made the diagnosis. Her response to B$_{12}$ therapy also proved the diagnosis to be correct, which is why a trial of aggressive injectable B$_{12}$ is always indicated when the patient's signs and symptoms indicate B$_{12}$ deficiency but lab results don't support the diagnosis.

CHAPTER 3 NOTES

1. Roach, E. Steve, and McLean, William T. Neurologic disorders of B$_{12}$ deficiency. *American Family Physician*, 1982, 25:111–115.

2. Heath, Thomas. Pernicious anemia: One man's journey through the baffling world of medical diagnosis. *Washington Post*, February 22, 2000, p. Z–12.

3. Schilling, R. F., and Williams, W. J. Vitamin B$_{12}$ deficiency: Under-diagnosed, overtreated? *Hospital Practice*, July 15, 1995, 47–54.

4. Wilhelm, H., Grodd, W., Schiefer, U., and Zrenner, E. Uncommon chiasmal lesions: demyelinating disease, vasculitis, and cobalamin deficiency. *German Journal of Ophthalmology*, 1993, 2:234–40.

5. Hotchkiss, J. Vitamin B$_{12}$—A Controversial Vitamin (conference presentation). June 2001, *Society for Orthomolecular Medicine*, San Francisco.

6. Kumar, S. Vitamin B$_{12}$ deficiency presenting with an acute reversible extrapyramidal syndrome. *Neurol India*, 2004;52:507–509.

7. Kumar, S. Recurrent seizures: An unusual manifestation of vitamin B$_{12}$ deficiency. *Neurol India* [serial online] 2004 [cited 2010 Jan 19];52:122–3. Available from: http://www.neurologyindia.com/text.asp?2004/52/1/122/6721.

8. Turner, M. R., Talbot, K. Functional vitamin B$_{12}$ deficiency. *Pract Neurol* 2009; 9:37–45.

9. Kalita, J., Misra, U. K. Vitamin B$_{12}$ deficiency neurological syndromes: correlation of clinical, MRI and cognitive evoked potential. *J Neurol* 2008;255:353–9.

10. Matrana, M. R., Gauthier, C., Lafaye, K.M. Paralysis and pernicious anemia in a young woman. *J La State Med Soc* 2009 Jul-Aug;161(4):228–32.

11. Isajiw, G. To peg or not to peg: A case of a hospice referral for vitamin B$_{12}$ deficiency. *The Linacre Quarterly* 76(2) May 2009:212–217.

12. Paul, I., Reichard, R. R. Subacute combined degeneration mimicking traumatic spinal cord injury. *Am J Forensic Med Pathol* 2009;30:47–48.

13. Svenson, J. Case Report: Neurologic disease and vitamin B$_{12}$ deficiency. *American Journal of Emergency Medicine* (2007) 25, 987.e3-987.e4.

14. Carmel, R., Watkins, D., Goodman, S. I., and Rosenblatt, D. S. Hereditary defect of cobalamin metabolism (cblG mutation) presenting as a neurologic disorder in adulthood. *New England Journal of Medicine* 1988, 318(26):1738–41.

15. Trojano, M., and Paolicelli, D. The differential diagnosis of multiple sclerosis: Classification and clinical features of relapsing and progressive neurological syndromes. *Neurological Sciences* 2001 Suppl 2:S98–102.

16. Schilling, R. F., and Williams, W. J. Vitamin B$_{12}$ deficiency: Underdiagnosed, overtreated? *Hospital Practice*, July 15, 1995, 47–54.

17. Ibid.

18. Norman, E. J. Cobalamin (vitamin B$_{12}$) deficiency identified in young, Caucasian women. *Blood*, 2000, 96(11):8b.

19. Payinda, G., and Hansen, T. Vitamin B(12) deficiency manifested as psychosis without anemia. *American Journal of Psychiatry* 2000, 157:660–61.

20. Physician information posted on the Neurology and Neurosurgery Forum, in answer to a question. Questions on the forum are answered by physicians from the Cleveland Clinic, a major U.S. hospital.

21. Goodkin, D. E., et al. Serum cobalamin deficiency is uncommon in multiple sclerosis. *Archives of Neurology* 1994, 51:1110–14.

22. yvonnekai.blogspot.com/2010/11/service-dog.html.

23. Kira, Jun-ichi, Tobimatsu, Shozo, and Goto, Ikuo. Vitamin B$_{12}$ metabolism and massive-dose methyl vitamin B$_{12}$ therapy in Japanese patients with multiple sclerosis. *Internal Medicine* 1994, 33:82–86.

24. Sandyk, R., and Awerbuch, G. I. Vitamin B$_{12}$ and its relationship to age of onset of multiple sclerosis. *International Journal of Neuroscience* (England) Jul–Aug 1993, 71: p93–9.

25. Kira, J., Tobimatsu, S., and Goto, I. Vitamin B$_{12}$ metabolism and massive-dose methyl vitamin B$_{12}$ therapy in Japanese patients with multiple sclerosis. *Internal Medicine* 1994, 33:82–86.

26. Matrana, M. R., Gauthier, C., Lafaye, K. M. Paralysis and pernicious anemia in a young woman. *J La State Med Soc* 2009 Jul-Aug;161(4):228–32.

27. *Adams and Victor's Principles of Neurology* (2001) 7th Ed. Maurice Victor and Allan H. Ropper, Ch. 41—Diseases of the Nervous System due to Nutritional Deficiency, pp. 1218–1223;McGraw-Hill.

4

Am I Losing My Mind? When B_{12} Deficiency Causes Mental Illness

"Deficiency of essential nutrients like folic acid and vitamin B_{12} is an obvious risk factor for both disorders with cognitive impairment and depression."
—C. G. Gottfries, M.D.[1]

"Current research suggests that low levels of vitamin B_{12} are associated with dementia and depression…. Vitamin B_{12} deficiency has also been associated with psychosis, bipolar disorder, and catatonia."
—Psychiatrist Glenn Catalano, M.D., and colleagues[2]

"I have gained a distinct sense that we physicians, neurologists, and psychiatrists have been miserly with our B_{12} diagnoses and treatments."
—John Dommisse, M.D.[3]

In the last chapter, we explained how B_{12} deficiency attacks the nerves, stripping them of their protective myelin coating and disrupting the communication between cells in the brain and other parts of the nervous system. This damage, as we noted, can make you lose your balance, develop multiple sclerosis-like symptoms, or suffer shooting pains or numbness in your feet, hands, arms, or legs. It can also make your memory fuzzy, cause cognitive difficulties, and even mimic Alzheimer's disease.

But the damage that B_{12} depletion causes can affect your nervous system in other ways as well. Because the nerve cells in your brain control how you feel, think, and behave, B_{12} deficiency can cause severe mental illness, including depression, paranoia, and even symptoms resembling schizophrenia. A deficiency of B_{12} is not the cause of *most* cases of mental illness, but it clearly plays a powerful role in a number of cases—and particularly in cases involving depression or bipolar disorder (manic depression).

One problem is that we don't know the true incidence of B_{12} deficiency in mental illness, because most physicians don't screen for it and no major studies have been done to document its incidence. Studies in the past have shown the incidence related to depression to be around 20 percent, which is highly significant—especially since these studies do not include patients falling in the gray zone.

The middle-aged man had been happy and healthy most of his life, but sometime after his fiftieth birthday his behavior changed radically. He became hyperactive, and he no longer slept more than a few hours each night. Worse, he developed the strange flights of thought and grandiose ideas typical of people in the manic phase of bipolar disorder.

> B$_{12}$ deficiency can cause severe mental illness, including depression, paranoia, and even symptoms resembling schizophrenia.

After four years, however, the man began suffering very different symptoms: He became anxious and sad, stopped eating, and was tired all the time. Eventually, he began having paranoid thoughts about his wife.

Finally, the man encountered a new physician who checked his B$_{12}$ levels, which were so low that his plasma B$_{12}$ was "undetectable." Further tests revealed that he had pernicious anemia (an autoimmune disease), and the new doctor started him on regular B$_{12}$ shots.

"His mental state improved dramatically within a few days," physicians P. M. Verbanck and O. LeBon report in the Journal of Clinical Psychiatry. *"By the end of the first week of treatment, the only remaining symptom was the paranoid delusions." These slowly subsided, disappearing completely after six months of treatment.*[4]

The patient described above had bipolar disorder because his B$_{12}$ levels were so low that his brain couldn't function correctly. In his case, the problem stemmed from pernicious anemia, but people with dangerously low B$_{12}$ due to other causes are equally at risk of developing severe depression or bipolar disorder.

How dramatically can B$_{12}$ deficiency increase your risk of developing severe, life-threatening depression? Researchers at the National Institute on Aging, evaluating a group of disabled women over the age of sixty-five, found that B$_{12}$ deficiency *doubled* the risk of severe depression in this group. The researchers, noting that these were independent women living in the community, report, "It should be an alarming sign that we found [a significant rate of B$_{12}$-deficiency-caused depression] in this population."[5]

In a related study, Dutch researchers screened nearly four thousand older individuals for depression, and then compared the laboratory tests results of those with depressive symptoms to non-depressed control group members. The researchers report that high homocysteine levels, vitamin B$_{12}$ deficiency, and to a lesser extent folate deficiency were all related to depressive disorders. When they controlled for other factors, the effects of homocysteine and folic acid levels were less prominent, but low B$_{12}$ levels were still strongly associated with depression.[6]

People over sixty are at the highest risk for depression due to B$_{12}$ deficiency, but anyone, at any age, can be a victim. Moreover, B$_{12}$ deficiency appears to put individuals at especially high risk for psychotic depression, which involves terrifying symptoms such as hallucinations and paranoia. Researchers evaluating fifty-three patients suffering from major depression found that the average B$_{12}$ concentration of those with psychotic depression was severely low (92–176 pg/ml), indicating gross deficiency, while those with non-psychotic depression had serum B$_{12}$ levels ranging from 156 to 310 pg/ml.[7] All fifty-three patients in this study suffered from B$_{12}$ deficiency, with some patients' serum B$_{12}$ registering in the gray zone.

Because psychotic depression so often drives its victims to commit murder or suicide, it's particularly critical that doctors check any depressed patients with symptoms of psychosis for low B$_{12}$. Prompt treatment of psychotic depression stemming from B$_{12}$ deficiency can lead to almost immediate recovery, even in the most severe cases.

Two young Bedouin women, brought to an Israeli hospital at different times, were experiencing terrible hallucinations. One, an eighteen-year-old, believed that a giant, hideous monster was trying to strangle her. The other, a twenty-three-year-old, heard threatening voices and suffered both daytime and nighttime hallucinations involving human figures trying to hurt her. Both women were depressed, anxious, and suffering from a severe lack of sleep. They'd been treated with antipsychotic drugs, but the medications didn't work.

Doctors at Ben-Gurion University measured the women's B$_{12}$ levels and found that both were profoundly deficient. Interestingly, neither showed the blood abnormalities typical of B$_{12}$ deficiency, apparently because both ate diets rich in folic acid (which, as we've explained, can mask the blood signs of low B$_{12}$).

The doctors started both women on injected B$_{12}$. One recovered completely within six weeks, and the other within eight weeks. Both are now taking daily high-dose oral supplements of B$_{12}$ and have no symptoms one year later.

The doctors report, "Although these women were not vegetarians, dietary analysis showed that their daily diet was based predominantly on bread, vegetables, and canned food, with a minimal intake of meat or dairy products."[8] This diet is very similar in B$_{12}$ content to that consumed by many American vegetarians and vegans who forgo meat and dairy products and to that of many dieters who follow diets that limit meat, milk, and cheese.

Depression, however, isn't the only mental illness that B$_{12}$ deficiency can cause. As we noted in Chapter 2, it can cause dementia as well, and research and case studies reported in the literature show that B$_{12}$ deficiency can also lead to delusions, hallucinations and other schizophrenia-like symptoms, obsessive-compulsive symptoms, and a wide range of other psychiatric problems. The following is a sampling of cases taken from medical journals:

- Physician G. Daynes reported many years ago that in his own practice as medical director of a hospital in South Africa, he successfully treated eight women whose postpartum psychosis stemmed from B$_{12}$ deficiency. (Postpartum psychosis is the disorder involved in the well-publicized case of Andrea Yates, who murdered her five children, and the condition is linked to many other suicides and murders.) His patients' recoveries led him to recommend that all women with postpartum psychosis receive large doses of B$_{12}$. "Where the postpartum psychosis is not primarily caused by lack of vitamin B$_{12}$, the giving of the preparation will do no harm," he noted, "so it seems to me that in all such cases it should be given as soon as possible."[9] (One note: We recommend testing patients before treatment is initiated, to determine if B$_{12}$ deficiency truly is causing or contributing to symptoms.)

- Doctors in Australia, evaluating a patient diagnosed with anxiety disorder and conversion disorder (a psychiatric diagnosis applied when doctors believe that a patient is converting emotional distress into physical symptoms, such as paralysis or blindness), discovered that she didn't have a psychiatric illness at all. She had a physical illness, B$_{12}$ deficiency, caused by her illegal use of "whipped cream bulbs" containing nitrous oxide (a popular recreational drug—see Chapter

8). When the doctors gave her three injections of B$_{12}$, her mental and physical symptoms disappeared almost completely.[10] This case illustrates the need for doctors to screen all young people with psychiatric symptoms or suspected histories of drug abuse for B$_{12}$ deficiency.

- Doctors in Massachusetts, treating a twenty-year-old woman who'd attempted suicide three months earlier, discovered the reason for the woman's urges to kill herself: She had autoimmune pernicious anemia. She now receives regular injections of B$_{12}$, which have eliminated her depression and suicidal thoughts.[11]

- Dr. Frederick Goggans and colleagues reported the case of an elderly man who suddenly developed severe mania, believing that his hometown was planning a large celebration in his honor, including appearances by Hollywood celebrities. "He became so physically energized," the doctors noted, "that six younger men were required to restrain him at the time of admission to the hospital." Lab tests showed a drastically low B$_{12}$ level, and his doctors eventually diagnosed pernicious anemia and treated him with B$_{12}$ injections. He recovered quickly, and at his six-month checkup he was doing fine.[12]

One telling fact is that around 90 percent of patients we identify with vitamin B$_{12}$ deficiency in the ER are on antidepressants, which reveals that their primary care doctors and other specialists failed to screen for B$_{12}$ deficiency as a reason for their depression. We seldom see patients coming into the ER complaining of post-partum depression, because these women typically seek help from their obstetricians or avoid seeking help at all. However, in 2006, two patients presented to the ER for post-partum depression; both were on antidepressants and were found to be B$_{12}$-deficient. Their obstetricians never considered B$_{12}$ deficiency, yet these doctors didn't hesitate to write their patients prescriptions for antidepressants. One of the women was so desperate she purposely crashed her car into a brick wall.

Routine B$_{12}$ screening of psychiatric patients could help to identify people like these, well before their declining B$_{12}$ levels lead to mental illness—and there are far more such people than doctors realize. In one recent study, researchers measured the serum B$_{12}$ levels of patients admitted to a general hospital and exhibiting psychiatric symptoms. (It should be noted that the researchers *excluded* all patients already diagnosed with B$_{12}$ deficiency.) They divided the patients into three categories: those with normal/high B$_{12}$, those with levels below 400 pg/mL (a level many researchers suggest should be the minimum), and those with levels lower than 200 pg/mL (the level the United States considers the acceptable threshold for serum B$_{12}$, although this number is undoubtedly far too low).

Of the 115 patients with depression or other mood disorders, the researchers reported nearly a third had B$_{12}$ levels below the first cutoff point of 400 pg/mL, and seven had levels below 200, indicating overt deficiency.

TESTS THAT COULD SAVE A MOTHER'S SANITY—AND A CHILD'S LIFE

More research is needed to determine the incidence of B$_{12}$ deficiency in women with postpartum depression or postpartum psychosis. In the meantime, we believe that all women diagnosed with postpartum mental illness should undergo screening, including serum B$_{12}$ and urinary MMA tests.

Pregnancy can dramatically worsen a pre-existing B$_{12}$ deficiency, because B$_{12}$ is transferred to the growing fetus throughout pregnancy, and prenatal vitamins contain only sixteen micrograms of this nutrient (compared to the 1,000 micrograms needed to treat a deficiency). Pregnant women at greatest risk for deficiency include vegans and vegetarians, those with autoimmune pernicious anemia or malabsorption syndromes such as Crohn's disease (an inflammatory intestinal disease) or celiac disease, and those with a history of gastric bypass for weight loss, strict dieting, anorexia, or bulimia. However, any woman who develops symptoms of mental illness following pregnancy needs B$_{12}$ screening.

It is crucial for doctors to identify the root causes of postpartum depression or psychosis—causes that appear to include B$_{12}$ deficiency in some cases—because, as the tragic case of Andrea Yates shows, more than one life may be at stake.

Note: Again, serum B$_{12}$ levels falling in the gray zone need to be treated. Also, doctors need to be aware that some women may fail to achieve normal B$_{12}$ levels using high-dose oral B$_{12}$ supplements or other commercially sold over-the-counter B$_{12}$ products (patches, gels, etc.).

Of the thirty-four patients with cognitive spectrum disorders, one-fifth had levels below 400 pg/mL, and two had levels below 200.

The researchers note that "the societal costs of mood disorders and cognitive disorders are staggering," with depression treatment alone costing tens of billions of dollars annually in the United States; and they say that given the inexpensiveness of testing patients for B$_{12}$ or folate deficiency, "Our findings do support the need for early identification of vitamin B$_{12}$ and folate deficiencies before clinically significant physical and mental symptoms appear."[13]

In another recent study, researchers reviewed laboratory data from psychiatric patients and also measured B$_{12}$ levels in a random sampling of patients whose dietary habits were documented. They report that 20 percent of the patients had vitamin B$_{12}$ deficiency (serum vitamin B$_{12}$ < 200 pg/mL), and 10 percent had levels below 160 pg/mL, indicating profound deficiency. "Our findings confirm that vitamin B$_{12}$ deficiency is not uncommon in psychiatric patients, even when exposed to adequate nutrition," they conclude, adding, "The true prevalence may be even greater since low serum levels may underestimate the actual extent of vitamin B$_{12}$ deficiency."[14]

Similarly, when Dr. H. Hermesh and colleagues studied thirty patients with obsessive-compulsive disorder, they found that 20 percent of them had abnormally low levels of B$_{12}$.[15] It's important to note that these studies are not including patients whose serum B$_{12}$ falls in the gray zone.

WHEN DID DOCTORS DISCOVER THE LINK BETWEEN B$_{12}$ AND MENTAL ILLNESS?

The answer to this question is over a century ago—which makes it all the more surprising that most doctors fail to routinely consider B$_{12}$ deficiency as a cause of psychiatric patients' symptoms.

Physicians Melvin Hector and John Burton note in a journal article[16] that in the early 1900s, doctors discovered that pernicious anemia (one form of B$_{12}$ deficiency) caused symptoms including apathy, decreased ability to do mental work, loss of memory, restlessness, irritability, indifference, emotional instability, disorientation and confusion, loss of inhibition, dementia, delirium, depression, delusions and hallucinations, confabulation, hysteria, neurasthenia, paranoia, and mania. These psychiatric manifestations were termed "megaloblastic madness," because people who had enlarged red blood cells (macrocytosis) caused by B$_{12}$ deficiency often appeared to have gone "mad."

In the late 1920s, when doctors first learned to treat pernicious anemia by giving patients large amounts of raw liver, multiple case reports showed that these very same psychiatric symptoms abated in treated patients. Similar reports of psychiatric symptoms caused by deficient B$_{12}$ and successfully treated by administering the vitamin, appeared on a regular basis over the remainder of the 1900s. Yet at the turn of a new century, when we have the benefit of more than one hundred years of research and documentation proving that B$_{12}$ deficiency causes psychiatric illness, very few mentally ill patients are being evaluated for underlying B$_{12}$ deficiency, and only a minute percentage receive the adjunctive urinary MMA test that can also assist in diagnosis.

In 1989, as a nursing school project, one of us (Sally) analyzed psychiatrists' patterns of testing for B$_{12}$ deficiency in a psychiatric facility. Of thirty-one inpatients seen during this study, only seven (23 percent) received serum B$_{12}$ tests, and *no* patients under the age of sixty were tested. Eight (or 26 percent) of the patients exhibited blood smear evidence of B$_{12}$ deficiency, but none of these patients' doctors ordered serum B$_{12}$ tests. One elderly paranoid and demented patient who finally received testing, and proved to be drastically deficient in B$_{12}$ (107 pg/ml), had been admitted to the same facility the previous year for the same symptoms, but had been discharged without doctors ever suspecting the cause of his problems. By the time he received a diagnosis during his second visit, it was too late to help him. He'd lived for a year in a nursing home after his first visit, when doctors described him as having "paranoid psychosis with dementia and multi-infarct dementia"—an accurate label, but one that did nothing to explain *why* he suffered from psychosis and dementia, or to correct the problem before it became irreversible. Of the remaining six patients who were screened for B$_{12}$ deficiency, three patients had serum B$_{12}$ levels in the gray zone.

At least back in 1989, some doctors would occasionally test older adults. In 2010, more than twenty years later, serum B$_{12}$ is not being universally screened for in psychiatric facilities. Currently, a psychiatric patient must be medically cleared for inpatient mental health admission. Tests include a complete blood count, basic metabolic panel, and comprehensive drug screen—but no tests for B$_{12}$ or B$_{12}$ markers.

The cost of such oversights, in terms of human suffering, is inestimable. The cost in health-care dollars is significant as well. Compare, for instance, the cost of B$_{12}$ treatment (which, as we've noted, averages about $36 dollars per year) to the cost of the commonly prescribed psychiatric drugs Ativan ($1,134 per year), Paxil ($1,503 per year), Prozac ($2,331 per year), or Risperdal ($3,388 per year)—not to mention the cost of psychiatric admissions or repeated emergency room visits. An ER visit to get medically cleared for psychiatric admission costs on average around $1,600. The daily room rates for inpatient mental health treatment at two local facilities in the Midwest are $1,067 to $1,368, which doesn't include the psychiatrist's fee. Can you imagine the financial savings for patients, insurance companies, and the government if B$_{12}$ deficiency were screened for, identified, and treated early?

The woman who came to our emergency department complaining of abdominal bloating and spine pain had a reputation with her doctors. Some thought she was crazy. Others labeled her as a drug-seeker, faking mental and physical illnesses in order to get prescriptions for drugs.

Her medical record, however, told a far different story. She'd undergone intestinal bypass surgery for weight-loss fifteen years earlier, impairing her body's ability to obtain B$_{12}$. Her medical records contained four years worth of lab tests, showing enlarged red blood cells, a classic sign of B$_{12}$ deficiency. She'd been through numerous surgeries, many of them no doubt involving nitrous oxide, which can destroy B$_{12}$ stores (see Chapter 8). She had a history of hypothyroidism, often found in association with autoimmune pernicious anemia. Her neurological and psychiatric symptoms—poor balance, numbness and tingling, gait abnormalities, depression, and anxiety—are textbook symptoms of a deficiency of B$_{12}$.

This sad and frightened woman had seen thirteen different doctors (primary care doctors, an internist, a neurologist, a psychiatrist, a gastroenterologist, and numerous ER physicians) in the previous three years, but not one identified her real problem. Some merely placed her on multivitamin and folic acid supplements, assuming that her enlarged red blood cells stemmed from folic acid deficiency due to a poor diet or alcohol abuse. Others dismissed her problems as "all in her head." And all left her in agonizing pain, both mental and physical, and forced her to continue her search for a drug or doctor capable of saving her from her misery. Our emergency department staff finally did save her by testing her B$_{12}$ level. It was 146 pg/ml,

Psychiatric Symptoms that Can Be Associated with B₁₂ Deficiency

Note: A number of these symptoms overlap with dementia, which we discuss in Chapter 2.

Among the most common psychiatric symptoms seen in people with B₁₂ deficiency are the following:

- confusion/disorientation

- memory loss

- depression

- suicidal ideations

- mania

- anxiety

- paranoia

- irritability

- apathy

- personality changes

- inappropriate sexual behavior

- delusions

- hallucinations

- violent/aggressive behavior

- schizophrenic symptoms

- sleep disturbances

- insomnia

- changes in taste, smell, vision, and sensory/motor function that can be mistaken for psychiatric problems *a level low enough to explain all of the symptoms that had ruined a decade of her life.*

In addition to causing mental illness in people with no history of psychiatric disease, B_{12} deficiency can cause a dramatic worsening of symptoms in people already diagnosed with mental disorders. Often, doctors dismiss these worsening symptoms as "just another phase" of the existing condition, or they treat them with ever-heavier doses of psychiatric drugs that do nothing at all to treat depleted B_{12} levels.

In August 2010, we saw a forty-six-year-old woman who was brought to the ER by ambulance because of severe psychosis. She had a history of psychiatric illness, was on numerous psychiatric medications, and had been in and out of psychiatric hospitals. She had a history of bipolar disorder and paranoid schizoaffective disorder. Her family was afraid she was a danger to herself as well as others. For her safety, she required restraints during her ER visit.

This woman needed B_{12} deficiency ruled out. The ER physician was reluctant, saying, "she already has a diagnosis." But the patient was tested in the ER, and was found to be severely B_{12} deficient. Her serum B_{12} was 127 pg/ml. She was macrocytic but not anemic, and her RBC-folic acid level was normal. Interestingly, her serum MMA was normal (0.16 μmol/L), yet her homocysteine was extremely elevated (90 μmol/L). (This is yet another example of how the serum MMA test has severe limitations—see Chapter 11.)

This patient received her first B_{12} shot in the ER, and we instructed the psychiatric facility to continue a series of B_{12} shots. Her other physicians were notified as well, so she could have continued follow-up treatment as an outpatient.

This woman's case illustrates an important point. If you've been diagnosed with any mental disorder, or your symptoms suddenly become much worse or return after a period of remission, it's important to rule out B_{12} deficiency as a cause—*even if your doctors say that B_{12} has nothing to do with your preexisting illness.* As psychiatrist Sydney Walker once noted, "Having one illness doesn't protect you from having another." In fact, mental disorders can make you more vulnerable to B_{12} deficiency, because they increase the odds that you're eating poorly or taking drugs that can compromise your B_{12} metabolism.

If your new symptoms do stem from a B_{12} problem, treating these symptoms with psychiatric drugs will simply allow the damage to your brain and nervous system to continue, with possibly fatal consequences. Correcting this deficiency, conversely, can often result in prompt and dramatic improvement.

Some psychiatric patients are lucky to have doctors who look for root causes when new symptoms arise. One was a middle-aged man who'd suffered a head injury decades earlier, resulting in behavior changes that his doctors successfully controlled with medication.

One day, the man suddenly became lethargic and began slurring his speech. By the time his caregivers brought him to the emergency department, he was in a stupor, exhibiting depression and oddly slowed movements, a mask-like flat expression, and abnormally slow speech.

Diagnosing him as catatonic, his doctors could have assumed that his problems stemmed from his earlier head injury and simply added more drugs to his treatment plan—or admitted him to a psychiatric hospital, where he might have languished for the rest of his life. Instead, they ran tests, discovered that he was severely B₁₂ deficient, and treated him with B₁₂ injections.

After two weeks in the hospital, they reported the man "was speaking spontaneously in sentences, had a wide emotional range, and was interacting with the other patients.... He was able to ambulate on his own, with improved balance and coordination.... There were no psychotic or depressive symptoms seen."[17]

In a similar case reported by different doctors, a schizophrenic man who'd been in remission for four years began displaying psychotic symptoms after a bout of pneumonia. His doctors could have said, "It's just a relapse." Instead, they tested his B₁₂ levels, which proved to be low. Within five days of B₁₂ therapy, the man's symptoms disappeared and he could once again lead a normal life.[18]

TAKING THE LEAD IN GETTING TESTED

The medical profession underestimates the role of B₁₂ deficiency in mental illness, rarely suspecting this disorder in patients with depression, anxiety, bipolar disorder, or other psychiatric problems. So, if you suffer from psychiatric symptoms, or you're caring for a spouse, child, or other loved one with a mental illness, **it's up to you to insist on thorough B₁₂ testing**. Our hope is that in the near future, testing for B₁₂ deficiency will become mandatory for all psychiatric patients—but until that time, you're on your own.

If your psychiatrist is reluctant to test you or your loved one, it may be necessary to consult other doctors, including your family physician or other specialists, in order to find one who is willing to order the tests. (Conversely, we sometimes find that psychiatrists are more willing than other doctors to order B$_{12}$ testing. For instance, the fifty-one-year-old woman we discussed in the previous chapter—who was diagnosed with multiple sclerosis, and eventually developed severe mental illness and tried to throw herself out of a moving car—received her diagnosis from a psychiatrist, after her other specialists missed the call.) When you do find a doctor who agrees to evaluate you or a loved one for B$_{12}$ deficiency, make sure the tests include a serum B$_{12}$ level. Do *not* assume that a doctor will order this test, because it is not part of most standard psychiatric evaluations or admissions, and it is not required for medical clearance.

> The medical profession underestimates the role of B$_{12}$ deficiency in mental illness.

Be *assertive* in insisting on these tests, and be sure that you get treatment—lifelong treatment, when necessary—if a deficiency is detected or your B$_{12}$ level is in the gray zone. We see far too many patients who've suffered unnecessarily for months or years, when a few tests and B$_{12}$ therapy could have cured their psychiatric symptoms completely. With your own sanity, or the well-being of a loved one at stake, why take a chance?

CHAPTER 4 NOTES:

1. Gottfries, C. G. Late life depression. *European Archives of Psychiatry and Clinical Neuroscience* 2001, 251(Suppl 2):57–61.

2. Catalano, G., Catalano, M. C., O'Dell, K. J., Humphrey, D. A., and Fritz, E. B. The utility of laboratory screening in medically ill patients with psychiatric symptoms. *Annals of Clinical Psychiatry* 2001, 13(3):135–140.

3. Dommisse, J. Letter re "Case report: The psychiatric manifestation of B$_{12}$ deficiency." *Primary Psychiatry* 1996, 3(1):50–5. Cited at www.johndommissemd.com.

4. Verbanck, P., and LeBon, O. Changing psychiatric symptoms in a patient with vitamin B$_{12}$ deficiency. *Journal of Clinical Psychiatry* 1991, 52(4):182–3.

5. Penninx, B. W., et al. Vitamin B$_{12}$ deficiency and depression in physically disabled older women: Epidemiologic evidence from the

Women's Health and Aging Study. *American Journal of Psychiatry* 2000 May;157(5):715–21.

6. Tiemeier, H., van Tuijl, H. R., Hofman, A., Meijer, J., Kiliaan, A. J., and Breteler, M. M. Vitamin B$_{12}$, folate, and homocysteine in depression: The Rotterdam Study. *American Journal of Psychiatry* 2002, 159(12):2099–101.

7. Levitt, A., and Joffe, R. Vitamin B$_{12}$ in psychotic depression. *British Journal of Psychiatry* 1988, 153:266–7.

8. Masalha, R., Chudakov, B., Muhamad, M., Rudoy, I., Volkov, I., and Wirguin, I. Cobalamin-responsive psychosis as the sole manifestation of vitamin B$_{12}$ deficiency. *Israeli Medical Association Journal* 2001, 3:701–3.

9. Daynes, G. Cyanocobalamin in postpartum psychosis. *South African Medical Journal* 1975, 49(34):1373.

10. Brett, A. Myeloneuropathy from whipped cream bulbs presenting as conversion disorder. *Australia and New Zealand Journal of Psychiatry* 1997, 31(1):131–2.

11. Middleman, A. B., and Melchiono, M. W. A routine CBC leads to a non-routine diagnosis. *Adolescent Medicine* 1996, 7(3):423–6.

12. Goggans, F. C. A case of mania secondary to vitamin B$_{12}$ deficiency. *American Journal of Psychiatry* 1984, 141(2):300–1.

13. Catalano, G., Catalano, M. C., O'Dell, K. J., Humphrey, D. A., and Fritz, E. B. The utility of laboratory screening in medically ill patients with psychiatric symptoms. *Annals of Clinical Psychiatry* 2001, 13(3):135–140.

14. Silver, H. Vitamin B$_{12}$ levels are low in hospitalized psychiatric patients. *Israeli Journal of Psychiatry and Related Sciences* 2000, 37(1):41–5.

15. Hermesh, H., Weizman, A., Shahar, A., and Munitz, H. Vitamin B$_{12}$ and folic acid serum levels in obsessive compulsive disorder. *Acta Psychiatrica Scandinavia* 1988, 78(1):8–10.

16. Hector, M., and Burton, J. What are the psychiatric manifestations of vitamin B$_{12}$ deficiency? *Journal of the American Geriatric Society* 1988, 36:1105-12.

17. Catalano, G., Catalano, M. C., Roenberg, E. I., Embi, P. J., and Embi, C. S. Catatonia: Another neuropsychiatric presentation of vitamin B$_{12}$ deficiency? *Psychosomatics* 1998, 39(5):456.

18. Buchman, N., Mendelsson, E., Lerner, V., and Kotler, M. Delirium associated with vitamin B$_{12}$ deficiency after pneumonia. *Clinical Neuropharmacology* 1999, 22(6):356–8.

5

Stroke, Heart Disease, and Other Vascular Problems:
The B_{12}-Homocysteine Connection

"High homocysteine can increase the risk of heart attack
as much as high cholesterol."
—Abbott Laboratories[1]

Scientists investigating the causes of cardiovascular disease are zeroing in on one culprit in particular—a risk identified more than thirty years ago, but ignored by doctors until recently. It's homocysteine, an amino acid that can wreak havoc on your cardiovascular system. High homocysteine levels put you at risk for coronary artery disease, heart attacks, strokes, deep vein thromboses (blood clots), and other deadly vascular problems. In fact, homocysteine has been dubbed "the cholesterol of the next century."[2]

What does this have to do with vitamin B_{12}? A great deal, because B_{12} allows another nutrient, folic acid, to convert homocysteine into a nontoxic amino acid. When your B_{12} levels drop to unhealthy levels, this process breaks down, and your homocysteine levels rise sharply—along with your risk of heart attack or stroke.

WHAT IS HOMOCYSTEINE AND WHY IS IT SO BAD FOR YOU?

The story of homocysteine begins with the food you eat. That food contains twenty amino acids, one of which is methionine.

Your body breaks down methionine into smaller particles, one of which is a molecule called SAMe. SAMe, in turn, breaks down into smaller substances, one of which is homocysteine. When everything's working right, this homocysteine quickly gets recycled back into methionine with the help of vitamin B$_{12}$ and folic acid, following two pathways (see below). Any excess homocysteine winds up in your liver, which breaks it down with the help of vitamins B$_{12}$, B$_6$, and folic acid. But if you're deficient in any one of these vitamins, this normal cycle is disrupted and homocysteine accumulates in your blood, with no place to go.

TWO MAJOR ENZYMATIC PATHWAYS IN HUMANS

1. The first pathway continuously recycles homocysteine (Hcy) back into methionine. This reaction is also essential for the conversion of folate: methyltetrahydrofalte (MTHF) to → tetrahydrofolate (THF).

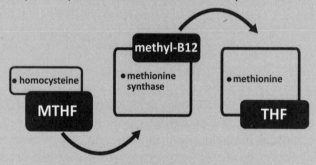

   In B$_{12}$ deficiency, MTHF accumulates along with an increase in Hcy. Both the enzyme *methionine synthase* and the coenzyme *methyl-B$_{12}$* are needed for this reaction to occur. The recycling of Hcy is important for the building of thousands of compounds and proteins that are necessary for healthy cells, tissues, and organs. Homocysteine is also detoxified and made harmless through a process called transsulfuration, which requires vitamin B$_6$, magnesium, and SAMe.

2. Both the enzyme methylmalonyl CoA mutase and the coenzyme adenosyl-B$_{12}$ are needed for this vital reaction to occur. In vitamin B$_{12}$ deficiency, methylmalonic acid accumulates resulting in abnormal fatty acid production, which is believed to be injurious to neuronal membranes.

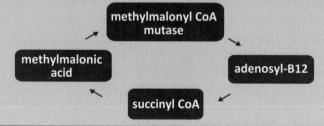

WHAT'S THE RISK OF ELEVATED HOMOCYSTEINE?

Mild or moderate elevation of homocysteine can be caused either by genetic defects or by nutritional deficiency of B_{12}, folic acid, or B_6. It is an independent risk factor for stroke, heart attack, other blood clots, and peripheral artery disease. B_{12} expert Ralph Green, M.D. notes, "For each 5 μmol/L increment in total plasma homocysteine (approximately 1 standard deviation of the mean for the normal population), there is a corresponding increase of about 40% in the relative risk of developing coronary artery disease. This increase is comparable to the risk associated with the same proportional increment in cholesterol and equates homocysteine and cholesterol as risk factors for ischemic heart disease. The relative risk/odds ratio for cerebrovascular and peripheral arterial disease associated with elevated homocysteine appears even greater than it is for coronary artery disease."[4]

That's dangerous, because homocysteine, while it's a "good guy" when it's rapidly transformed into beneficial substances, is a "bad guy" when left on its own. Excess homocysteine causes your blood vessels to lose their elasticity, making it harder for them to dilate and damaging their inner lining. That damage, in turn, allows cholesterol, collagen, and calcium to attach to the inner walls of your blood vessels, where they can form sticky deposits called atherosclerotic plaques. These plaques narrow your arteries and drastically increase your risk of suffering deadly disorders, such as coronary artery disease, heart attacks, strokes, "mini strokes" (transient ischemic attacks, or TIAs), blood clots (pulmonary embolism, deep vein thrombosis), carotid and renal artery stenosis (narrowing), or aneurysms (ballooning of damaged blood vessels). In addition, elevated homocysteine levels alter your biochemistry in ways that appear to promote abnormal blood clotting.[3]

> High homocysteine levels put you at risk for coronary artery disease, heart attacks, strokes, and other deadly vascular problems. B_{12} allows folic acid to convert homocysteine into a nontoxic amino acid.

Homocysteine is also an "oxidant" that decreases the production of nitric oxide*—a substance crucial to healthy blood vessel function.

---

* Nitric oxide, by the way, should not be confused with the anesthetic agent nitrous oxide. The two names sound alike, but there is no relationship.

Decreased nitric oxide, in turn, is strongly linked to both atherosclerosis and high blood pressure.

Initially, researchers wondered if high homocysteine, rather than causing cardiovascular disease, simply occurred as a side effect. Studies show, however, that elevated homocysteine *precedes* the onset of disease.[5] This strongly indicates that homocysteine, rather than just being a marker for cardiovascular disease, actively contributes to the disease process.

Five to 10 percent of the population, and as many as 30 to 40 percent of senior citizens, have elevated homocysteine levels.[6] The older you are, the more likely you are to have high homocysteine. Men tend to have higher levels than women, smokers often have higher levels than non-smokers, and genes play a major role in influencing your homocysteine level. Certain medications, too, can affect homocysteine status, as can impaired kidney function. But in people without kidney problems, the primary cause of the problem, no matter what other factors are involved, is a low level of folate and/or vitamin B$_{12}$, or, to a lesser degree, a low level of vitamin B$_6$.

WHY FOLATE CAN'T DO THE JOB BY ITSELF

Increasing numbers of doctors are aware of the dangers of high homocysteine, and of the benefits of folic acid therapy. Unfortunately, few of these doctors fully understand the critical role that vitamin B$_{12}$ plays in detoxifying homocysteine. This is a serious oversight, because people with high homocysteine levels often respond fully *only* when they're given large amounts of B$_{12}$ as well. The reason: People who are deficient in B$_{12}$ can't assimilate folic acid properly, and as a result, much of the folic acid is trapped in an inaccessible form. Thus, testing for B$_{12}$ deficiency (and treatment if needed) must always be part of a homocysteine-lowering program.

Yet, many cardiologists prescribe only folic acid to patients with high homocysteine levels, and many others merely augment this folic acid regimen with a multivitamin containing small amounts of B$_{12}$. This is often ineffective, because a few micrograms of B$_{12}$ won't correct a significant deficiency. If you have high homocysteine levels, your doctor needs to test you to determine if a vitamin B$_{12}$ deficiency exists. Proper treatment of high homocysteine may include high doses of folic acid, vitamin B$_{12}$ and vitamin B$_6$.

Jean, a fifty-seven-year-old insurance agent, exercised regularly, avoided cigarettes, ate a diet high in folic acid, and took folate supplements in order to keep her cardiovascular system healthy—but, as she eventually learned, it wasn't enough.

Because Jean was experiencing some symptoms of B_{12} deficiency that hadn't been noticed by her family physician or her other doctors, we ordered several tests for low B_{12}. In addition, Jean's homocysteine level was measured. All of her tests (B_{12}, MMA, homocysteine, gastrin, and parietal cell antibody) came back grossly abnormal.

As it turned out, Jean had autoimmune pernicious anemia. Even though she took folic acid supplements and ate a diet rich in this nutrient, her homocysteine level was high because she had a B_{12} deficiency. Her complete blood count was normal because her blood cells could use excess folic acid instead of B_{12}. (This is why folic acid supplements can mask B_{12} deficiency.)

While folic acid made Jean's complete blood count appear normal and fooled her initial doctors into missing her true diagnosis, her cells couldn't use folic acid to convert homocysteine to methionine—a process that requires B_{12}. That's why her homocysteine levels soared, putting her at risk for cardiovascular disease and other medical problems.

A POWERFUL CONNECTION

How strong is the link between high homocysteine and cardiovascular disease? Several years ago, Israeli researchers decided to find out by comparing the homocysteine levels of people whose fathers had suffered heart attacks to the levels of people whose fathers had no such history. In addition, the researchers compared homocysteine levels of people in Jerusalem, where the rate of heart attacks is high, with the levels of people in the United States, where the heart attack rate is lower.

The researchers found that male children of heart attack victims had significantly higher homocysteine levels than control group members. When they charted the homocysteine levels of all of the study subjects, they found that people in the top 20 percent were far more likely than other subjects to be in the "parental heart attack" group.

In addition, men in Jerusalem had much higher homocysteine levels than the U.S. men—a logical explanation for their higher heart attack rate. The researchers add that the difference in homocysteine levels between men in the two countries "was largely attributable to *lower plasma vitamin B_{12} levels* [emphasis added] in the Israeli population."[7]

In a different study, conducted as part of the prestigious large-scale Physicians' Health Study, researchers compared doctors who'd suffered heart attacks during a five-year period to those with healthy hearts. The researchers analyzed homocysteine levels using plasma samples the doctors donated at the beginning of the study.

After controlling for age and smoking habits, the researchers reported, "Moderately high levels of plasma homocysteine are associated with subsequent risk of myocardial infarction [heart attack] independent of other coronary risk factors." Men in the top 5 percent of homocysteine level were more than three times as likely as other subjects to suffer heart attacks. The researchers concluded, "Because high levels can often be easily treated with vitamin supplements, homocysteine may be an independent, modifiable risk factor."[8]

Even more dramatic findings appeared in the *New England Journal of Medicine* some years ago. Norwegian researchers followed 587 patients with existing coronary artery disease and reported that within about five years of undergoing treatment, 11 percent of the patients had died. "We found a strong, graded relation between plasma homocysteine levels and overall mortality," the researchers reported, with around 4 percent of patients in the low-homocysteine group dying as compared to nearly one quarter of those in the high-homocysteine group. The strong correlation remained even after the researchers controlled for other risk factors.

"Our results," the researchers said, "should serve as an additional strong incentive to the initiation of intervention trials with homocysteine-lowering therapy."[9] So should similar results from a study of more than 400 patients who'd suffered heart attacks or unstable angina. In this study, the long-term death rate from cardiac disease was more than twice as high for patients in the upper two quintiles of homocysteine level as it was for other patients.[10]

Still more evidence of the dangers of high homocysteine comes from a "meta-analysis"—a study that pools data from multiple studies in order to increase statistical power. Physician David Wald and colleagues evaluated seventy-two genetic studies analyzing the effects of a common gene variant that raises homocysteine levels, as well as twenty prospective studies analyzing the association between serum homocysteine levels and disease risk. "The genetic studies and the prospective studies do not share the same potential sources of error, but both yield similarly highly significant results—strong evidence that the association between homocysteine and cardiovascular disease is causal," the researchers concluded.[11]

Even in young people, research shows high homocysteine is a threat. A recent large-scale study found that elevated homocysteine nearly doubles the risk of stroke in women between the ages of fifteen and forty-four. The researchers commented, "The magnitude of the increase in stroke risk was similar to that of smoking a pack of cigarettes per day."[12]

Dozens of additional studies corroborate these findings, implicating high homocysteine as one of the most powerful cardiovascular risk factors ever identified. Luckily, it's a problem that is easy to treat—and the treatment can begin lowering homocysteine levels almost immediately. One recent study, lasting only eight weeks, tested the effects of folic acid alone, B_{12} alone, and folic acid plus B_{12} in lowering the homocysteine levels of patients who'd suffered ischemic strokes. The researchers found that all three approaches worked, but that "the combination therapy yielded the most remarkable result,

> Even in young people, research shows high homocysteine is a threat.

i.e., plasma total homocysteine was reduced by 38.5 percent."[13] A similar British study found a 23 percent decrease in homocysteine levels after six weeks of treatment with folic acid and B_{12}.[14] Evidence indicates that equally impressive results can be achieved by the majority of people who stick with the vitamin regimen.

DOES IT HELP TO LOWER HIGH HOMOCYSTEINE LEVELS?

The short answer is: almost certainly yes. Because the medical community's interest in homocysteine's role in cardiovascular disease is new, doctors are still collecting information about how effective a tool homocysteine-lowering therapy will be. Some studies show no effects of lowering homocysteine levels, but data from other studies indicate that the treatment can dramatically lower the risk of death or debility. Among the findings are the following:

- Swiss researchers offered homocysteine-lowering therapy to half of a group of 553 patients who'd undergone angioplasty to correct coronary artery stenosis (narrowing of the arteries). After one year, the researchers reported, the incidence of "major adverse events"—deaths, nonfatal heart attacks, or the need for repeat angioplasty—was one-third lower in the treatment group.[15]

- In a separate six-month double-blind study (a study in which neither the doctor nor the patient knows which treatment is being given), the same Swiss research group administered folic acid, B$_{12}$ and B$_6$ (a combination they call "folate treatment"), or a placebo to 205 patients who'd undergone successful coronary artery angioplasty. They reported that the rate of restenosis—that is, re-narrowing of the arteries after the angioplasty opened them—was significantly lower in the treatment group than in the placebo group (19.6 percent vs. 37.6 percent), and that this group had less than half the need for a repeated procedure on the targeted lesion. The researchers concluded, "This inexpensive treatment, which has minimal side effects, should be considered as adjunctive therapy for patients undergoing coronary angioplasty."[16*]

- Irish researchers studied patients with a genetic disease called ho-mocystinuria, which causes extremely high levels of homocysteine. Normally, half of people with this disease suffer a heart attack or other "vascular event" by the time they're thirty years old. The re-searchers placed 158 patients on homocysteine-lowering therapy and report that by the time the patients reached an average age of forty-two, twelve patients had collectively experienced seventeen episodes of pulmonary embolism, heart attack, deep vein thrombosis, or other serious vascular problems. "Without treatment," the researchers noted, "112 vascular events would have been expected."[17] In a simi-lar study, Australian researchers reported a 90 percent reduction in

---

* A more recent study (Lange, et al., *New England Journal of Medicine*, 2004), which concluded that B vitamin supplementation was ineffective in preventing restenosis, is mis-leading because the researchers actually found that patients with elevated homocysteine levels—the primary group for which the therapy would be expected to be effective—in-deed did show a decreased level of restenosis. So did women (who are at higher risk than men for pernicious anemia) and diabetics (who are at heightened risk for undiagnosed B$_{12}$ deficiency because many are on the B$_{12}$-lowering drug metformin—and because people with Type 1 diabetes are at elevated risk for other autoimmune disorders, such as perni-cious anemia). Thus, in the three groups most likely to have high homocysteine and/or low B$_{12}$ levels, B vitamin therapy did indeed reduce the rate of restenosis—even though the amount of B$_{12}$ used in this study was inadequate. These findings clearly point out the need to screen patients to determine their individual needs and develop logical and improved treatment plans. In addition, studies using different forms of B$_{12}$ (not cyanoco-balamin) as well as different routes for improved absorption need to be studied.

Why the Thirty-Year Wait?

Cardiovascular disease is the nation's leading killer and a major cause of disability. In 2009, approximately 785,000 Americans had a new heart attack, and approximately 470,000 had a recurrent attack. The Centers for Disease Control and Prevention (CDC) notes, "About every 25 seconds, an American will have a coronary event, and about one every minute will die from one."[19] Thus, it's amazing that the discovery of the homocysteine/cardiovascular disease link, more than four decades ago, didn't immediately result in a flurry of research and treatment efforts.

Why the gap between discovery and implementation? The answer involves politics, greed, and ignorance.

In the 1960s, Dr. Kilmer McCully, a pathologist at Harvard Medical School, was studying a group of children who'd suffered strokes or blood clots—problems we associate with adults. These children, it turned out, had inborn errors of metabolism that led to extremely high homocysteine levels, which, in turn, put the children at high risk for "adult" cardiovascular problems.

As Dr. McCully studied these children, he began to wonder: Is this same substance, homocysteine, responsible for premature strokes and atherosclerosis in adults, as well? Do adults who suffer heart attacks at forty or strokes at fifty—decades before these problems arise in less susceptible people—have some form of inherited metabolic error, much like children who suffer strokes or develop atherosclerosis? Eventually, his data led McCully to conclude that adults whose homocysteine levels climbed for a variety of reasons (poor diet, malabsorption, veganism, gastrointestinal surgeries, etc.), or those whose genetic makeup left them vulnerable to deficiencies of folic acid, vitamin B_{12}, or vitamin B_6, could be at drastically increased risk for cardiovascular disease. He concluded, further, that simple vitamin therapy could spare many of these people from the ravages of heart attacks, strokes, and blood clots.

McCully announced his conclusions to the medical world in 1969. At the time, however, doctors were firmly proclaiming that another substance, cholesterol, was the key risk factor for cardiovascular disease—and that's where the research money, and the drug company dollars, were going. When McCully argued that cholesterol was not the main culprit in heart disease, he was vilified. "My laboratory was removed from the department to another part of the hospital," McCully recalls. "It was made clear to me that I should look elsewhere for support." He left Harvard and his research was swept under the rug, although he quietly continued his crusade to make the world aware of the homocysteine/cardiovascular disease link.

Now, more than thirty years later, researchers around the world are proving this link, and McCully's old colleagues are admitting that he was far ahead of his time. "There is a tremendous avalanche of publications," says McCully. "Now about twenty to thirty publications per month are being published. One estimate I saw is there are now over 1,500 publications on homocysteine and vascular heart disease."[20]

Notes the *Journal of Longevity*, "Dr. McCully's research has been a turning point in health science. If he hadn't been so persistent in the face of criticism by his peers, this entire facet of cardiovascular health—the influence of homocysteine—might have remained hidden and many instances of circulatory problems might have remained mysteries."[21]

cardiovascular events in people with homocystinuria who received homocysteine-lowering therapy.[18]

- Researchers in the United Kingdom and Norway evaluated eighty-nine men, ranging in age from thirty-nine to sixty-seven, with existing coronary artery disease, to determine if oral B vitamins would have an effect on the health of their arteries. After eight weeks of treatment with folic acid and vitamin B$_{12}$, the subjects' plasma homocysteine levels dropped significantly compared to levels in similar men taking a placebo. In addition, the arteries of men taking the vitamins dilated more efficiently in response to blood flow demands. These findings, the researchers concluded, "support the view that lowering homocysteine, through B vitamin supplementation, may reduce cardiovascular risk."[22]

These reports are exciting, because they indicate that homocysteine-reducing vitamin therapy—an inexpensive, simple, and safe treatment—may significantly reduce the rate of cardiovascular disease. What's more, these studies used low-dose oral B$_{12}$, which is less effective than high-dose B$_{12}$, in patients with existing deficiencies. In addition, they used oral tablets rather than B_{12} lozenges or injections, and used cyanocobalamin rather than the bioactive form methylcobalamin.

Unfortunately, most current studies neglect to include serum B_{12} levels in the gray zone or to perform urinary MMA testing of subjects, both of which must be a part of future studies in order for researchers to fully understand how B_{12} factors into this equation. Given the fact that folic acid, vitamin B_{12}, and vitamin B_6 are virtually risk-free treatments, however, people who discover that their homocysteine levels are high shouldn't take any chances.

"I have always had a very personal interest in heart disease," physician Tedd Mitchell wrote in an article for USA Today's *weekend magazine.*[23] *"My grandfather died in his 50s of a massive heart attack. And my father had a quadruple bypass in his 50s. This definitely gives me a 'positive' family history of coronary artery disease."*

Mitchell once wondered why his relatives, who had no apparent risk factors—they were nonsmokers, with no high blood pressure, diabetes, high cholesterol, or obesity—were targets for cardiovascular disease at an early age. Then he read about homocysteine, and he decided to have his own level checked. "Lo and behold," he says, "it was significantly elevated." As a result of the studies he's read, he's altered his life-style: Every day, he takes supplements of folic acid, vitamin B_{12}, and vitamin B_6. "I'm happy to report," he adds, "my homocysteine level is now normal."

While many treatments for cardiovascular disease involve potentially dangerous drugs or surgeries, this is one case in which the expected incidence of significant adverse effects is zero. Moreover, while the field of cardiovascular medicine is rife with controversy, this is one instance in which mainstream and holistic doctors are in total agreement about the choice of treatment. To demonstrate just how universal the recommended treatment protocol is, the website of a major drug company explains, "Homocysteine can be easily controlled by providing your body with folic acid, vitamin B_6, and vitamin B_{12} at amounts exceeding the recommended daily allowances."[24] It's difficult to find many examples of major drug companies telling you to take vitamins!

Although we don't yet know who will benefit and to what degree, homocysteine-lowering therapy may prove to be one of the most powerful and simple preventive measures we can implement for people at risk for cardiovascular disease. While we currently tell patients, "Stop smoking, exercise, lose weight, and lower your cholesterol," a quarter of heart attack victims have none of these risk factors.[25] Similarly, thousands of people each year suffer at early ages from strokes, blood clots, or related problems, even though they're seemingly in excellent health. Many of these people carry very common gene variants that can cause their homocysteine to rise to dangerous levels. For these people in particular, early and accurate testing for high homocysteine and low B$_{12}$ levels might mean the difference between dying young and leading a long, healthy life.

The twenty-one-year-old woman[26] who came to the emergency department of a Canadian hospital suffered from a deadly problem that a young woman shouldn't have: a blood clot lodged in a vein within her kidney. It's a problem that's rare even in older adults, and usually occurs in people who've had kidney transplants or suffered a blow to the abdomen.

However, the young patient had two risk factors for vascular disease. First, she'd recently started taking oral contraceptives, which slightly increase the risk of developing blood clots. And second, she had very high levels of homocysteine, along with a low serum B$_{12}$ level (140ng/L) indicative of a severe deficiency. Further investigation also revealed that she carried two copies of a particular variant of the MTHFR (methylene tetrahydrofolate reductase) gene that is linked to elevated homocysteine levels in as much as 10 percent of the population.

*The doctors told the woman to stop taking her birth control pills, gave her drug treatments to dissolve the clot, and started her on oral folic acid, oral B$_{12}$, and B$_{12}$ injections. Her homocysteine levels dropped markedly over time, almost assuredly reducing her risk of a future clot dramatically.**

If early testing for high homocysteine ever becomes commonplace, it's possible that such life-threatening vascular events in young people will become far more rare. That's because we may be able to identify hundreds

---

* Her levels never became completely normal, a problem that her doctors attribute to noncompliance with the folic acid regimen, but which could also stem from the fact that she was switched from injected B$_{12}$ to very low levels of oral B$_{12}$ (25 mcg). In our opinion, given the woman's genetic vulnerability, her original documented B$_{12}$ deficiency, and her high risk of future blood clots, she should have remained on injected B$_{12}$ for life. Six months after treatment, her serum B$_{12}$ was only 255 ng/L or 255 pg/ml (reference range 180–500 ng/L), indicating a need for continued B$_{12}$ injections. This case is an example of under-treating B$_{12}$ deficiency. Daily high-dose B$_{12}$ lozenges may be tried, but the patient must be monitored. Patients may use a combination therapy of high-dose B$_{12}$ lozenges and bi-monthly injections.

MORE THAN JUST A VASCULAR RISK

In this chapter, we've focused on homocysteine's deleterious effects on your heart and blood vessels. However, high homocysteine can put you at risk for other serious or even fatal medical problems as well. Elevated homocysteine levels are now linked to:

- cognitive impairment (difficulty thinking)

- dementia

- Alzheimer's disease

- depression

- fetal neural tube defects (linked to high maternal homocysteine levels)

In addition, preliminary evidence suggests an association between high homocysteine levels and:

- inflammatory bowel disease

- osteoporosis

- age-related presbyopia (farsightedness)

- complications in both type 1 and type 2 diabetes.[27]

of thousands of people who can be treated with vitamins at a very early age, before they ever begin to develop the blood vessel lesions that can cause premature heart attacks, blood clots, or strokes. Identifying B_{12} deficiencies that can lead to high homocysteine levels would also have huge health benefits.

Yet as a practicing physician and nurse, we do not see cardiologists including B_{12} in their cardiac work-ups. Moreover, the few cardiologists who order Hcy tests typically treat high levels only with folic acid. And we don't see internists or general practitioners testing for B_{12} deficiency or ordering homocysteine levels, although they have no problem ordering numerous lipid profiles for cholesterol. What we *do* see are hundreds of cardiac patients coming through the emergency department who have been prescribed high-dose folic acid, but no B_{12}.

In the spring of 2010, Bob, a fifty-six-year-old executive, arrived at the emergency department (ED) with chest pain. He had a history of a previous heart attack, non-insulin dependent diabetes, GERD, depression, and five car-diac stents. His last two cardiac stents had been inserted six weeks previously.

Bob was borderline anemic and his red blood cells were normal in size. He'd complained of numbness and tingling in his feet, but his doctors had told him this was due to his diabetes. He'd been taking a proton-pump inhibitor for five years, an anti-depressant for three years, and a cholesterol-lowering agent and multi-vitamin prescribed by his cardiologist for the past five years.

Bob was very symptomatic for B$_{12}$ deficiency and scored high on the Cobalamin Deficiency Risk (CDR) score (see Appendix M). Reviewing Bob's previous visits, admissions, and out-patient lab draws, the ED doctor saw that Bob was never screened for B$_{12}$ deficiency, nor was his homocysteine checked. The ED physician ordered tests including serum B$_{12}$, MMA, and Hcy levels.

The test results showed that Bob had normal renal function, and his lipid profile was picture-perfect. However, he had a significant B$_{12}$ deficiency (serum B$_{12}$ 198 pg/ml) and very elevated Hcy at 27μmol/L. The evidence indicated that Bob's unaddressed B$_{12}$ deficiency, causing hyperhomocystine-mia, led to his significant coronary artery disease and poor health.

HIGH HOMOCYSTEINE AND PREGNANCY: RISKS TO BOTH MOTHER AND CHILD

We've talked about the risks of high homocysteine to the adult heart, but it can also damage an unborn child. In addition, it can contribute to the development of a very common and a potentially fatal cardiovascular complication in pregnant women.

It's well established that high levels of homocysteine in pregnant women are linked to an increased risk of neural tube defects (see Chapter 6). That's why doctors give pregnant women supplemental folic acid, and why they should give them supplemental vitamin B$_{12}$ as well.

In addition, high maternal homocysteine levels are a strong risk factor for preeclampsia, a potentially fatal pregnancy complication characterized by high blood pressure, swelling of the hands and face, and protein in the urine. One study, using blood samples taken early in pregnancy, compared fifty-six women who later developed severe preeclampsia to matched control group members who did not develop this complication. The samples from the women who later suffered from preeclampsia contained significantly higher homocysteine levels than samples from problem-free women, with those in the highest 25 percent having an almost three times greater risk of developing preeclampsia than other subjects.[28]

Homocysteine and kidney disease

One group of people who nearly always develop dangerously high homocysteine levels are individuals in end-stage renal disease (ESRD). These people's kidneys no longer function, and they are significantly debilitated, but with dialysis treatment they can live relatively normal lives for years. Their high homocysteine, however, puts them at vastly increased risk for strokes, heart attacks, and other vascular problems.

For the most part, doctors trying to lower the homocysteine levels of patients on dialysis resort to high doses of folic acid. This is because dietary folate is the strongest predictor of plasma homocysteine levels in patients with ESRD. But, as we've noted, folic acid can't lower homocysteine in the absence of sufficient vitamin B_{12}.

It's not surprising, therefore, that folate supplementation of patients with ESRD rarely reduces homocysteine to normal levels. To see if adding vitamin B_{12} to the treatment regimen would increase its effectiveness, doctors recently performed a prospective trial involving twenty-four dialysis patients with normal or higher-than-normal folate and B_{12} levels. The patients received either standard therapy (folic acid, vitamin B_6, and a small dose of oral B_{12}) or standard therapy augmented with injected B_{12}.

The researchers found that the injected B_{12} reduced plasma homocysteine levels by an average of 32 percent, even though the patients initially appeared to have adequate B_{12} stores. "Patients with higher baseline plasma homocysteine concentrations," they add, "had the greatest response." They conclude, "Patients with considerable persisting hyperhomocystinemia, despite high-dose folic acid therapy, are likely to respond to the addition of hydroxocobalamin [B_{12}], irrespective of their serum vitamin B_{12} concentrations."[29]

In a similar study in Japan, twenty-one hemodialysis patients were randomly assigned to receive folic acid supplements, vitamin B_{12} injections plus folic acid, or a combination of folic acid, vitamin B_6, and injected vitamin B_{12}. At the end of the three-week study, the researchers reported,

"Treatment resulted in normalization of fasting homocysteine levels in all 14 patients treated by the combined administration of methylcobalamin (B$_{12}$) and supplementation of folic acid, regardless of whether there was supplementation of vitamin B$_6$." They add, "The benefit of methylcobalamin administration on lowering plasma homocysteine levels in hemodialysis patients was remarkable."[30]

There is evidence, too, that homocysteine—in addition to its role in damaging blood vessels—acts, through an entirely different mechanism, as a potent uremic toxin that disrupts normal cellular function.[31] These findings should prompt doctors who treat patients with kidney problems to monitor homocysteine and MMA* levels, and to provide oral folic acid and high-dose methyl B$_{12}$ at the first sign of a problem. In our opinion, all dialysis patients should receive high-dose methyl-B$_{12}$ lozenges and/or injections. What we do not know (because no one has done a study and published it in a scientific journal) is if methyl-B$_{12}$ oral pills and lozenges are as effective as methyl-B$_{12}$ injections, and if hydroxo-B12 injections are as effective as methyl-B12 injections (using the same amount and frequency). Research in this area would be of great benefit to patients with kidney disease.

Alessandra Perna, M.D. and colleagues point out that chronic renal failure patients "have a high mortality rate, attributable mainly to cardiovascular disease: 9 percent per year, which is 30 times the risk in the general population, and even after age adjustment, cardiovascular disease mortality remains 10 to 20 times higher."[32] It is imperative, for the sake of renal disease sufferers and their families, that we study the likely role that homocysteine plays in this astronomical incidence of heart and blood vessel disease, and investigate as well the role that injected B$_{12}$ can potentially play in helping to reduce these patients' cardiovascular risk.

The relationship between kidney disease and high homocysteine, by the way, raises other interesting questions that should be investigated by researchers. One is the "chicken and egg" type of question: Which comes first, kidney disease or the high homocysteine levels seen in dialysis patients? Elevated homocysteine damages the lining of veins and arteries throughout the body, including those in the kidneys. What percentage of patients genetically prone to high homocysteine levels end up in renal

---

* In patients with kidney failure, urine MMA testing needs to be done, rather than serum MMA. Serum MMA can give falsely high values in patients with renal insufficiency, or in those who've experienced significant blood loss or dehydration.

failure because excess homocysteine has been scarring and injuring their kidneys for years? Doctors expect to see high homocysteine levels in patients with kidney failure, but never contemplate the probability that in many cases, elevated homocysteine might be a culprit rather than merely a side effect.

The bottom line: If you're at risk, get tested

It's clear to us, given the evidence that high homocysteine is a powerful risk factor for vascular disease in both young and old people, that screening should become commonplace for people at risk for cardiovascular problems. We believe that homocysteine testing should also become routine for senior citizens, pregnant women, and people with the following risk factors:

- Type I or Type II diabetes
- extended use of medications that can raise homocysteine levels, including certain lipid-lowering drugs, metformin, levodopa, certain anticonvulsants, and possibly androgens
- renal disease
- autoimmune disease
- thyroid disease
- any of the risk factors we've outlined for B_{12} deficiency

If you're overweight or have hyperlipidemia, don't let your doctor forgo homocysteine testing on the basis that "we already know the reasons for your cardiovascular troubles." Some doctors assume that obesity and high blood lipids are adequate explanations for cardiovascular problems, but the presence of these risk factors doesn't rule out the possibility of others.

Patients with high homocysteine levels should be evaluated for underlying B_{12} deficiency, and should be treated with standard doses of folic acid and vitamin B_6, and high-dose B_{12}. Even people in the upper range of what's considered normal should be started on homocysteine-lowering therapy, because levels only 12 percent above the highest normal level are linked to a threefold increase in the risk of heart attack.[33]

There's no downside to treatment, because the vitamins are completely harmless, and they cost only a few dollars out-of-pocket. Conversely, failing to treat high homocysteine levels correctly, or to investigate whether they stem from B_{12} deficiency, can be very dangerous—both to your wallet and to your health.

In a 2009 article in Thrombosis Journal[34], doctors describe a twenty-seven-year-old man who came to a Chicago hospital complaining of ongoing and progressive lower extremity weakness, numbness, and abnormal sensations in both legs.

On the second day of his admission, still with no diagnosis, the man began complaining of crushing chest pain and shortness of breath and started sweating profusely. His EKG showed he was suffering a heart attack, and he underwent emergency angioplasty. The surgeon found a large blood clot in his left coronary artery and inserted a stent.

Doctors started the man on aspirin, a blood thinner, and other cardiac medications. The next day, his echocardiogram showed reduced left ventricular function of 45 percent. Despite the successful cardiac stent placement, he continued to complain of difficulty breathing and shortness of breath.

A CT of the man's chest revealed multiple small blood clots in his left lower lung. His blood work revealed macrocytic anemia and elevated LDH, which are classic signs of B_{12} deficiency. His serum B_{12} was very low at 158 pg/ml, and he had normal serum folate. His homocysteine was severely elevated at 105 μmol/L.

> **Few doctors consider the B_{12}-homocysteine connection when treating cardiac or occlusive vascular disorders.**

At this point, the man's doctors tested him for pernicious anemia. They found that he was positive for anti-intrinsic factor antibodies and started him on B_{12} therapy. Seven days after his heart attack, a repeat echocardiogram showed normal left ventricular function. After ten days of B_{12} therapy, his homocysteine decreased dramatically from 105 μmol/L to 12.9 μmol/L. His neurological signs and symptoms gradually improved, and after his hospital stay, he was transferred to a physical therapy rehabilitation center, not only to address his cardiovascular event, but to address the original neurological problems caused by chronic severe B_{12} deficiency.

Cases like this man's are not rare. In fact, similar cases of pernicious anemia causing major blood clots have been reported world-wide.[35-38] Yet few doctors consider the B_{12}-homocysteine connection when treating

---

RETHINKING FORTIFIED CEREALS

The United States and Canada fortify many foods with folic acid, and Great Britain may be working on implementing a similar plan. British researchers recently conducted a study in which fifty-three healthy adults received increasing doses of folic acid over a six-month period. At the beginning of the study, the subjects' levels of homocysteine dropped in response to this nutrient. But as the folic acid dosage increased, homocysteine levels dropped less in response to this vitamin and more in response to vitamin B_{12}.

This finding, the researchers say, "suggests that a fortification policy based on folic acid and vitamin B_{12}, rather than folic acid alone, is likely to be much more effective at lowering...homocysteine concentrations, with potential benefits for reduction of risk of vascular disease."[39]

Only recently have scientists studied the potential ill effects of adding excess folic acid to grain and cereal in the presence of B_{12} deficiency. Ponnusamy Saravanan and Chitranjan S. Yajnik note that in 1997, Canada introduced mandatory folic acid fortification, and the prevalence of B_{12} deficiency has since increased. "In addition, neural tube defects attributable to B_{12} deficiency have tripled in the same period."[40] In the U.S., data from the National Health and Nutrition Examination Survey III (conducted after folic acid fortification) revealed that in the presence of B_{12} deficiency, high folic acid is associated with anemia and cognitive impairment in older adults. In the Pune Maternal Nutrition Study, Saravanan and Yajnik showed that "children born to mothers with the combination of 'high folic acid and low B_{12}' had higher truncal adiposity and insulin resistance." They cite research showing that B_{12} deficiency is increasing in countries with mandatory folic acid fortification and affecting all ages. "Studies on the prevalence of vitamin B_{12} deficiency during pregnancy and in women of childbearing age, plus the effects of B_{12} supplementation are therefore urgently needed," the British researchers add.[41]

Fortifying foods with B_{12} may sound good; however, it is not as easy as it sounds. Unlike folic acid, B_{12} is difficult to absorb and would

---

require very large doses in the grain to correct a deficiency. There is also the problem with the current daily recommended intake (DRI) or recommended daily allowance (RDA) for vitamin B$_{12}$, which, in our opinion, it is much too low for health and prevention of disease. Lastly, the U.S. uses cyanocobalamin rather than the active form of B$_{12}$ (methylcobalamin). Until all of these issues are worked out, we believe B$_{12}$ fortification would be a great waste of economic resources and would offer a false sense of protection for many people.

cardiac or occlusive vascular disorders. Thus, **it's up to patients and their families to be assertive** and insist on B$_{12}$ and homocysteine testing.

Also, if you undergo homocysteine-lowering therapy, insist that your doctor first obtain a baseline B$_{12}$ and urinary MMA. As we've noted, folic acid therapy corrects the anemia and enlarged blood cells that doctors generally look for when checking for B$_{12}$ deficiency, but does nothing to stop the neurological damage caused by depleted B$_{12}$ stores. Thus, if you're significantly deficient and your B$_{12}$ levels aren't checked first, folic acid therapy can mask the symptoms of your B$_{12}$ deficiency and allow its devastating neurological consequences—including neuropathy, dementia, and mental illness—to proceed to the point at which they become irreversible. In addition, you may fail to lower your homocysteine to healthy levels, thus placing yourself at continued risk for vascular disease.

The following statement, by hematologist A. C. Anthony, is typical of the warnings given in hematology textbooks: "Be certain B$_{12}$ deficiency does not exist when administering folic acid…. Failure to recognize [B$_{12}$] deficiency as the etiology [origin] of neurologic disease and treatment of [B$_{12}$] deficiency with folate…represent significant extremes of deviation from the dictum *primum non nocere* [first, do no harm]."[42]

Equally important, B$_{12}$ testing will allow your doctor to tailor your homocysteine-lowering program to your individual needs. In some cases, high-dose oral B$_{12}$ supplements will be sufficient. In others, injected B$_{12}$ will be necessary. Your doctor can't merely guess how much B$_{12}$ is enough for you, or rely on products marketed as homocysteine-lowering medications.

CHAPTER 5 NOTES:

1. Abbott Laboratories, http://www.abbott.com.my/t_healthv_main.html.

2. "Hot health tips," USC Care Medical Group, http://www.usc.edu/health/uscp/hhtsuddenheart.html.

3. Nygard, O., Nordrehaug, J. E., Refsum, H., Ueland, P. M., Farstad, M., and Vollset, S. E. Plasma homocysteine levels and mortality in patients with coronary artery disease. *New England Journal of Medicine* 1997, 337:230–6.

4. Carmel, R., Green, R., Rosenblatt, D. S., and Watkins, D. Update on cobalamin, folate, and homocysteine. *Hematology* 2003(1):62–81

5. O'Callaghan, P. and Graham, I. Update on homocysteine. *Heartwise* (Irish Heart Foundation), Winter 2000.

6. Booth, G. L., and Wang, E. E. Preventive health care 2000 update: Screening and management of hyperhomocysteinemia for the prevention of coronary artery disease events. The Canadian Task Force on Preventive Health Care. *Canadian Medical Association Journal* 2000, 163(1):21–9.

7. Kark, J. D., Sinnreich, R., Rosenberg, I. H., Jacques, P. F., and Selhub, J. Plasma homocysteine and parental myocardial infarction in young adults in Jerusalem. *Circulation* 2002, 105(23):2725–9.

8. Stampfer, M. J., Malinow, M. R., Willett, W. C., Newcomer, L. M, Upson, B., Ullmann, D., Tishler, P. V., and Hennekens, C. H. *Journal of the American Medical Association* 1992, 268(7):877–81.

9. Nygard, O., Nordrehaug, J. E., Refsum, H., Ueland, P. M., Farstad, M., and Vollset, S. E. Plasma homocysteine levels and mortality in patients with coronary artery disease. *New England Journal of Medicine* 1997, 337:230–6.

10. Stubbs, P. J., Al-Obaidi, M. K., Conroy, R. M., Collinson, P. O., Graham, I. M., and Noble, M. Effect of plasma homocysteine concentration on early and late events in patients with acute coronary syndromes. *Circulation* 2000, 102:605–10.

11. Wald, D. S., Law, M., and Morris, J. K. Homocysteine and cardiovascular disease: Evidence on causality from a meta-analysis. *British Medical Journal* 2002, 325:1202

12. Kittner, S. J., Giles, W. H., Macko, R. F., Hebel, J. R., Wozniak, M. A., Wityk, R. J., Stolley, P. D., Stern, B. J., Sloan, M. A., Sherwin, R., Price, T. R., McCarter, R. J., Johnson, C. J., Earley, C. J., Buchholz, D. W., and Malinow, M.

R. Homocyst(e)ine and risk of cerebral infarction in a biracial population: The stroke prevention in young women study. Stroke 1999, 30(8):1554–60; and, "Study links vitamin B deficiency to risk of stroke in younger women." *Doctor's Guide*, August 30, 1999, http://www.docguide.com.

13. Sato, Y., Kaji, M., Kondo, I., Yoshida, H., Satoh, K., and Metoki, N. Hyperhomocysteinemia in Japanese patients with convalescent stage ischemic stroke: Effect of combined therapy with folic acid and mecobalamine. *Journal of the Neurological Sciences* 2002, 202(1–2):65–8.

14. MacMahon, M., Kirkpatrick, C., Cummings, C. E., Clayton, A., Robinson, P. J., Tomiak, R. H., Liu, M., Kush, D., and Tobert, J. *Nutrition, Metabolism, and Cardiovascular Diseases* 2000, 10(4):195–203.

15. Schnyder, G., Roffi, M., Flammer, Y., Pin, R., and Hess, O. M. Effect of homocysteine-lowering therapy with folic acid, vitamin B(12), and vitamin B(6) on clinical outcome after percutaneous coronary intervention. The Swiss Heart Study: a randomized controlled trial. *Journal of the American Medical Association* 2002, 288(8):973–9.

16. Schnyder, G., Roffi, M., Pin, R., Flammer, Y., Lange, H., Eberli, F. R., Meier, B., Turi, Z. G., and Hess, O. M. Decreased rate of coronary restenosis after lowering of plasma homocysteine levels. *New England Journal of Medicine* 2001, 345(22):1593–600.

17. Yap, S., Boers, G. H., Wilcken, B., Wilcken, D. E., Brenton, D. P., Lee, P. J., Walter, J. H., Howard, P. M., and Naughten, E. R. Vascular outcome in patients with homocystinuria due to cystathionine beta-synthase deficiency treated chronically: a multicenter observational study. *Arteriosclerosis, Thrombosis, and Vascular Biology* 2001, 21(12):2080–5.

18. Ueland, P. M., Refsum, H., Beresford, S. A. A., and Vollset, S. E. The controversy over homocysteine and cardiovascular risk. *American Journal of Clinical Nutrition* 2000, 72:324–32.

19. Statistics are from the Centers for Disease Control and Prevention. February is American Heart Month: http://www.cdc.gov/features/heart-month/

20. Quotes are from Dr. McCully's discussion with Richard Passwater, Ph.D., at NutritionFocus.com, http.//www.nutritionfocus.com/nutrition_library/homocysteine.html, and from Bucco, Gloria, "Kilmer McCully, M.D., connects homocysteine and heart disease," *Nutrition Science News*, July 1999.

21. Yutsis, P. Homocysteine or cholesterol: Which is more deadly? *Journal of Longevity*, http://www.journaloflongevity.com/JOLWeb/Archives/86/deadly.html.

22. Chambers, J. C., Ueland, P. M., Obeid, O. A., Wrigley, J., Refsum, H., and Kooner. J. S. Improved vascular endothelial function after oral B vitamins. An effect mediated through reduced concentrations of free plasma homocysteine. *Circulation* 2000, 102:2479–83.

23. Mitchell, Tedd. At the heart of a family mystery. USAweekend.com, February 25, 2001.

24. http://www.abbott.com.my/t_healthv_main.html.

25. Ibid.

26. This woman's case appears in Chan, H. H. W., Douketis, J. D., and Nowaczyk, M. J. M. Acute renal vein thrombosis, oral contraceptive use, and hyperhomocysteinemia. *Mayo Clinic Proceedings* 2001, 76:212–214.

27. References for information in this chart include: Herrmann, W. and Knapp, J-P. Hyperhomocysteinemia: A new risk factor for degenerative diseases. *Clinical Laboratory* 2002, 48:471–81; Krumdieck, C. L. and Prince, C. W. Mechanisms of homocysteine toxicity on connective tissues: Implications for the morbidity of aging. *Journal of Nutrition* 2000, 130(2S Suppl):365S–368S; Romagnuolo, J., Fedorak, R. N., Dias, V. C., Bamforth, F., and Teltscher, M. Hyperhomocysteinemia and inflammatory bowel disease: Prevalence and predictors in a cross-sectional study. *American Journal of Gastroenterology* 2001, 96(7):2143–9; Kark, J. D., Selhub, J., Bostom, A., Adler, B., and Rosenberg, I. H. Plasma homocysteine and all-cause mortality in diabetes. *The Lancet* 1999, 353:1936–7; and Agullo-Ortuno, M. T., Albaladejo, M. D., Parra, S., Rodriguez-Manotas, M., Fenollar, M., Ruiz-Espejo, F., Tebar, J., and Martinez, P. Plasmatic homocysteine concentration and its relationship with complications associated to diabetes mellitus. *Clinica Chimica Acta* 2002, 326(1–2):105–12.

28. Cotter, A. M., Molloy, A. M., Scott, J. M., and Daly, S. F. Elevated plasma homocysteine in early pregnancy: a risk factor for the development of severe preeclampsia. *American Journal of Obstetrics and Gynecology* 2001, 185(4):781–5.

29. Elian, K. M., and Hoffer, L. J. Hydroxocobalamin reduces hyperhomocysteinemia in end-stage renal disease. *Metabolism* 2002, 51(7):881–6.

30. Koyama, K., Usami, T., Takeuchi, O., Morozumi, K., and Kimura, G. Efficacy of methylcobalamin on lowering total homocysteine plasma con-

centrations in haemodialysis patients receiving high-dose folic acid supplementation. *Nephrology, Dialysis, Transplantation* 2002, 17(5):916–22.

31. Perna, A. F., Castaldo, P., Ingross, D., and De Santo, N. Homocysteine, a new cardiovascular risk factor, is also a powerful uremic toxin. *Journal of Nephrology* 1999, 12:230–40.

32. Ibid.

33. Chambers, J. C., Ueland, P. M., Obeid, O. A., Wrigley, J., Refsum, H., and Kooner, J. S. Improved vascular endothelial function after oral B vitamins: An effect mediated through reduced concentrations of free plasma homocysteine. *Circulation* 2000, 102:2479–83.

34. Melhem, A., Desai, A., Hofmann, M. A. Acute myocardial infarction and pulmonary embolism in a young man with pernicious anemia—induced severe hyperhomocystinemia. *Thromb J.* 2009 May 13; 7:5.

35. Calera, A., Mora, J., Kotler, M., Eiger, G. Pulmonary embolism in a patient with pernicious anemia and hyperhomocystinemia. *Chest.* 2002 Oct;122(4): 1487–8.

36. Kupeli, E., Cengiz, C., Cila, A., Karnak, D. Hyperhomocystinemia due to pernicious anemia leading to pulmonary thromboembolism in a heterozygous mutation carrier. *Clin Appl Thromb Hemost.* 2008 Jul;14(3):365–8.

37. Leemann, B., Boughanem, N., Schnider, A. Ischemic, an uncommon complication of Biermer disease (pernicious anemia). *Rev Neurol (Paris).* 2006 Oct;162(1):1007–10.

38. Goette A. et al. Aortic thrombus and pulmonary embolism in a patient with hyperhomocystinemia. *Nat Clin Pract Cardiovasc Med.* 2006 Jul;3(7):396–9.

39. Quinlivan, E. P., McPartlin, J., McNulty, H., Ward, M., Strain, J. J, Weir, D. G., and Scott, J. M. Importance of both folic acid and vitamin B$_{12}$ in reduction of risk of vascular disease. *Lancet* 2002, 359(9302):227–8.

40. Saravanan, P., Yajnik, C. S. Role of maternal vitamin B$_{12}$ on the metabolic health of the offspring: a contributor to the diabetes epidemic? *Br J Diabetes Vasc Dis* 2010;10: 109–114.

41. Ibid.

42. Antony, A. C. Megaloblastic anemias. In R. Hoffman, et al., *Hematology: Basic Principles and Practice*, 3rd edition, 2000, Philadelphia: Churchill Livingstone.

6

Lost Children: When B_{12} Deficiency Causes Developmental Disabilities or Learning Problems

"My baby became symptomatic, not me. The result was irreversible brain damage in my breast-fed child."
—A B_{12}-deficient mother

If you're a parent, protecting your child from danger is your biggest concern. But no matter how cautious you are, there's one danger that you may not recognize: the risk that your child may suffer, both physically and mentally, from a B_{12} deficiency. Low B_{12} levels severely damage the brains of hundreds of children each year, and new research shows that subclinical mental deficits may occur in tens of thousands more.

In some cases, children suffer irreversible brain damage because they have inborn defects of B_{12} metabolism that doctors fail to identify. In other cases, environmental factors—primarily diet—are to blame. The most common cause of B_{12} deficiency in infants and young children is maternal dietary deficiency, which typically begins to cause symptoms in breastfed babies between the ages of four and eight months.[1] Unfortunately, doctors know far too little about either acquired or inborn B_{12} problems. Parents, as well, often aren't aware that breast-feeding their babies during infancy, and feeding them healthy meals when they're older, won't guarantee they'll be safe. In fact, ironically, it's often the most health-conscious mothers who put their children at greatest risk.

Lisa smiled, sat up, and said "Mama" and "Dada" right on schedule, but when she turned eight months old, something went terribly wrong.

She stopped talking. She couldn't stand up or grasp her toys. She stopped responding with smiles and coos to the people around her. Eventually, she couldn't even sit up without help. Her arms writhed in a snakelike way, a sign that B$_{12}$ deficiency was affecting her brain and nervous system. Her eyes fixed on people, but didn't follow them when they moved. She was frail and short, and her head was abnormally small for her age.

Lisa's doctors must have weighed many different diagnoses as she regressed in front of their eyes: autism, Rett syndrome, Tay-Sachs' disease, or a tumor or infection. But they missed an easy call, and in doing so they nearly robbed her of the chance to lead a normal life.

When Lisa was fourteen months old, her parents took her to a new doctor who took note of the fact that she'd been breast-fed by a vegetarian mother who ate few of the animal products that contain B$_{12}$. A test of the mother's B$_{12}$ level came back low at 226 pg/ml (considered "normal" by the lab, but actually in the "gray zone" we've discussed)—and Lisa's levels were depleted. Immediate treatment with B$_{12}$ led to rapid improvement in Lisa's symptoms, and she quickly grew taller and put on weight. Nine years later, the doctor reported, she was completely normal.[2]

Lisa owes her functioning brain and body to this doctor, who spotted and aggressively treated her B$_{12}$ deficiency just in time to prevent a permanent brain injury. If he'd missed the diagnosis, as her previous doctors had, Lisa would most likely be mentally retarded and wheelchair-bound for the rest of her life.

> **The most common cause of B$_{12}$ deficiency in infants and young children is maternal dietary deficiency.**

Other mothers and their children, however, are not as lucky. In November 2009, we received an e-mail from a mother in the Midwest whose baby, Megan, began showing signs of developmental delay at six months of age. Her doctors, uneducated about B$_{12}$ deficiency, decided to "wait and watch," thinking that she might have some form of cerebral palsy, outgrow her symptoms, or perhaps develop autism.

As the months passed, Megan continued to miss developmental milestones and she continually grew weaker. Over the next seven months, Megan continued to fall behind.

At thirteen and a half months of age, Megan was referred to a pediatric developmental specialist, and more tests were ordered. An MRI showed brain atrophy (shrinkage), a classic sign of B$_{12}$ deficiency in infants. The urinary organic acid profile showed grossly elevated MMA and revealed Megan's severe underlying B$_{12}$ deficiency. This led Megan's doctors to check her serum B$_{12}$, which was only 64 pg/ml, as well as her Hcy, which was severely elevated at 46 μmol/L.

Sadly, unlike the child we discussed earlier, Megan will never fully recover. Her brain and nervous system are permanently injured, and she will more than likely require life-long care. She is now two years and seven months old, cannot walk or talk yet, and has myoclonic seizures. She is now babbling and cruises while holding onto furniture, which places her developmentally at around nine months of age.

Megan's devastating symptoms occurred because her mother had an undiagnosed B$_{12}$ deficiency and breast-fed her. Megan's mom was not a vegetarian, but suffered from a B$_{12}$ deficiency that her OB/GYN never caught. Why? Because most doctors don't check the B$_{12}$ status of pregnant and nursing moms, which is an enormous and costly mistake.

Megan's mom notes that she was asymptomatic—which was remarkable, given her deficiency—but her serum B$_{12}$ was very low at 140 pg/ml. Even though this would be considered subclinical B$_{12}$ deficiency (see Chapter 11), it clearly demonstrates that a low serum B$_{12}$ in a pregnant or nursing mother cannot sustain normal brain growth and development, and can cause life-long injury and disability.

The rapid decline that Megan experienced is very common in infants with low B$_{12}$ levels. In adults, B$_{12}$ deficiency is often insidious, taking its toll over years or even decades. In children, however, a severe deficiency can strike with terrifying swiftness. Within months, a happy, babbling, cooing, crawling infant can be reduced to a child who appears half-conscious and can barely lift its head. Babies and toddlers affected by severe B$_{12}$ deficiency begin to lose their speech and social skills, and they become apathetic and irritable. They often refuse to eat, and they regress to the point where they can no longer sit, crawl, stand, or walk. Their heads and bodies grow too slowly, and they fail to gain weight, becoming thin and weak. Brain scans frequently show atrophy of the cerebral cortex.

If caught in time, B$_{12}$ deficiency can be corrected quickly, and affected infants and toddlers can regain all of their skills and receive a good prognosis for a full recovery. Sadly, however, many cases aren't diagnosed until children become permanently learning-disabled or even mentally retarded. And many cases, involving much milder and harder-to-detect symptoms, are never diagnosed at all.

Some children are genetically destined to develop B$_{12}$ deficiency, a problem we'll discuss later in this chapter and more extensively in Chapter 12. Thousands of other children have borderline or even dangerously low B$_{12}$ levels because of what they eat (or, more correctly, what they *don't* eat). And many others have a "second-hand" deficiency, starting in their earliest days of life, because their mothers had deficient levels of B$_{12}$ during pregnancy or while breast-feeding—the primary reason for B$_{12}$ deficiency in infants and young children.[3]

When mothers are deficient in B$_{12}$, the damage to their babies starts in the womb. You've probably heard of neural tube defects (NTDs), which are very common, severe birth defects occurring when the brain or spinal cord fails to form correctly. Low levels of folic acid increase the risk for NTDs, which is why doctors now ensure that their pregnant patients get plenty of this vitamin. However, research also strongly implicates low B$_{12}$ levels as a factor in NTDs[4], which isn't surprising, since folic acid and B$_{12}$ work hand in hand. (You'll remember from earlier chapters that for the body to use folic acid, vitamin B$_{12}$ must be present.)

Women with B$_{12}$ deficiency or a low intake of vitamin B$_{12}$ are at higher risk of giving birth to children with potentially disabling or fatal birth defects. As reported in the journal *Pediatrics*[5] in March 2009, women with vitamin B$_{12}$ deficiency in early pregnancy were up to five times more likely to have a child with NTDs, such as spina bifida, than women with high levels of B$_{12}$.

Other researchers reported a three-fold increase in the risk of NTDs in mothers who had vitamin B$_{12}$ status in the lowest quartile, regardless of folic acid fortification. They concluded that vitamin B$_{12}$ fortification in conjunction with folic acid supplementation may reduce NTDs more effectively than folic acid fortification alone.[6]

In addition, studies show that children of severely B$_{12}$-deficient mothers exhibit abnormal behavior stemming from dysfunction of the basal ganglia (a part of the brain that helps control movement and emotional regulation) and pyramidal tracts (pathways linking the motor cortex to the spinal cord).[7] Studies of animals also link B$_{12}$ deficiency to an increased risk of stillbirth and infant death, as well as to low birth weight in newborns.[8]

Even women with adequate stores of B$_{12}$ can damage their unborn babies' brains if they fail to take in enough B$_{12}$ in their diet. Because only newly-absorbed vitamin B$_{12}$ readily crosses the placenta, the vitamin B$_{12}$ stockpiled by the mother's body is largely ineffective in protecting the health of the fetus.[9]

Worse, the danger of second-hand B$_{12}$ deficiency doesn't end the day a baby is born. Mothers with depleted B$_{12}$ stores who exclusively breast-feed their babies unknowingly put them at great risk for developmental disability or even death. This is a common cause of B$_{12}$ problems in infants; one study, for instance, found that half of a group of six infants diagnosed with crippling B$_{12}$ deficiency became ill after being nursed by vegetarian mothers. (The other half were born to mothers with undiagnosed pernicious anemia, an autoimmune disease.)[10]

Vegetarian and vegan mothers are devastated and feel tremendous guilt when their children suffer harm due to B$_{12}$ deficiency, but in reality, most of these tragedies are the fault of doctors who fail to screen pregnant and nursing mothers for this deficiency—and who then often misdiagnose these women's children as mentally retarded or autistic, rather than considering B$_{12}$ deficiency when the infants lose their speech, social skills, and motor skills.

> **Women with B$_{12}$ deficiency or a low intake of vitamin B$_{12}$ are at higher risk of giving birth to children with potentially disabling or fatal birth defects.**

Because B$_{12}$ occurs naturally only in animal products, a vegan diet, which excludes eggs and dairy products as well as meat and fish, provides virtually no natural B$_{12}$. A vegetarian diet, while it can include eggs and cheese, may provide too little B$_{12}$, especially if a mother has any of the risk factors that make her vulnerable to B$_{12}$ deficiency (see Chapter 1). A macrobiotic diet, which excludes most animal protein with the exception of fish, also can lead to B$_{12}$ depletion. And even vegan, vegetarian, or macrobiotic-diet mothers who take B$_{12}$ supplements can easily become deficient if they take too low a dose—a common occurrence—or if they have trouble absorbing the vitamin.

Another problem occurs when mothers on no-animal-protein diets take ineffective supplements. Studies show that vegetarian formulations of B$_{12}$ supplements don't always dissolve well, meaning that even a correct dosage of the vitamin can pass through the gastrointestinal tract largely undigested.[11] In addition, many vegans supplement their diets with spirulina (an algae), tempeh (fermented soy), or nori (a seaweed) in the belief that these plant foods contain vitamin B$_{12}$—a widely accepted idea based on laboratory tests that showed significant amounts of the vitamin in these plants. Newer research, however, shows that the tests are primarily detecting "pseudo-vitamin B$_{12}$" analogues that may actually block the uptake of real B$_{12}$.[12]

Pseudo-B$_{12}$ also shows up as real B$_{12}$ in blood tests, meaning that spirulina-consuming vegetarians with "normal" B$_{12}$ levels may actually be severely deficient. Nutritionist Stephen Byrnes recently wrote, "In my own practice, I recently saved two vegans from death from anemia by convincing them to eat generous amounts of dairy products. Both of [them] thought their B$_{12}$ needs were being met by tempeh and spirulina. They weren't."[13]

Vegetarian and vegan mothers also are the most likely to breast-feed for long periods of time, which puts nursing children at high risk of B$_{12}$ deficiency if the mothers don't supplement their diets correctly. Children can be severely crippled by B$_{12}$ deficiency, even if their breast-feeding vegan mothers have "normal" B$_{12}$ levels, because, as in the case of pregnancy, the mother's body will not mobilize existing stores of B$_{12}$ efficiently in order to make up for a dietary deficiency. "Consequently," hematologist Julian Davis and his colleagues say, "even mothers who have only recently become vegans and who have no hematologic or biochemical evidence of vitamin B$_{12}$ deficiency may place their nurslings at risk for this vitamin deficiency."[14] Adding to this risk, babies who are B$_{12}$-deficient often become anorexic and reject solid foods, leading mothers to breast-feed them even longer and further worsen their B$_{12}$ deficiency.

Note: Pregnant and nursing mothers need to be treated in the gray zone—optimal serum B$_{12}$ levels should be 1,000 pg/ml or greater.

A GROWING BUT IGNORED RISK FOR VEGETARIANS

The 2008 study "Vegetarianism in America," published by *Vegetarian Times*, revealed that 3.2 percent of U.S. adults (7.3 million people) follow a vegetarian diet. About 0.5 percent of the U.S. population (1 million people) are vegans who consume no animal products. Ten percent of U.S. adults (22.8 million) said they largely follow a vegetarian-inclined diet.

Vegetarian, vegan, and macrobiotic diets are growing in popularity, particularly among young people and particularly among females of childbearing age. Given the overall healthfulness of vegan/vegetarian diets, this is a good thing, *except* when the people following these otherwise-healthy diets fail to get enough B$_{12}$.

Unfortunately, that's a common occurrence. Among the findings of researchers are the following:

- "Serum vitamin [B$_{12}$] levels are significantly lower in subjects consuming alternative nutrition, with deficiency observed in 24 percent of vegetarians and 78 percent of vegans vs. 0 percent in omnivores."[15]

- "The increased MMA concentration suggested a 25 percent frequency of functional vitamin B$_{12}$ deficiency [in vegetarians]."[16]

- "The prevalence of hyperhomocystinemia [a strong indicator of B$_{12}$ deficiency, if kidney disease and thyroid disease are not present] was higher in vegetarians (53.3 percent) than in controls (10.3 percent)."[17]

- "Evidence indicates that over 80 percent of those people who have been vegans for two years or more are deficient in cobalamin [B$_{12}$] as determined by a serum cobalamin below 250 pg/ml and/or an elevated level of urinary MMA."[18]

These findings should place obstetricians and pediatricians on alert. As the numbers of vegetarian and vegan women grow, so too, almost inevitably, will the problem of babies suffering from preventable brain and nervous system damage when their mothers are not educated about proper B$_{12}$ supplementation. The solution is simple: Doctors, dietitians, and other health professionals must ensure that women following a vegetarian or vegan diet receive in-depth information about the necessity for B$_{12}$ supplements, accurate information about which supplements work and which don't, and regular tests of their serum B$_{12}$ and urinary MMA levels during pregnancy and nursing.

None of this is a criticism of meat-free diets, which—because they are low in fat, high in phytochemicals and antioxidants, and generally low in artificial colorings and additives—tend to be very healthful. If they contain plenty of supplemental B$_{12}$, vegan or vegetarian or macrobiotic diets can help the heart and reduce the risk of cancer and diabetes. But without adequate B$_{12}$, the same diets can be a death sentence—not only for adults, but for the children they love.

OTHER MOTHERS, OTHER RISKS

While vegan or vegetarian mothers are the most likely to be low in B$_{12}$, even mothers who eat large amounts of meat and other animal products may be B$_{12}$-deficient and not know it. Women at highest risk include those with undiagnosed pernicious anemia, those who've undergone gastrointestinal surgery (including weight-loss surgeries, such as gastric bypass), those with family histories of pernicious anemia, those who eat poorly during pregnancy, and those with autoimmune or malabsorption disorders (e.g., gluten enteropathy). But a woman who has none of these risk factors, and appears completely healthy, can still be starving her baby of B$_{12}$.

A recent study, in fact, showed that one third of infants develop elevated MMA levels by six weeks of age, a possible sign of inadequate levels of B$_{12}$. "Notably," the researchers say, "we studied consecutive pregnancies in healthy, well-nourished mothers who consumed an omnivorous, non-vegetarian diet, and even in this population we found biochemical evidence of cobalamin [B$_{12}$] deficiency."[19]

This finding was particularly true for infants who were not firstborns. This indicates, the researchers say, that "the prevalence of impaired cobalamin status in the neonatal period may be underestimated"—a mistake that could lead to tens of thousands of children suffering subtle but permanent neurologic damage.

This is why we believe that at-risk women who are pregnant need to have a serum B$_{12}$ and urinary MMA test, particularly if they plan to nurse their babies.* Testing is especially important for pregnant teens, who often eat poor diets; a recent study of fifty-eight pregnant adolescents showed that twenty-five had suboptimal serum B$_{12}$ levels.[20]

In addition, any infant with an unexplained developmental disability should be screened immediately for B$_{12}$ deficiency (and the mother should be screened as well). Babies and toddlers diagnosed quickly are highly likely to make full recoveries, while those who go months or years without a diagnosis are likely to suffer permanent neurological damage and become mentally retarded. (One note: Young children who do get early diagnoses sometimes receive only partial or inadequate treatment, which can lead to partial or sub-optimal recoveries.) The nervous system develops most rapidly during the first two years, and the brain reaches full growth and maturity by age six, so

> **Any infant with an unexplained developmental disability should be screened immediately for B$_{12}$ deficiency.**

---

* Serum B$_{12}$ levels are reported to give false positive test results during pregnancy (low serum B$_{12}$ levels in the absence of deficiency), a finding we question. As a result, B$_{12}$ deficiency is unrecognized and underappreciated in pregnancy, placing both mother and child at great risk.

the early months and years are the most critical for detection and correction of B$_{12}$ deficiency.

Jamie developed normally until he became lethargic and irritable at four months of age. When Jamie was eight months old, a doctor noted his small head size, and his inability to sit unsupported or lift his head when placed on his back or tummy. Jamie also moved his limbs in an abnormal, snake-like motion, and his eyes failed to fix on a toy or follow movements.

Tests showed that Jamie's mother had pernicious anemia and a severely low serum B$_{12}$ level of 128 pg/ml. Unaware of her deficiency, she'd breast-fed Jamie, thinking she was providing him with the best diet possible.

"The child's response to vitamin B$_{12}$ supplements was remarkable," his doctors say, "with an improvement in head growth up to the 90th percentile, disappearance of the [abnormal movements], and improved development." However, follow-up tests five years later showed that the boy suffered from borderline intellectual retardation—a permanent consequence of his early lack of B$_{12}$.[21]

CHILDHOOD AND ADOLESCENCE: B$_{12}$ DEFICIENCY AND LEARNING PROBLEMS

Every year, several million parents put their children on vegetarian, vegan, or macrobiotic diets. At the same time, millions of adolescents choose, either for health reasons or for philosophical reasons, to forgo meat and animal products.

Again, this is a valid decision—*if* these children and teens obtain the right amounts of supplemental B$_{12}$ (as well as adequate levels of iron and other nutrients), and if they have no medical problems that prevent them from absorbing B$_{12}$ properly. Research indicates, however, that a large number of non-meat-eating children aren't getting enough vitamin B$_{12}$ either in their diets or from supplements, and that their brains aren't functioning optimally as a result.

In 1985, Dr. Wija van Staveren and colleagues began following a group of infants being raised on vegan diets. Because these diets contain no animal products, they are extremely low in vitamin B$_{12}$. Testing the children in their early years, the researchers noticed subtle but significant impairments in the psychomotor functioning of the vegan children as compared to those eating meat and dairy products.

Told of these findings, many parents of the vegan children participating in the study chose to switch their children to diets containing milk, eggs, and in some cases meat. On average, the children began eating animal products at around the age of six. When the children reached adolescence, the researchers again compared them to a group of children raised from birth on diets including animal products. Each of the forty-eight formerly-vegan children and the twenty-four control children took a ninety-minute battery of tests that measured their cognitive skills, and the researchers measured their serum B$_{12}$ and MMA levels.

Many of the children raised until age six on vegan diets were still B$_{12}$-deficient, even after years of eating at least some animal proteins. "We found a significant association between cobalamin [B$_{12}$] status and performance on tests measuring fluid intelligence, spatial ability, and short-term memory," van Staveren and colleagues say, with the formerly-vegan children scoring lower than the control group members in each case.

The deficit in the early-vegan children's fluid intelligence is particularly troubling, the researchers say, "because it involves reasoning, the capacity to solve complex problems, abstract thinking ability, and the ability to learn. Any defect in this area may have far-reaching consequences for individual functioning."

Most of the children switched from vegan diets had B$_{12}$ intakes close to the Recommended Dietary Allowance at the time of the follow-up study, yet many of them continued to suffer from B$_{12}$ deficiency. "Because these subjects consumed a diet extremely low in cobalamin [B$_{12}$] from birth up to the age of six years," the researchers say, "their cobalamin stores may never have reached an optimal level and moderate intakes may not have been sufficient for obtaining normal serum cobalamin status."[22*]

There are three lessons to be learned from this study. One is that an alarming percentage of people who put their children on vegetarian, vegan, and macrobiotic diets are failing to do the right thing when it comes to B$_{12}$ supplements. Another is that children on these diets need to have their serum B$_{12}$ and urine MMA status checked regularly, and they need B$_{12}$ injections if high-dose oral supplements aren't keeping their levels of the vitamin high enough. And a third lesson is that if your

---

* It's puzzling that although the parents of the children in this study were highly educated, and researchers detected the children's low cobalamin status in infancy, a number of these children's personal physicians apparently did not conduct regular B$_{12}$ testing during childhood, or provide B$_{12}$ injections when needed—the only likely explanation for the children's continuing deficiency. We would consider this to be substandard or negligent medical care for children with identified deficiencies.

child becomes B_{12}-deficient, simply switching him or her to a diet higher in B_{12} and offering a multivitamin supplement is not enough. Children with B_{12} deficiency need higher-than-normal amounts of the vitamin in order to replenish their depleted stores, just as adults do, and the standard vitamin formulas that parents typically buy are not up to the job. (For example, Flintstones children's multivitamins—which are similar to most oral vitamin preparations for children—contain only six micrograms of B_{12}, compared to the 1,000 micrograms needed daily if oral B_{12} is taken to correct a deficiency.)

SYMPTOMS: FROM SUBTLE TO SEVERE

Like the children in the study by Dr. van Staveren and colleagues, many B_{12}-deficient children have symptoms too subtle to be picked up by most doctors, or even by parents. Their mental symptoms—memory deficits, slight declines in fluid IQ, fatigue, mood changes—may be written off as behavior problems, "growing pains," or even mild learning disabilities. As a consequence, the children may wind up on Ritalin or other drugs rather than receiving a proper diagnosis.

In some cases, however, the symptoms seen in children and teens are dramatic, resembling those of middle-aged adults or senior citizens with drastic B_{12} depletion. Symptoms can range from muscle weakness and learning problems to paralysis, psychiatric disorders, or even blindness. And as with adults, children can undergo drastic neurological deterioration, even when standard blood tests show no signs of macrocytic anemia.

The first thing fourteen-year-old "F. C." noticed was that his calf hurt when he stood up. The pain grew worse and worse, and soon he began stumbling and falling. Eventually, he needed help walking.

Examining F. C., a physician learned that the boy suffered from fatigue and daytime sleepiness. F. C. was small for his age and thin, weighing only eighty-eight pounds, and his heart beat too slowly. He seemed "flat" emotionally, and he answered the doctor's questions in monosyllables, cooperating momentarily and then becoming withdrawn.

Learning that F. C. was a longtime vegan and a picky eater, the doctor suspected B_{12} deficiency. Tests showed a serum B_{12} level in the gray zone, but massively elevated MMA and homocysteine levels, indicating severe B_{12} depletion.

When the doctor gave F. C. B$_{12}$ injections, the teen regained his ability to walk. In addition, when the mental deficits caused by F. C.'s low B$_{12}$ levels disappeared, his aloofness and lack of emotion vanished, and he once again responded normally to his friends and family. F. C.'s MMA and homocysteine levels were normal at follow-up, but he continued to show neurologic abnormalities eighteen months after diagnosis and treatment—a result of nerve injury caused by late-diagnosed B$_{12}$ deficiency.[23]

A related case was reported in December 2007 in the Toronto Sun. *The thirteen-year-old boy profiled by the newspaper nearly died because his doctors and pediatric specialists couldn't diagnose his mysterious neurological disorder. But it wasn't mysterious; it was simply a vitamin B$_{12}$ deficiency that went undiagnosed and untreated for nearly a year.*

The reporter who interviewed the boy's family wrote that they "look back on a year that resembled an endless episode of House, *where dumbfounded diagnosticians struggled to figure out what was wrong with him. For eight long months, J.J. was in and out of the Hospital for Sick Children in Toronto while he slowly lost his ability to walk, write, and, most crushingly for the young artist, his remarkable talent to draw."*

The reporter adds, "By the time his parents rushed him back to the hospital in August, they were at their wits' end with no answers in sight. Their son was in a wheelchair, deep yellow from jaundice, and his stymied pediatrician worried J.J.'s organs were shutting down. No one could figure out why."

The answer became clear when doctors checked J.J.'s serum B$_{12}$: it was a record-setting zero. As a result, of his chronic misdiagnosis, J.J.'s simple B$_{12}$ deficiency progressed to the point where it injured his myelin and nerves.

The boy received a diagnosis of subacute combined degeneration of the spinal cord, secondary to pernicious anemia. A year after treatment, he was being home-schooled and needed to use a walker. His ability to concentrate was impaired, and he had trouble using his hands and legs. B$_{12}$ is essential for bone-forming cells called osteoblasts, and J.J. was found to have osteoporosis in his spine with multiple fractures.[24]

While children eating vegan or vegetarian diets are the most likely to have deficient B$_{12}$ levels, they aren't the only young people prone to develop a deficiency. The same risk factors that apply to adults—any history of gastrointestinal disease (particularly Crohn's disease) or ileal surgery, the presence of any autoimmune disorder (especially thyroid disease), celiac disease or gluten intolerance, the presence of iron deficiency, use of B$_{12}$-lowering medications, any unexplained neurological or mental symptoms, or any exposure to nitrous oxide (either during surgery or dental work, or as a drug of abuse)—apply to children and teens, and should lead parents and doctors to suspect possible B$_{12}$ deficiency. Teens with bulimia or anorexia should also be checked for B$_{12}$ deficiency, because they are prone to nutritional deficiencies.

Most pediatric cases involving neurological damage are due to acquired B$_{12}$ deficiency; however, many cases involve children eating vegan, vegetarian, or macrobiotic diets. Parents who implement such diets can avoid these tragedies by researching the issue of B$_{12}$ supplementation thoroughly, and having their children's serum B$_{12}$ and urinary MMA levels (and their own, if they are pregnant or nursing women) tested regularly. It's also crucial for doctors and patients to realize that a serum B$_{12}$ in the gray zone (200–450 pg/ml) must always be treated. As Joel Fuhrman, a physician and a practicing vegetarian, says, "It is entirely irresponsible for a health professional not to recommend B$_{12}$ supplementation in some form or frequent monitoring of MMA with blood tests for those who do not consume any animal products in their diets. No controversy exists."[25] This is true for all vegetarians and vegans, and it's particularly true in the case of the youngest and most vulnerable—the babies and children who trust their parents, and their doctors, to protect their health.

In addition to the risks we've covered, poor B$_{12}$ status increases the odds of preterm birth, intrauterine growth retardation, and recurrent miscarriage (more on this in Chapter 9).[26] Thus, adequate B$_{12}$ is critical before conception, during pregnancy, and during breast-feeding. A serum B$_{12}$ falling in the "gray zone" is not adequate for prenatal or postnatal care. Moreover, prenatal vitamins do not contain enough B$_{12}$ to correct a deficiency or beginning deficiency, and a growing fetus in the womb needs plentiful amounts of B$_{12}$, which pregnancy can deplete (see Chapter 12).

DEVELOPMENTAL DISORDERS: THE B$_{12}$ LINK

Not all cases of B$_{12}$ deficiency in infancy stem from an inadequate diet. A number of children suffer, instead, from genetic flaws that impair some aspect of the complex process of B$_{12}$ metabolism. In fact, there are ten different inherited defects that are known to impair the pathways of B$_{12}$ metabolism and transport in humans. Seven alter cellular utilization and coenzyme production, and the other three affect absorption and transport. All of these disorders can severely damage a child—especially if they aren't detected early.

In a 2002 issue of Discover, *physician Mark Cohen describes the frantic phone call he received from a mother one day. The woman's daughter, Jennifer, at three and a half years of age, suffered from a developmental disability of unknown origin, and doctors diagnosed her as autistic because she showed little affection, played only by herself, showed no imagination, and did not speak normally.*

The day Jennifer's mother called, the little girl had been fine at school. When she came home, however, her mother said, "She sat down to play, and when she stood up, she couldn't walk right, like she was dizzy. And she just doesn't seem to be herself."

She took Jennifer to Dr. Cohen's office, where he spotted troubling signs and symptoms: The toddler lurched when she walked, fell several times, turned her head to the right to look at objects, and used her left but not her right hand.

"I think this little girl has had a stroke," Dr. Cohen said. An MRI, indeed, revealed a stroke caused by a blood clot, and further tests revealed a "sky high" homocysteine level. The diagnosis: homocystinuria, an inborn error of metabolism that often involves a disruption in the B$_{12}$ pathway. When homocystinuria is identified early, treatment will prevent strokes and other damage.

When Jennifer received treatment for her disorder, she began smiling and interacting, started playing with toys, began learning sign language, and no longer appeared autistic. She has not suffered another stroke since treatment began.

A happy ending? Not really. Jennifer almost assuredly wouldn't have suffered her first stroke, or developed autistic behaviors, if her pediatrician would have screened her for vitamin B$_{12}$ deficiency. Jennifer had signs and symptoms of B$_{12}$ deficiency (developmental delay, poor speech, poor socialization), but her doctors (like most pediatricians and pediatric specialists) were uneducated on this disorder. Her disorder could have been identified early on if any of the specialists who saw Jennifer over the three and a half years of her life had ordered tests for B$_{12}$ deficiency or inborn errors of B$_{12}$ metabolism.[27]

---

* B$_{12}$ (hydroxocobalamin) therapy is essential only in specific forms of homocystinuria. Because homocystinuria can also stem from an inborn error in the metabolism of B$_6$ or folic acid, not all children respond to B$_{12}$; some require treatment of bioactive folate, vitamin B$_6$, a combination of vitamins, betaine, and/or alterations in the protein or amino acid content of their diet (see Chapter 12).

In most cases, children with inborn errors of B$_{12}$ metabolism develop severe symptoms within the first few months of life. Sometimes, however, symptoms—typically difficulty in walking, and mental and cognitive problems—don't appear until the affected children reach toddlerhood, childhood, the teen years, or even early adulthood. These late-onset errors of metabolism may not be picked up during newborn screening. Thus, any infants, children, teens, or young adults who develop neurologic symptoms should be tested for B$_{12}$ deficiency and inborn errors of B$_{12}$ metabolism.

Such testing rarely occurs, however, because few doctors are familiar with these conditions. Says genetic pediatric researcher Piero Rinaldo, M.D., "As a matter of fact, you cannot diagnose what you don't know, and unfortunately a large proportion of cases remain undiagnosed because these disorders are not yet included in mainstream medical practice."[28] This oversight can have fatal medical consequences—and devastating legal consequences as well.

In 1989, Patricia Stallings rushed her infant son, Ryan, to the emergency department after he became lethargic, vomited his food, and developed trouble breathing. Lab tests ordered by the hospital's doctors showed the presence of ethylene glycol (a substance found in antifreeze) in Ryan's blood. Believing that Stallings had tried to poison Ryan, the authorities placed him in foster care, allowing Patricia only brief visits, during which she could hold and feed him. Shortly after one of these visits, Ryan became desperately ill and was rushed to the hospital, where he died. Suspecting Stallings of again poisoning her son, police arrested her. A jury convicted her of first degree murder, and Patricia went to prison. At the time, she was pregnant with her second son, a child who would be the key to her freedom.

Patricia's second child, David, entered foster care immediately after his birth. Shortly afterward, he began developing symptoms eerily similar to Ryan's. David's doctors diagnosed him with methylmalonic acidemia, an inborn error of B$_{12}$ metabolism, and immediately began appropriate treatment. Concerned that he might have sent an innocent woman to prison, the attorney who prosecuted Patricia Stallings consulted with several doctors and finally asked Dr. Piero Rinaldo (the researcher cited earlier in this chapter) to investigate. Dr. Rinaldo conclusively determined that Ryan's symptoms, like his brother's, stemmed from methylmalonic acidemia. The two labs that analyzed Ryan's blood had used older gas chromatography techniques that confused one of the substances elevated in Ryan's disorder with ethylene glycol.

The prosecutor dismissed the charges against Patricia Stallings, but by then she'd lost a year of her life for the "crime" of having a baby with an inborn error of B$_{12}$ metabolism. Worse yet, Rinaldo says, the incorrect treatment implemented by Ryan's doctors in response to the misdiagnosis of poisoning most likely contributed to his death.

As in Patricia Stallings' case, inborn errors of B$_{12}$ metabolism can affect more than one child in a family. One recent report in the medical literature[29] describes two siblings, a sixteen-year-old girl and her twenty-four-year-old sister, who both suffered from methylmalonic acidemia. The younger sister became psychotic, developed severe neuropathy, and eventually was placed on a ventilator, but she recovered fully after a correct diagnosis and treatment. Her older sister suffered for two years with painful, progressive spinal cord damage before being accurately diagnosed. (The older sister's case is another example of a B$_{12}$-related problem that could easily be misdiagnosed as multiple sclerosis.) Another report by a separate group of researchers[30] describes two siblings who died as a result of undiagnosed methylmalonic aciduria, one misdiagnosed as having metabolic acidosis due to new-onset diabetes and the other misdiagnosed as having Reye's syndrome.

Clinicians should consider inborn errors of B$_{12}$ metabolism as a possibility in patients who are critically ill with unclear clinical and biochemical findings, particularly when there is a suspicious family history. Detecting such errors early can save lives and prevent disability, and, thus, prevent multiple tragedies.

SPECULATION: IS THERE AN AUTISM/B$_{12}$ CONNECTION?

Children with autism, a once-rare developmental disorder that is now becoming alarmingly common, exhibit severe speech and language problems, aloofness or abnormal social interaction, repetitive and ritualistic behavior (such as obsessively lining up toys), and in many cases self-injurious or aggressive behavior.

Some cases of autism have known causes: for instance, prenatal rubella infection, meningitis during early development, or specific genetic disorders. In general, however, autism is simply a *description* rather than an actual diagnosis, because the cause of a child's autistic symptoms is rarely identified. In fact, autism appears to have multiple causes, and preliminary clinical evidence strongly indicates that some of these causes involve un-diagnosed vitamin B$_{12}$ deficiency or inborn errors of B$_{12}$ metabolism.

Vitamin B$_{12}$ is vital for proper brain function, growth and develop-ment. Classic B$_{12}$ deficiency in infants and young children frequently causes symptoms similar to those seen in autism, including aloofness, loss of speech and social skills, and movement abnormalities (see Chapter 12).

Increasingly, doctors are finding that many autistic children improve remarkably when they receive B$_{12}$ injections. British researcher Dr. Ray Bhatt, for instance, has reported remarkable improvement in autistic children treated with vitamin B$_{12}$, saying, "The number who have ben-efited is a surprise."[31] Sidney Baker, M.D., a leading autism expert, notes that parents often see positive changes within "hours to days" after beginning B$_{12}$ injections, and recommends that all autistic children be screened for vitamin B$_{12}$ deficiency. "But even those without the MMA marker often respond dramatically to B$_{12}$," he says.[32] It would be interesting to know how many of these responders have serum B$_{12}$ levels in the gray zone.

> Classic B$_{12}$ deficiency in infants and young children frequently causes symptoms similar to those seen in autism.

Arnold Brenner, M.D., who has conducted trials of injected B$_{12}$ on a number of autistic patients, says the benefits seen in his patients included decreases in hyperactivity, improvements in speech, and a reduction in anger and rage reactions. Brenner says that while two of his patients had borderline levels of B$_{12}$, most who improved had normal or even high levels, and "there are no clear biological markers as to who may benefit."[33]

It is of interest that while two of Dr. Brenner's patients (as well as their mothers) were found to exhibit overt B$_{12}$ deficiency, the remainder presented with normal or even elevated levels of B$_{12}$, and none exhibited elevations in plasma homocysteine. (Unfortunately, urinary MMAs were not performed.)[34*] We ourselves have identified several children diag-nosed with autism who had serum B$_{12}$ levels greater than 500 pg/ml but

---

* Very little formal research has been done to date on the autism/B$_{12}$ connection. The only article found on MEDLINE regarding the relationship between B$_{12}$ and autism was from 1981, entitled "Folic Acid and B$_{12}$ in Autism and Neuropsychiatric Disturbances of Childhood," in the *Journal of the American Academy of Childhood Psychiatry*. The authors, T. L. Lowe, et al., concluded that there was no evidence of low serum B$_{12}$ or folate levels or low CSF folate in children with autism, nor did autistic children's values differ from the normal population. This study is severely flawed and outdated, however, because neither MMAs nor Hcys were performed.

whose urinary MMA results were elevated and abnormal. All of these children responded well to either hydroxocobalamin or methyl-B_{12} injections. (We believe the range of the gray zone for children should be set higher than for adults.)

One physician who specializes in treating autism, James Neubrander, M.D., reports tremendous success in treating autism, pervasive developmental disorder (PDD), and Asperger's syndrome with methylcobalamin injections. Dr. Neubrander conducted a study in which he administered injectable methylcobalamin to eighty-five children diagnosed with autism spectrum disorders. Parents of 50 percent of the children reported improvement in fifteen or more symptoms.[35]

Of the eighty-five children Dr. Neubrander studied, sixty-seven had urinary MMAs performed, and forty-nine had homocysteine levels performed. Thirteen of the sixty-seven children who received MMA testing, or 19 percent, had elevated MMAs, indicating true vitamin B_{12} deficiency. Five of the forty-nine children who received homocysteine testing, or 10 percent, had elevated homocysteine, indicating B_{12}, B_6, or folic acid deficiency or possibly an inborn error of metabolism. These abnormal results could stem from nutritional deficiencies as a result of inadequate intake, from diseases of the gastrointestinal tract, from defects in B_{12} transport, or from inborn errors of B_{12} metabolism. This study clearly indicates that some children are being misdiagnosed as autistic, when there is demonstrable evidence that they have a functional B_{12} deficiency.

In June 2004, Dr. Neubrander reported (via personal communication) that he has now treated approximately 500 children diagnosed on the autism spectrum with subcutaneous methylcobalamin injections, and that nine out of ten exhibited significant improvement in symptoms. The primary symptoms parents reported as improved were language and communication, 71 percent; awareness, 65 percent; cognition and higher levels of reasoning, 52 percent; engagement, 43 percent; eye contact, 37 percent; better behavior, 35 percent; ability to focus, 35 percent; greater understanding, 35 percent; vocalization, 35 percent; and "trying new things," 33 percent.

Because 90 percent of the children responded to injectable methylcobalamin, with responses ranging from mild to dramatic, Neubrander concluded that "the current 'gold standard' lab tests documenting B_{12} deficiency, as we presently define it, have no predicative value as to which children may or may not respond to methylcobalamin therapy."[36]

However, despite Dr. Neubrander's findings, we strongly believe that all autistic children need to be tested before beginning methylcobalamin treatment to ascertain which of them have true B$_{12}$ problems. Documentation will assist us in finding out the true incidence of B$_{12}$ deficiency in autism, provide important data for future research, and aid in the development of needed protocols and update B$_{12}$ parameters in children.

Autism is a complex disorder, involving genetic, infectious, autoimmune, and environmental factors, and it's highly unlikely that vitamin B$_{12}$ plays a role in every case. But we agree with the view of the late Dr. Bernard Rimland, director of the Autism Research Institute and a leading international expert on the link between vitamin deficiencies and autism, who commented, "In my view, vitamin B$_{12}$ represents one of the most promising, and least-well investigated, modalities for treating autistic children."[37]

For our family, the issue of B$_{12}$ and autism took a personal turn in 1996 when my nephew Billy was born. At first a cuddly baby, Billy became resistant to hugs and cuddles as he grew older. He walked late, at fourteen months, and still wasn't talking at a year and a half.

Billy's parents took him for a speech evaluation that revealed a significant delay. Billy began speech therapy and started attending special classes at age three, but he was so disruptive that his preschool teachers couldn't handle him, finally placing him full-time in a class for autistic children. Billy avoided eye contact, rarely engaged in social interaction with other children or adults, did not play in a creative way, and did not initiate any speech or language but merely parroted what other people said (a behavior called echolalia, common in autism). A psychologist finally gave Billy a diagnosis—autism—and told his mother that there was no cure. His recommendation: "Make him comfortable."

Shocked by the grim outlook of the psychologist, Billy's mother took her son for additional testing by the school system and a pediatric neurologist, only to receive the same verdict: autism, with little hope for a normal or even near-normal life. Tests when Billy was four showed a slowed EEG—a sign of neurological abnormality—and a prominent rooting reflex (a reflex that is present in infants, but normally disappears around six months of age and is a sign of neurological damage when it occurs after that time).

When Billy was nearly four years old, his maternal grandmother was diagnosed with pernicious anemia. At this time, I prompted Billy's mother and

*father to have him tested for B$_{12}$ deficiency. We knew that his tests would
be skewed, because his mother had started Billy on daily liquid B vitamins
when he was just over three years old. (He had initially demonstrated small
improvements in language and behavior when taking these vitamins, but
his progress had leveled off.) Billy's serum B$_{12}$ levels came back high, and
his Hcy level came back normal, but his serum MMA came back borderline
high (0.4 μmol/L). This was fascinating, because with his high B$_{12}$ intake,
his plasma MMA should have been in the very low range.*

*As a result of this finding, Billy's family decided to do a trial of injected
B$_{12}$ (hydroxocobalamin). They did not inform family and friends, or Billy's
teachers, because they wanted to receive unbiased feedback about the
results—if any.*

*Within two weeks, the people around Billy witnessed dramatic changes.
Billy started looking directly at people. His enunciation, voice tone, and
verbal expressiveness improved, and he even developed a sense of humor.
He started showing imagination in his play, parking his toy truck next to
him at snack time and tucking in his stuffed bear in at night. He could hold
a pencil, using it to draw and color, and his "chicken scratches" turned into
legible letters. He stopped walking on his toes, and he no longer walked and
ran with an abnormal posture. Moreover, his once-prominent abnormal
rooting reflex disappeared.*

*From kindergarten through the seventh grade, Billy made steady progress,
although he continued to require a specialized classroom. He is now thirteen
years old and will be entering the eighth grade soon. This year, he will be in
a normal classroom without aides. His grades are outstanding, and he has
earned a 4.0 grade point average in all subjects. In the spring of 2010, he
took a state-wide test in math and scored at a college level.*

*Billy does still have some limitations. He's slow in processing informa-
tion, and his mother reports that it takes him a long time to complete his
homework or move from one problem to the next. In addition, he needs to
reread material over and over to comprehend it. He also has some social
impairments and has difficulty making friends and having age-appropriate
conversations. Fortunately, he has three brothers who give him lots of help in
this area.*

*Billy continues to receive hydroxocobalamin B$_{12}$ injections every three
weeks, but he no longer takes the other high-dose liquid B-vitamin supplements, which proved unhelpful in his case. While he continues to have some*

significant challenges, his dramatic turnaround proved that he didn't suffer from incurable autism; he suffered from a B$_{12}$ deficiency, probably both genetically and environmentally influenced (due to nitrous oxide exposure), that could be treated and at least partially (and perhaps wholly) cured with B$_{12}$ therapy.

Of course, not all children diagnosed with autism spectrum disorder have a B$_{12}$ deficiency or defect, but we believe that a significant percentage do. Given the response of autistic patients to B$_{12}$ treatment and the documentation of elevated MMA and Hcy by Dr. Neubrander, as well as our own experience, it appears the number may be around 25 percent, and perhaps even higher.

How many children like Billy could be helped by B$_{12}$ testing and treatment? Currently we have no way of knowing, because to date no formal research has examined this question. But with autism now affecting as many as one in 110 children according to a recent CDC study, it is a question we urgently need to answer.

Meanwhile, any child labeled with an autism spectrum disorder should be evaluated for B$_{12}$ deficiency, using serum B$_{12}$, urinary MMA and plasma homocysteine tests. Because a number of autistic children with normal test results respond strongly to B$_{12}$, we also strongly recommend that every autistic child—regardless of test results—receive a trial of injected hydroxo-B$_{12}$ or methyl-B$_{12}$. Not every child will benefit, but for those who do, the benefits may be remarkable.

We advocate testing before any B$_{12}$ therapy because 1) it is critical to know if B$_{12}$ deficiency was the cause of the developmental delay or autistic-like behavior; 2) it is important to know how severe the deficiency was (if present); 3) if B$_{12}$ deficiency is found, the underlying cause needs to be identified; 4) life-long treatment may be necessary; and 5) documenting the incidence will help clinicians to develop needed protocols. (See Chapter 12: The Autism-B$_{12}$ Connection: When Low B$_{12}$ Causes Pediatric Brain Injury.)

RED FLAGS OF B$_{12}$ DEFICIENCY IN INFANTS, CHILDREN, AND TEENAGERS

If your child exhibits any of the following signs or symptoms, insist that your doctor order urinary MMA and serum B$_{12}$ tests:

- movement problems, including difficulty in walking or writing
- mental changes—irritability, altered mood, poor memory, "flat" emotional tone, autistic-like withdrawal
- vision problems/abnormalities
- slowed weight and height gain
- leg pains or other abnormal sensations
- fatigue
- loss of previously acquired speech, language, motor, and/or social skills
- loss of appetite
- an abnormally small head circumference in infants or toddlers
- apathy, lethargy, or irritability
- involuntary movements, such as arm waving in infants or toddlers
- tics
- gray hairs/premature graying
- areas of hypopigmented skin in a Caucasian child and/or vitiligo, or areas of hyperpigmented skin in an African-American child
- a rooting reflex after eight months of age (this reflex is usually absent after six months of age)
- a history of any surgery (including dental surgeries) involving nitrous oxide. This substance, used as an anesthetic agent and often administered during dental work or surgeries such as insertion of ear tubes in children with chronic ear infections, can inactivate the body's stores of B$_{12}$ and cause severe neurological damage (see chapters 8 and 12).

- failure to thrive (poor appetite, poor growth and/or weight gain, general poor health)

- chronic constipation

- a diagnosis of developmental delay, autism, cerebral palsy, mental retardation, or other neurological disorder

- severe food allergies or sensitivities

- a diagnosis of celiac disease or gluten enteropathy

- a thyroid disorder or other autoimmune disorder

- a history of stroke or a diagnosis of atherosclerosis

- a diagnosis of any psychiatric or behavioral disorder or problem (schizophrenia, depression, bipolar disorder, suicidal behavior, conduct disorder, anxiety disorder, attention deficit hyperactivity disorder, learning disability, etc.)

- a diagnosis of Downs Syndrome

CHAPTER 6 NOTES:

1. Muhammad, R., Fernhoff, P., et al. Neurologic impairment in children associated with maternal dietary deficiency of cobalamin—Georgia, 2001. *MMWR Weekly*, January 31, 2003/52(04);61-64.

2. Graham, S. M., Arvela, O. M., and Wise, G. A. Long-term neurologic consequences of nutritional vitamin B$_{12}$ deficiency in infants. *Journal of Pediatrics* 1992, 121:710–4.

3. Muhammad, R., Fernhoff, P., et al. Neurologic impairment in children associated with maternal dietary deficiency of cobalamin—Georgia, 2001. *MMWR Weekly*, January 31, 2003/52(04);61-64.

4. Steen, M. T., Boddie, A. M., Fisher, A. J., Macmahon, W., Saxe, D., Sullivan, K. M., Dembure, P. P., and Elsas, L. J. Neural-tube defects are associated with low concentrations of cobalamin (vitamin B$_{12}$) in amniotic fluid. *Prenatal Diagnosis* 1998, 18(6):545–55; and, Dawson, E. B., Evans, D. R., and Van Hook, J. W. Amniotic fluid B$_{12}$ and folate levels associated with neural tube defects. *American Journal of Perinatology* 1998, 15(9):511–4; and, Thorand, B., Pietrzik, K., Prinze-Langenohl, R., Hages,

M., and Holzgreve, W. Maternal and fetal serum and red blood cell folate and vitamin B$_{12}$ concentrations in pregnancies affected by neural tube defects. *Zeitschrift für Geburtshilfe und Neonatologie* 1996, 200(5):176–80; and, Kirke, P. N., Molloy, A. M., Daly, L. E., Burke, H., Weir, D. G., and Scott, J. M. Maternal plasma folate and vitamin B$_{12}$ are independent risk factors for neural tube defects. *Quarterly Journal of Medicine* 1993, 86(11):703–8; and, Weeks, E. W., Tamura, T., Davis, R. O., Birch, R., Vaughn, W. H., Franklin, J. C., Barganier, C., Cosper, P., Finley, S. C., and Finley, W. H. Nutrient levels in amniotic fluid from women with normal and neural tube defect pregnancies. *Biology of the Neonate* 1992, 61(4):226–31.

5. Molloy, A. M., et al. Maternal vitamin B$_{12}$ status and risk of neural tube defects in a population with high neural tube defect prevalence and no folic acid fortification. *Pediatrics* 2009;123:917-923.

6. Thompson, M. D., et al. Vitamin B-12 and neural tube defects: the Canadian experience. *Am J Clin Nutr* 2009;89(suppl):697S-701S.

7. Ramakrishna, T. Vitamins and brain development. *Physiological Research* 1999, 48(3):175–87.

8. Shojania, A. M. Folic acid and vitamin B$_{12}$ deficiency in pregnancy and in the neonatal period. *Clinics in Perinatology* 1984, 11(2):433–59.

9. Davis, J. R., Goldenring, J., and Lubin, B. H. Nutritional vitamin B$_{12}$ deficiency in infants. *American Journal of Diseases of Children* 1981, 135:566–567.

10. Graham, S. M., Arvela, O. M., and Wise, G. A. Long-term neurologic consequences of nutritional vitamin B$_{12}$ deficiency in infants. *Journal of Pediatrics* 1992, 121:710–4.

11. Crane, M. G., Register, U. D., Lukens, R. H., and Gregory, R. Cobalamin (CBL) studies on two total vegetarian (vegan) families. *Vegetarian Nutrition: An International Journal* 1998, 2(3):87–92.

12. Watanabe, F., Katsura, H., Takenaka, S., Fujita, T., Abe, K., Tamura, Y., Nakatsuka, T., and Nakano, Y. Pseudovitamin B(12) is the predominant cobamide of an algal health food, spirulina tablets. *Journal of Agricultural and Food Chemistry* 1999, 47(11):4736–41. See also: Vegetarian Society UK fact sheet, "Vitamin B$_{12}$," http://www.vegsoc.org/info/b12.html.

13. Byrne, S. "The myths of vegetarianism," *Nexus Magazine*, 2002 (online).

14. Davis, J. R., Goldenring, J., and Lubin, B. H. Nutritional vitamin B$_{12}$ deficiency in infants. *American Journal of Diseases of Children* 1981, 135:566–567.

15. Krajcovicova-Kudlackova, M., Blazicek, P., Babinska, K., Kopcova, J., Klvanova, J., Bederova, A., and Magalova, T. Traditional and alternative nutrition—levels of homocysteine and lipid parameters in adults. *Scandinavian Journal of Clinical and Laboratory Investigation* 2000, 60(8):657–64.

16. Herrmann, W., Schorr, H., Purschwitz, K., Rassoul, F., and Richter, V. Total homocysteine, vitamin B(12), and total antioxidant status in vegetarians. *Clinical Chemistry* 2001, 47(6):1094–101.

17. Bissoli, L., Di Francesco, V., Ballarin, A., Mandragona, R., Trespidi, R., Brocco, G., Caruso, B., Bosello, O., and Zamboni, M. Effect of vegetarian diet on homocysteine levels. *Annals of Nutrition and Metabolism* 2002, 46(2):73–9.

18. Crane, M. G., Register, U. D., Lukens, R. H., and Gregory, R. Cobalamin (CBL) studies on two total vegetarian (vegan) families. *Vegetarian Nutrition: An International Journal* 1998, 2(3):87–92.

19. Bjorke Monsen, A. L., Ueland, P. M., Vollset, S. E., Guttormsen, A. B., Markestad, T., Solheim, E., and Refsum, H. Determinants of cobalamin status in newborns. *Pediatrics* 2001, 108(3):624–630.

20. Gadowsky, S. L., Gale, K., Wolfe, S., Jory, J., Gibson, R., and O'Connor, D. Biochemical folate, B$_{12}$, and iron status of a group of pregnant adolescents accessed through the public health system in southern Ontario. *Journal of Adolescent Health* 1995, 16:465–474.

21. Graham, S. M., Arvela, O. M., and Wise, G. A. Long-term neurologic consequences of nutritional vitamin B$_{12}$ deficiency in infants. *Journal of Pediatrics* 1992, 121:710–4.

22. Louwman, M., van Dusseldorp, M., van de Vijver, F. J. R., Thomas, C. M. G., Schneede, J., Ueland, P. M., Refsum, H., and van Staveren, W. A. Signs of impaired cognitive function in adolescents with marginal cobalamin status. *American Journal of Clinical Nutrition* 2000, 72:762–9.

23. Licht, D. J., Berry, G. T., Brooks, D. G., and Younkin, D. P. Reversible subacute combined degeneration of the spinal cord in a fourteen-year-old due to a strict vegan diet. *Clinical Pediatrics* 2001, 40(7):413–5.

24. *Toronto Sun*, "Boy paralyzed by 'forgotten disease.'" December 17, 2007 by Michele Mandel.

25. Fuhrman's quote appears on www.breathing.com/articles/vitamin-b12-vegan.htm.

26. Murphy, M.M., et al Longitudinal study of the effect of pregnancy on maternal and fetal cobalamin status in healthy women and their off-spring. *J. Nutr* (2007)137:1863-1867.

27. Cohen M. The toppling toddler. *Discover* 2001, 22(11), online.

28. Dr. Rinaldo is quoted in "Spotlight on Childhood Diseases," on the Mayo Clinic website (Mayoclinic.com).

29. Roze, E., et al. Neuropsychiatric disturbances in presumed late-onset cobalamin C disease. *Archives of Neurology* 2003, 60(10):1457–62.

30. Ciani, F., et al. Lethal late onset cblB methylmalonic aciduria. *Critical Care Medicine* 2000, 28:2119–21.

31. Bhatt is cited in "Vitamin disorder may be key to autism," *London Daily Telegraph*, August 17, 1995.

32. Baker, Sidney, personal communication.

33. Brenner, Arnold, "Vitamin B₁₂ and the autism spectrum," letter to physicians and parents, June 26, 1996.

34. Brenner, A., open letter to physicians, 1996.

35. Presentation to the Defeat Autism Now! (DAN!) Conference, 2003.

36. Ibid.

37. Rimland, B. R. personal communication, 2002.

7

Vitamin B_{12} and Cancer, Impaired Immune Function, and Autoimmune Disease

"Diets sufficient in methyl enhancers folate, choline, and B_{12} have proved to prevent cancer not only in animals but in humans as well."
—Paul Frankel, Ph.D., *The Methylation Miracle* (1999)[1]

Avoiding cancer isn't just a matter of luck and genes. While your genes influence your cancer risk, your lifestyle and your diet also play a powerful preventive role—and here again, vitamin B_{12} appears to be crucial.

B_{12} is a critical element in the construction of DNA, and is essential for the production of red blood cells. In addition, it's needed for a healthy immune system. As we'll explain in this chapter, evidence indicates that healthy B_{12} levels can protect you against destructive processes that can contribute to cancer and to other deadly diseases as well.

THE GROWING DATA ON B_{12} DEFICIENCY AND CANCER

It's long been known that pernicious anemia, one form of B_{12} deficiency, is linked to an increased risk of gastric cancer. In this case, both the cancer and the anemia stem from an autoimmune process in which the body attacks its own cells, causing damage to parietal cells in the stomach. These cells are then unable to produce intrinsic factor (needed to metabolize B_{12}) and hydrochloric acid (needed for normal gastric function and absorption of B_{12}). The result: both B_{12} deficiency and damaged cells that are prone to turn cancerous.

It's less well known, however, that deficient B_{12} levels appear to be a risk factor for other forms of cancer that have nothing to do with pernicious anemia. Thus, people with B_{12} deficiency due to *any* cause—poor diet, malabsorption, metabolic defects, gastric bypass, gastrointestinal surgeries, overexposure to nitrous oxide, use of medications that lower B_{12} levels, etc.—could be unknowingly putting themselves at risk of developing cancer.

One of the strongest associations that scientists are identifying is between breast cancer and B_{12} deficiency. Researchers at Johns Hopkins measured the B_{12} in blood samples taken from women who'd donated blood, comparing samples from 195 women who'd later developed breast cancer to samples from 195 cancer-free women. Among postmenopausal women, the researchers found, those whose B_{12} levels fell into the lowest fifth were *two to four times* more likely to develop breast cancer than those in the upper four-fifths.[2]

> **Why do deficient B₁₂ levels appear to promote the development of cancer?**

This finding is exciting, because increasing vitamin B_{12} intake is an easy lifestyle change to make. Even women who resist other lifestyle alterations that can lower breast cancer risk, such as increasing exercise, reducing alcohol intake, and reducing fat intake, could potentially reduce their breast cancer risk simply by taking high-dose B_{12} supplements (if they show no evidence of problems in metabolizing B_{12}) or receiving B_{12} injections.[*]

In addition to breast cancer, other cancers are being tentatively linked by scientific studies to deficient levels of vitamin B_{12}. Among these are cervical cancer, lung cancer, and oral cancer (see box in this chapter).

Why do deficient B_{12} levels appear to promote the development of cancer? One reason is that the body needs ample B_{12} in order for folate to work, and one of folate's crucial jobs is to synthesize the nucleotide "building blocks" of DNA. When folate is trapped in an unusable form due to a lack of B_{12}, it can't do this job correctly.

This leads to an imbalance in the supply of DNA building blocks, forcing the body to make changes in DNA structure that can make the DNA more vulnerable to breakage. Broken DNA strands can lead to mutations that, in turn, can lead to cancer. Research shows that chromosome

---

[*] When folic acid "trapping" occurs, Hcy is not converted into methionine, and Hcy levels begin to rise. The accumulation of Hcy in the blood is toxic to blood vessels, causing plaque formation which leads to occlusive vascular disorders such as coronary artery disease (CAD), myocardial infarctions (MI), cerebral vascular accidents (CVA), transient ischemic attacks (TIA), pulmonary embolisms (PE), deep vein thromboses (DVT), and carotid and renal artery stenosis.

COULD B$_{12}$ DEFICIENCY INCREASE YOUR RISK OF CANCER?

Are you at greater risk of developing cancer if your B$_{12}$ levels are too low? Research findings indicate that the answer is "yes." Among the reports are the following conclusions:

- Researchers looking at B$_{12}$ levels in women with and without cervical cancer found that both folic acid and B$_{12}$ appeared to exert protective effects.[4]

- A study of human papillomavirus (HPV) infection—an infection strongly linked to the development of cervical cancer—found that women with lower levels of B$_{12}$ circulating in their blood tended to have more persistent HPV infection.[5]

- A recent study showed that the risk of invasive cervical cancer is greatly elevated for women with high levels of homocysteine, an amino acid that damages the body when it accumulates in excess (see Chapter 5). High homocysteine levels are in turn linked to low levels of folate, vitamin B$_{12}$, and/or vitamin B$_6$.[6]

- Studying cancerous lung tissue and adjacent non-cancerous cells taken from patients with lung cancer, researchers found that folate and B$_{12}$ levels were significantly lower in cells that had turned cancerous than in adjacent, non-cancerous cells.[7]

- Researchers in Alabama studied women who were at high risk for oral cancer because they chewed tobacco or betel. Women who ate fewer servings of animal products were more likely to have pre-malignant lesions than those who ate more animal-based foods, and those eating low amounts of both animal products and vegetables were at highest risk[8]—not a surprising finding, since the B$_{12}$ from animal products and the folate from vegetables work hand-in-hand.

---

breakage is strongly correlated with deficiencies of either folate or B$_{12}$ (or with high levels of homocysteine, linked to B vitamin deficiencies), and that large dietary supplements of B$_{12}$ can minimize this breakage.[3]

In addition, B$_{12}$ deficiency can cause defects in a biological process called methylation, and these defects in turn can cause the wrong genes on chromosomes to "turn on" or prevent the right genes from being activated. Abnormal methylation patterns are characteristic of cells that are in the process of turning cancerous, and scientist Sang-Woon Choi notes that "genomic DNA hypomethylation is a common phenomenon in cancers in the colon, lung, stomach, uterus, and cervix." Abnormal hyper-methylation, too, is implicated in some cancers.

How important are proper methylation, and a diet high in the nutrients that your body needs for this process, in preventing cancer? One study showed that a diet high in folate, required for proper methylation, is asso-ciated with a nearly 40 percent drop in colon cancer risk. (You'll remem-ber that folate can do its job only in the presence of B$_{12}$, so if you're B$_{12}$-deficient, much of the folate in your body is useless.) Another found that high doses of folic acid and vitamin B$_{12}$ markedly reduce the numbers of precancerous cells in the sputum of cigarette smokers. Still another study, this one in Japan, found that smokers taking supplements of B$_{12}$ and fo-late showed a dramatic reversal of cell changes linked to the development of cancer.[9] There's also some evidence linking poor methylation or a diet low in the nutrients that promote methylation to liver cancer, childhood brain tumors, lymphoma, and pancreatic cancer.[10]

Poor methylation also results in high levels of the amino acid homo-cysteine, which can put you at risk not only for heart disease (see Chapter 5), but possibly also for cancer (and, in particular, for "female" cancers). Cancer researcher B. T. Zhu notes that the high homocysteine levels re-sulting from low B$_{12}$, folate, and/or B$_6$ levels can cause the body to break down estrogens abnormally, reducing levels of one tumor-inhibiting estrogen metabolite while leading to an accumulation of a different one that is "strongly procarcinogenic."

"This hypothesis," he says, "...predicts that adequate dietary intake of folate, vitamin B$_6$ and vitamin B$_{12}$ may reduce hyperhomocysteinemia-associated risk for hormonal cancer."[11]

Moreover, B$_{12}$ deficiency impairs the functioning of the immune sys-tem, and an immune system that isn't functioning right can't defend you as well against cancerous cells. In fact, the immune system problems that result from B$_{12}$ deficiency are linked not just to cancer, but also to a range of problems we'll discuss later in this chapter.

What Is Methylation?

Methylation is the process by which methyl groups (molecules consisting of one carbon atom and three hydrogen atoms) attach to different substances in the body, changing their function. One important job of methylation is to prevent potentially harmful genes from being expressed.

Paul Frankel, Ph.D., an expert on methylation, explains this in simple terms: "Imagine your genetic makeup as a blueprint for a house, and the methyl groups as coffee cups sitting on the blueprint. Since you can build only the part of the blueprint you see, when you put a cup in a different place, it covers up a different part of the house, and therefore that part is not made—or 'expressed' in genetic terms."[12]

As we age, our bodies become less able to correctly methylate DNA. The result: more and more DNA errors that can eventually lead to the expression of cancer-promoting genes. Deficiencies of vitamin B$_{12}$, folic acid, vitamin B$_6$, and choline dramatically increase the risk of improper methylation, as can a high alcohol intake.

It's critical to optimize your intake of methylation-promoting nutrients before a cancer can develop. Improving your methylation status after a cancer develops will improve the health of all of your cells, but unfortunately that includes cancerous cells as well as normal ones.

When B$_{12}$ deficiency causes false cancer scares

In addition to increasing your risk of cancer, B$_{12}$ deficiency can increase the odds that you'll receive an *incorrect* diagnosis of precancerous lesions, particularly if you're a woman. That's because B$_{12}$ deficiency causes the cells lining the cervix to become deformed. These cell changes can cause Pap smears to appear abnormal, often leading to additional tests or even to unnecessary surgeries.

Thus, the presence of what appear to be pre-malignant cells in a Pap smear should always lead doctors to include comprehensive B$_{12}$ testing as part of the diagnostic process. This should include treating a serum B$_{12}$ falling in the gray zone.

For one fifty-seven-year-old woman we know, the diagnosis of B₁₂ deficiency came at least eight years too late.

Luckily, the diagnosis came in time to spare her from dementia, paralysis, pain and suffering, and early death. Although her doctors initially labeled her arm tremor and numbness as essential tremor or possibly a symptom of multiple sclerosis, her son (a physician) ordered the tests I recommended for B₁₂ deficiency and discovered her real diagnosis: autoimmune pernicious anemia. As a result, she won't experience the inexorable mental and physical decline that so many people with undiagnosed B₁₂ deficiency suffer. But she wasn't spared from years of unnecessary worry, expense, and debility that preceded her diagnosis.

Clearly, her tremor should have led to testing for B₁₂ deficiency, because medical texts and articles (see Chapter 3) describe the neurological consequences of this deficiency—consequences that can include tremor and numbness. In addition, this woman suffered from Hashimoto's thyroiditis, an autoimmune disorder that is strongly associated with autoimmune pernicious anemia, and her mother had been diagnosed with pernicious anemia. The most basic and inexpensive test for low B₁₂, a serum B₁₂ level (ordered later by her son), clearly showed her deficiency. Other B₁₂ deficiency markers (MMA and Hcy) were also abnormal. Further testing revealed her autoimmune pernicious anemia.

But the problem could have been detected still earlier by other physicians, including the woman's gynecologist. She'd had abnormal Pap smears for eight years, which is not rare for B₁₂-deficient women because—as we've noted above—the cells that line the cervix don't form normally in the absence of adequate supplies of this vitamin. But her OB/GYN never tested her for B₁₂ deficiency. Instead, every six months, he ordered a repeat Pap smear (which also came back abnormal). Also, because of this woman's abnormal Pap smears, the doctor ordered a dilatation and curettage (D&C) and a loop electrosurgical excision procedure (LEEP), both unpleasant procedures. These treatments didn't eradicate her atypical cervical cells, and in addition, she suffered the mental anguish of repeated cancer scares and the strain of waiting for biopsy results. Her gynecologist urged her to get a hysterectomy, but she declined and opted for bi-yearly pap smears.

This woman was diagnosed with pernicious anemia in July of 2000, began receiving injections of B₁₂, and went back to her OB/GYN for a repeat Pap smear in October. This time, for the first time in eight years, the result was perfectly normal. This doesn't surprise us at all, because her untreated pernicious anemia made the cells irregular in the first place—and treating that disease caused the cells to become healthy again.

Suggesting that the test results "could be an error," her OB/GYN recommended that she continue to have biannual Pap smears. Instead, she waited a year before undergoing her next Pap smear, which once again came back perfectly normal. It is now ten years since she began receiving B₁₂ shots, and her Pap smears continue to show no abnormalities.

Not all stories, however, end as well. Here's one that didn't.

In 2010, we heard from a now 39-year-old woman named Jenna who was severely injured due to misdiagnosed B₁₂ deficiency following a gastric bypass. None of Jenna's doctors placed her on B₁₂ or monitored her B₁₂ status. Jenna had numerous signs and symptoms of B₁₂ deficiency over a four-year period, but all of her doctors failed to diagnose her. She also had abnormal pap smears showing atypical cells, which led her gynecologist to order biannual pap smears and perform a D&C and LEEP procedure.

Jenna's cells remained abnormal until her severe B₁₂ deficiency was finally diagnosed. If only one of her doctors (including her gynecologist) had known the signs and symptoms of B₁₂ deficiency, Jenna would not be severely disabled and permanently wheelchair-bound.

Jenna suffers from subacute combined degeneration of the spinal cord, caused by late-diagnosed vitamin B₁₂ deficiency. She has no feelings in her legs, and she has bladder dysfunction caused by nerve damage due to prolonged untreated B₁₂ deficiency. As a result, Jenna suffers from urinary retention, gets frequent urinary tract infections, and needs to be catheterized intermittently on a daily basis.

It's possible that the abnormal cervical cells seen in women with B₁₂ deficiency could eventually become cancerous, if the deficiency is not treated in time. (The strong association between B₁₂ deficiency and cervical cancer certainly suggests this.) Thus, doctors who consider possible B₁₂ deficiency in all patients with abnormal Pap smears will not only save B₁₂-deficient women time, money, and stress—they may also save some of these women's lives.

B$_{12}$'S EFFECTS ON IMMUNE FUNCTION

One consequence of an immune system damaged by low B$_{12}$ is cancer. But the immune system that's too low in B$_{12}$ can go awry in many ways, and the results can take many forms, most of them serious, and many potentially fatal.

For example, B$_{12}$ deficiency appears to make the body react abnormally to vaccines, a problem that can be life threatening. Evidence of this comes from a recent study of elderly hospital patients given a vaccine to protect against pneumonia. (This is the same shot that seniors routinely receive.) Half of the participants had very low B$_{12}$ levels, while the other half—matched for age and diagnosis—had higher levels.

> **Individuals who are B$_{12}$ deficient are vulnerable to adverse reactions to immunizations.**

Before receiving the vaccine, both groups of patients had similar levels of antibodies to pneumonia. Afterward, however, the group with high B$_{12}$ levels had much higher antibody levels than those with low B$_{12}$ levels. This indicates, the researchers say, that while vaccination leads to the formation of "memory cells" primed to combat disease, the development of these cells into an effective disease-fighting force depends in part on the level of vitamin B$_{12}$.

"These findings may be clinically significant," according to the researchers, "since the efficacy of the pneumococcal vaccine is only about 46 to 70 percent in the elderly, and a significant proportion of elderly patients have subclinical vitamin B$_{12}$ deficiency."[13]

Translation: If you're a senior citizen who's careful to get your pneumonia vaccination, you may be wasting your money if you're low in B$_{12}$, because the shot might not protect you at all. The same is true if you're younger and have a B$_{12}$ deficiency. We believe it is irresponsible to give immunizations to patients who are symptomatic or at risk for B$_{12}$ deficiency without identifying and treating them first.

Moreover, since any vaccination can adversely affect individuals with impaired immune systems, we speculate that B$_{12}$ deficiency may play a key role in some of the thousands of severe reactions to immunizations that occur each year. Individuals who are B$_{12}$ deficient are vulnerable to adverse reactions to immunizations, because their immune systems are impaired. This is an area that requires further serious study.

Poor Practice: Immunizing People Who Are B$_{12}$ Deficient

In June 2009, the World Health Organization (WHO) announced that a pandemic of H1N1 flu (swine flu) was underway. This flu, and other forms of flu as well, are particularly dangerous for people with weakened immune systems. These people may not develop full immunity after becoming infected, and thus may be more likely to get infected with the same influenza virus more than once.

To date, the swine flu does not appear to be much more dangerous than typical seasonal flu strains. However, it can be severely debilitating. For instance, in the fall of 2009, Suzy, a 32-year-old hospital nurse, came down with the swine flu. Suzy was very ill and missed work for four weeks. How could she develop such a severe case of the flu, when she'd been immunized three weeks earlier?

What the doctors didn't know was that Suzy had a vitamin B$_{12}$ deficiency at the time she was immunized. Suzy had undergone a gastric bypass for weight loss three years earlier. Her doctors never monitored her B$_{12}$ status, never placed her on B$_{12}$ prophylactically, and never educated her that she would eventually become B$_{12}$-deficient and would need lifelong B$_{12}$ therapy. It's our guess that Suzy—like the B$_{12}$-deficient seniors we talked about earlier—couldn't mount an effective defense against the flu virus, even after being vaccinated, because her immune system was impaired by her B$_{12}$ deficiency.

And here's another question that deserves study: Why does the flu hit some areas of the world harder than others? For instance, it was recently reported that people in Mexico had a higher death rate from the swine flu during the height of the epidemic than people in other countries. Many factors, including poorer nutrition and reduced access to medical care, probably played a role in this increased risk. However, it is of interest that B$_{12}$ deficiency is more prevalent in countries where diets are low in animal products. A study of school-aged children from Mexico found that 22% had severe B$_{12}$ deficiency (serum B$_{12}$ <140 pg/ml) due to B$_{12}$-deficient diets and malabsorption problems caused by bacterial overgrowth of the small intestine and Giardia lamblia infection.[14,15] This evidence suggests that B$_{12}$ status is a factor epidemiologists should consider as they track the effects of flu viruses across the globe.

HIV, AIDS, and B$_{12}$

AIDS (acquired immunodeficiency syndrome), a disease that cripples the immune system and leaves its victims defenseless against many infections and cancers, is caused by the human immunodeficiency virus, or HIV. Growing evidence shows that B$_{12}$ deficiency is extremely common in individuals with AIDS, and this deficiency may play a role in the progress of the disease.

One remarkable finding is that B$_{12}$ deficiency is linked to a more rapid onset of AIDS symptoms in people who've been infected with HIV. Researchers at Johns Hopkins discovered that whether or not participants were undergoing prescription drug treatment, "development of deficiency of vitamin A or vitamin B$_{12}$ was associated with a decline in CD4 cell count, while normalization of vitamin A, vitamin B$_{12}$ and zinc was associated with higher CD4 cell counts." The researchers conclude, "These data suggest that micronutrient deficiencies are associated with HIV-1 disease progression and raise the possibility that normalization might increase symptom-free survival."[16] A similar study, by a different research group, found that HIV-infected men with low serum B$_{12}$ levels "had significantly shorter AIDS-free time" than those with adequate B$_{12}$ levels.[17]

> Low B$_{12}$ levels are very common in HIV-infected individuals.

In related research, investigators discovered that under experimental conditions, several forms of vitamin B$_{12}$ (including methylcobalamin and hydroxocobalamin) inhibit HIV infection of blood cells. The researchers suggest that "these or related agents may be useful as anti-viral treatments" that target HIV.[18]

Low B$_{12}$ levels are very common in HIV-infected individuals, with up to a third showing signs of deficiency, and about half showing evidence of low B$_{12}$,[19] often in spite of normal serum B$_{12}$ levels. One reason for this deficiency is that patients with AIDS-related diarrhea absorb vitamin B$_{12}$ very poorly.[20] Another is that AIDS patients exhibit reductions in stomach acid, intrinsic factor, and holotranscobalamin II (substances needed to break down B$_{12}$, transport it to the intestine, and carry it to cells throughout the body).[21]

It is possible that B$_{12}$ plays a significant role in the neurological symptoms associated with AIDS. Almost a third of people with AIDS suffer from neuropathy, a painful tingling or numbness of the feet, legs, arms, or hands. This neuropathy is very similar to that seen in patients with a primary diagnosis of B$_{12}$ deficiency (see Chapter 3). HIV-related neuropathy can stem from a number of causes, including the use of medications such as Hivid, Videx, Zerit, Epivir, dapsone, Myambutol, isoniazid, Flagyl, Taxol, Thalomid, or Oncovin (some of which, by the way, also reduce B$_{12}$ levels). However, given the high incidence of B$_{12}$ deficiency in people with AIDS, depleted B$_{12}$ stores may very well contribute to a significant number of cases of HIV-related neuropathy.

Even in AIDS patients whose B$_{12}$ levels appear normal, the body's B$_{12}$ pathways can break down in ways that lead to neurological problems. One group of scientists recently studied patients with AIDS and myelopathy (nervous system damage), patients with AIDS but without myelopathy, and non-HIV-infected controls. The AIDS patients with myelopathy, but not those free of this symptom, showed defects in a crucial B$_{12}$ pathway. This is additional strong evidence that "hidden" B$_{12}$ problems are common in AIDS, and these problems could cause or worsen neurological symptoms in many AIDS patients.

Another terrifying symptom of AIDS is dementia, which often occurs in late stages of the disease. Here again, B$_{12}$ deficiency is part of the picture. As we explained in Chapter 2, B$_{12}$ deficiency is one cause of dementia in the elderly—so it makes sense that the rampant B$_{12}$ deficiency in AIDS patients may contribute to dementia in this group as well.

Future research will give us a better understanding of the relationship between AIDS symptoms and B$_{12}$ deficiency. In the meantime, because the B$_{12}$ pathways can break down at so many stages in AIDS, **we strongly recommend that anyone with HIV or AIDS receive B$_{12}$ screening**, especially when symptomatic. It also makes sense that AIDS patients should prophylactically receive high-dose B$_{12}$ therapy.

George, a thirty-eight-year-old diagnosed with AIDS, visited our ER three times in two months complaining of painful foot neuropathy. I reviewed his blood work and noted that no doctor had ordered a serum B$_{12}$ level, much less an MMA. Instead, his physicians had treated his painful neuropathy with Neurontin (which was ineffective), telling him there was nothing more they could do.

I told George to get his MMA and B$_{12}$ levels checked, but his doctors did not follow through on this advice. Recently, I came across his chart, and I *found that he'd returned to the ER two years after I'd last seen him. At the most recent visit, he was anemic, his blood smear showed signs of B$_{12}$ deficiency, and his gastroenterologist reported that an endoscopy of his stomach showed atrophic gastritis (inflammation and wasting of the stomach lining that drastically decreases stomach acid, impairing the body's ability to break B$_{12}$ apart from protein so it can be absorbed).*

George is still taking Neurontin, even though it barely takes the edge off his pain. His doctors also put him on Prevacid, which will reduce his stomach acid still further and worsen his already-serious B$_{12}$ depletion. Given his obvious B$_{12}$ deficiency, it is likely that this treatment will put him at risk for increasing motor problems, pain, and eventually dementia.

Another patient, Sam—a thirty-three-year-old diagnosed with AIDS—came to the ER complaining of left leg weakness, numbness, spasms, and uncontrollable pain. He was taking Zerit for neuropathy and was thin, weak, and pale. At his last admission (six months earlier), he was seen by

---

AIDS IN AFRICA: A B$_{12}$ LINK?

AIDS is a worldwide problem, but it strikes African nations the hardest. There are many reasons for this, including poverty and lack of health education. However, it's our guess that B$_{12}$ deficiency could possibly play at least some role in the AIDS crisis in African countries.

Many Africans eat a mostly vegetarian diet lacking in B$_{12}$.[22] In addition, most African women breast-feed their children, which is a good idea when maternal diets are adequate, but can lead to drastically low B$_{12}$ levels in children when mothers have B$_{12}$ deficiency. And malnutrition is rampant in many areas of Africa, with one study showing that children in a rural South African community had dietary intakes below 50 percent of the RDA for vitamin B$_{12}$ and a host of other nutrients.[23]

Given that B$_{12}$ deficiency impairs the immune system's ability to fight off infection, and may speed the development of AIDS in HIV-infected people, it is only logical to assume that the poor B$_{12}$ status of millions of Africans could play a role in this terrible epidemic. It would be wise for the public health officials combating this crisis to include, as part of their prevention strategy, efforts to improve the B$_{12}$ status of people throughout Africa.

a psychiatrist for depression. The doctor's notes revealed that Sam had difficulty concentrating and his memory was poor.

Sam was in a high-risk group for B₁₂ deficiency and was clearly symptomatic. His blood test results showed severe vitamin B₁₂ deficiency. His serum B₁₂ was only 132 pg/ml, and his Hcy was elevated at 36 μmol/L, placing him at great vascular risk. He was anemic, but not macrocytic. A CT of his brain showed atrophy, which the radiologist remarked was quite unusual for a person of his age—but brain atrophy is well documented in the literature on B₁₂ deficiency, especially in children.

B₁₂ DEFICIENCY AND AUTOIMMUNE DISORDERS

It seems strange that B₁₂ deficiency is involved in both under-activation and over-activation of the immune system. However, it's true, because one cause of vitamin B₁₂ deficiency is *pernicious anemia*, an autoimmune disorder in which the body attacks its own cells.

Most physicians incorrectly use the term *pernicious anemia*. This diagnosis is properly reserved for the autoimmune phenomenon that results in disease and dysfunction of the stomach (gastric atrophy, poor stomach acid production, intrinsic factor deficiency, and gastric autoantibodies directed against intrinsic factor and/or parietal cells). Therefore, a person who has a B₁₂ deficiency stemming from Crohn's disease, gastric bypass surgery, celiac disease, or dietary causes does not have "pernicious anemia." (However, patients as well as physicians need to understand that no matter what the cause of B₁₂ deficiency, it can be just as deadly or "pernicious" if not diagnosed and treated. Cobalamin deficiency is cobalamin deficiency, and all forms must be treated and their underlying causes identified.)

Autoimmune pernicious anemia is a condition in which the stomach lining that contains the parietal cells is destroyed through an autoimmune mechanism. The parietal cells secrete intrinsic factor, which is necessary for B₁₂ absorption. Without intrinsic factor, B₁₂ deficiency ensues. It is thought that this failure of intrinsic factor secretion is a result of gastric mucosal atrophy (wasting of the stomach lining). The gastric atrophy is caused by immune destruction of the acid- and pepsin-secreting portions of the stomach lining.

Pernicious anemia patients have poor gastric acid production and often complain of a bloated and prolonged full feeling after eating. Progressive destruction of the parietal cells causes decreased secretion of hydrochloric acid and enzymes required to release food-bound vitamin B$_{12}$. Over time, this leads to wasting and inflammation of the stomach lining and achlorhydria (no stomach acid). The destruction of the stomach lining is thought to be the end stage of the autoimmune process. Typically, antibodies to parietal cells and/or intrinsic factor are seen in pernicious anemia patients.

New research is questioning whether pernicious anemia is an autoimmune disorder or possibly caused by an infectious disease, Helicobacter pylori (H. pylori). Researchers are investigating the possibility that long-standing H. pylori leads to atrophic gastritis and is the catalyst for the induction of gastric autoimmunity. This new theory is still under debate.[24] Regardless of the cause, patients with autoimmune pernicious anemia need monitoring by esophagogastroduodenoscopy (EGD) because of their increased risk for gastric cancer and carcinoids (a type of neuroendocrine tumor). Chronic elevation of the hormone gastrin (which occurs in PA patients) may cause tumors called gastrinomas.

Approximately one in 25 patients with PA develops gastric carcinoids.[25] Researchers who followed PA patients for 6.7 years found that those with

---

DIAGNOSING PERNICIOUS ANEMIA: A NOTE FOR PHYSICIANS

The criteria for the diagnosis of autoimmune pernicious anemia (PA) include:

1. Presence of corpus-restricted atrophy, with or without a spared antrum, as shown by EGD of the stomach.

2. Presence of hyperplasia of enterochromaffin-like (ECL) cells.

3. Hypochlorhydria or achlorhydria (poor or no stomach acid).

4. Elevated fasting serum gastrin.

5. Decreased levels of pepsinogen I.

6. Anti-parietal cell antibody (is found in 90% of people with PA, but its specificity is only 50%).

7. Anti-intrinsic factor antibody (is very specific for PA, but has a low sensitivity of 50%).

chronic atrophic gastritis had an annual incidence risk of 0.14% for developing gastric cancer.[26]

Experts recommend that PA patients undergo routine endoscopic surveillance every two to five years, but PA patients complaining of weight loss, dysphagia, abdominal pain, dyspeptic symptoms, and/or iron deficiency require immediate EGD investigation. PA patients must be monitored at least yearly by clinical interview and physical exam to identify any new symptoms that may warrant an earlier EGD exam.

Because PA is an autoimmune disease, people with this condition are at increased risk of acquiring other autoimmune diseases, such as thyroid autoimmune disorders (up to 32%), type 1 diabetes (3–4%), and vitiligo (2–8%). Therefore, people with autoimmune disorders (and thyroid disorders in particular) should always be screened for pernicious anemia/B$_{12}$ deficiency. Conversely, people with true autoimmune pernicious anemia need to be screened yearly (or earlier if symptomatic) for thyroid disorders because of this increased association. Other autoimmune disorders associated with pernicious anemia include Addison's disease, premature ovarian failure, rheumatoid arthritis, lupus, hypoparathyroidism, hypogammaglobulinemia, agammaglobulinemia, ulcerative colitis, and idiopathic adrenocortical insufficiency.

IS LOW B$_{12}$ PUTTING YOU AT RISK FOR CANCER OR OTHER IMMUNE-RELATED PROBLEMS?

Research suggests that B$_{12}$ deficiency may increase any individual's risk for immune system dysfunction or cancer, but you may be particularly vulnerable if:

- You have an autoimmune disorder
- You have a family history of autoimmune disorders or impaired immune system function
- You have a family history of cancer, and in particular gastrointestinal or "female" cancers
- You have a history of abnormal Pap smears
- You carry the HIV virus or have AIDS

Chapter 7 Notes:

1. Frankel, P. *The Methylation Miracle*, New York: St. Martin's Press, 1999.

2. Wu, K., Helzlsouer, K. J., Comstock, G. W., Hoffman, S. C., Nadeau, M.R., and Selhub, J. A prospective study on folate, B$_{12}$, and pyridoxal 5'-phosphate (B$_6$) and breast cancer. *Cancer Epidemiology, Biomarkers and Prevention* 1999, 8(3):209–17.

3. Choi, Sang-Woon. Vitamin B$_{12}$ deficiency: A new risk factor for breast cancer? *Nutrition Reviews* 1999, 57(8):250–53.

4. Alberg, A. J., Selhub, J., Shah, K. V., Viscidi, R. P., Comstock, G.W., and Helzlsouer, K. J. The risk of cervical cancer in relation to serum concentrations of folate, vitamin B$_{12}$, and homocysteine. *Cancer Epidemiology, Biomarkers, and Prevention* 2000, 9(7):761–4.

5. Sedjo, R. L., Inserra, P., Abrahamsen, M., Harris, R. B., Roe, D. J., Baldwin, S., and Giuliano, A. R. Human papillomavirus persistence and nutrients involved in the methylation pathway among a cohort of young women. *Cancer Epidemiology, Biomarkers and Prevention* 2002, 11(4):353–9.

6. Weinstein, S. J., Ziegler, R. G., Selhub, J., Fears, T. R., Strickler, H.D., Brinton, L. A., Hamman, R. F., Levine, R. S., Mallin, K., and Stolley, P. D. Elevated serum homocysteine levels and increased risk of invasive cervical cancer in U.S. women. *Cancer Causes and Control* 2001, 12(4):317–24.

7. Piyathilake, C. J., Johanning, G. L., Macaluso, M., Whiteside, M., Oelschlager, D. K., Heimburger, D. C., and Grizzle, W. E. Localized folate and vitamin B$_{12}$ deficiency in squamous cell lung cancer is associated with global DNA hypomethylation. *Nutrition and Cancer* 2000, 37(1):99–107.

8. Carley, K. W., Puttaiah, R., Alvarez, J. O., Heimburger, D. C., and Anantha, N. Diet and oral premalignancy in female south Indian tobacco and betel chewers: A case-control study. *Nutr Cancer* 1994, 22(1):73–84.

9. All three studies cited in Frankel, P., *The Methylation Miracle*, New York: St. Martin's Press, 1999.

10. Frankel, P. *The Methylation Miracle*. New York: St. Martin's Press, 1999.

11. Zhu, B. T. Medical hypothesis: Hyperhomocysteinemia is a risk factor for estrogen-induced hormonal cancer. *International Journal of Oncology* 2003, 22(3):499–508.

12. Frankel, P. *The Methylation Miracle.* New York: St. Martin's Press, 1999.

13. Fata, F., Herzlich, B., Schiffman, G., and Ast, A. Impaired antibody responses to pneumococcal polysaccharide in elderly patients with low serum vitamin B₁₂ levels. *Annals of Internal Medicine* 1996, 124:299–304.

14. Rasmussen, S. A., Fernhoff, P. M., Scanlon, K. S. Vitamin B₁₂ deficiency in children and adolescents. *J Pediatr* 2001;138:10-17.

15. Allen, L. H., et al. Vitamin B₁₂ deficiency and malabsorption are highly prevalent in rural Mexican communities. *Am J Clin Nutr* 1995:62:1013-9.

16. Baum, M. K., Shor-Posner, G., Lu, Y., Rosner, B., Sauberlich, H. E., Fletcher, M. A., Szapocznik, J., Eisdorfer, C., Buring, J. E., and Hennekens, C. H. *AIDS* 1995, 9(9):1051–6.

17. Tang, A. M., Graham, N. M., Chandra, R. K., and Saah, A. J. Low serum vitamin B₁₂ concentrations are associated with faster human immunodeficiency virus type 1 (HIV-1) disease progression. *Journal of Nutrition* 1997, 127(2):345–51.

18. Weinberg, J. B., Shugars, D. C., Sherman, P. A., Sauls, D. L., and Fyfe, J. A. Cobalamin inhibition of HIV-1 integrase and integration of HIV-1 DNA into cellular DNA. *Biochemical and Biophysical Research Communications* 1998, 246(2):393–7.

19. Herbert, V., Fong, W., Gulle, V., and Stopler, T. Low holotranscobalamin II is the earliest serum marker for subnormal vitamin B₁₂ (cobalamin) absorption in patients with AIDS. *American Journal of Hematology* 1990, 34(2):132–9.

20. Bjarnason, I., Sharpstone, D. R., Francis, N., Marker, A., Taylor, C., Barrett. M., Macpherson, A., Baldwin, C., Menzies, I. S., Crane, R. C., Smith, T., Pozniak, A., and Gazzard, B. G. Intestinal inflammation, ileal structure and function in HIV. *AIDS* 1996, 10(12):1385–91.

21. Herzlich, B. C., Schiano, T. D., Moussa, Z., Zimbalist, E., Panagopoulos, G., Ast, A., and Nawabi, I. Decreased intrinsic factor secretion in AIDS: Relation to parietal cell acid secretory capacity and vitamin B₁₂ malabsorption. *American Journal of Gastroenterology* 1992, 87(12):1781–8.

22. Neumann, C. G. Livestock development and impact on diet quality and the growth and development of children. Consultative Group on International Agricultural Research, http://www.cgiar.org.

23. Faber, M., Jogessar, V. B., and Benade, A. J. Nutritional status and dietary intakes of children aged 2–5 years and their caregivers in a rural South African community. *International Journal of Food Science and Nutrition* 2001, 52(5):401–11.

24. Lahner, E, Annibale, B. Pernicious anemia: New insights from a gastroenterological point of view. *World J Gastroenterol.* 2009 November 7; 15(41):5121-5128.

25. Kokkola, A., et al. The risk of gastric carcinoma and carcinoid tumours in patients with pernicious anaemia. A prospective follow-up study. *Scand J Gastroenterol.* 1998;33:88-92.

26. Lahner, E., et al. Long-term follow-up in atrophic body gastritis patients: atrophy and intestinal metaplasia are persistent lesions irrespective of Helicobacter pylori infection. *Aliment Pharmacol Ther.* 2005;22:471-481.

8

Under the Knife: Why Low B_{12} Levels Make Surgery Dangerous

Imagine how it feels to hear that your tiny, beautiful four-month-old baby needs an operation. Luckily, the doctor tells you, the problem is correctable: The bones of her skull fused too early, and the surgeon needs to remove some tissue so her brain has room to grow.

On the day of the surgery, you kiss your daughter, who looks impossibly tiny and helpless as she's wheeled off to the operating room. You will the clock to move faster as the minutes tick by, telling yourself that nothing will go wrong, that she's going to be fine. Eventually, you breathe a sigh of relief when the surgeon comes through the doors and tells you that all went well.

But later on, you find out that it didn't. Your baby, happy and healthy before her surgery, stops smiling and loses her sparkle and playfulness. She also stops eating, grows "floppy" and unresponsive, and becomes so dehydrated that she needs emergency treatment. In the hospital, magnetic resonance imaging scans reveal brain atrophy (shrinkage). Tests show that your baby's B_{12} stores dropped to life-threatening levels after the anesthetic agent (nitrous oxide) used in her surgery severely worsened her undiagnosed B_{12} deficiency. Now she's desperately ill, and she may never fully recover.

No surgery, minor or major, is risk-free. Even if you're in the hands of the best doctors and the best operating room staffs, unpredictable crises can occur, and there's a chance you may become crippled or even die. It's a risk you're likely willing to take, if an operation can improve or even save your life.

Surgery can be vastly more risky, however, if you're one of the millions of Americans who suffer from undiagnosed B_{12} deficiency. In fact, if you're B_{12}-deficient, even the simplest of surgical or dental procedures can turn dangerous or even deadly—and your doctor or dentist isn't likely to recognize that you're at risk until it's too late.

The danger to B$_{12}$-deficient surgery patients involves a very common anesthetic agent, nitrous oxide (N$_2$O), used millions of times a year to reduce pain and sedate patients during surgical and dental procedures. You probably know this agent better as "laughing gas," because of its well-known ability to make you feel giggly, an effect that makes it a popular drug of abuse. For people with undiagnosed B$_{12}$ deficiency, however, there's nothing funny about N$_2$O's effects. That's because nitrous oxide has an unusual property: It inactivates vitamin B$_{12}$ in the body.

> If you're B$_{12}$ deficient, even the simplest of surgical or dental procedures can turn dangerous or even deadly.

Cobalamin (B$_{12}$) exists in three oxidative states (called +1, +2, and +3). When we eat food with B$_{12}$, take supplements, or even get an injection of B$_{12}$, the body must convert it into the active coenzymes (methylcobalamin and adenosylcobalamin) that are the only forms the body can use.

These coenzymes are in the +1 state. B$_{12}$ must be in this +1 form for it to have any biological activity. Nitrous oxide causes its harmful effects by irreversibly oxidizing the cobalt ion of vitamin B$_{12}$ from the +1 active state to the +2 and +3 inactive states.

$$N_2O \longrightarrow Co+ \longrightarrow Co++ \text{ and } Co+++$$

Therefore, if a person is already low in B$_{12}$, giving nitrous oxide quickly creates a critical B$_{12}$ deficiency that can be life-threatening.

If you're not B$_{12}$-deficient, the effects of N$_2$O typically aren't dangerous, because your body can renew its stores of B$_{12}$ within a few days. But if your B$_{12}$ levels are too low, you have an overt deficiency, or you have an undetected B$_{12}$ malabsorption problem, exposure to nitrous oxide during surgery can have devastating consequences—even if you're young or middle-aged, and even if you appear fine before undergoing your surgery.

The story that begins this chapter, based on a real-life case,[1] is a good example. This four-month-old baby appeared healthy and normal before her surgery, despite her undiagnosed B$_{12}$ deficiency. Now, as a result of the neurological damage she suffered when exposure to N$_2$O inactivated her already-low B$_{12}$ stores, she may be mentally disabled for life. Other B$_{12}$-deficient patients lose their ability to walk, suffer excruciating pain, become paralyzed or incontinent, or even develop full-blown dementia after exposure to N$_2$O.

Nitrous oxide's ability to wreak havoc on the mind and body of a B$_{12}$-deficient patient isn't a new discovery. Doctors first reported the phenomenon more than thirty years ago, and dozens of case studies are described in the medical literature. Moreover, it's not just a handful of patients who are at risk. Neurosurgeons Kathryn Holloway and Anthony Alberico say, "N$_2$O is very dangerous in the B$_{12}$-deficient patient. Because B$_{12}$ deficiency is not uncommon and N$_2$O use is ubiquitous, the potential exists in every [surgical] practice for this complication to occur." Thus, they stress, "The surgeon should…look for evidence of B$_{12}$ deficiency in every patient."[2]

Unfortunately, most surgeons don't, and the consequences of this failure can be horrific.

A sixty-nine-year-old retired butcher undergoes what should be a routine surgery for a benign prostate problem. Within two weeks, he finds it increasingly hard to walk, and his legs become numb.

About this time, he develops gallbladder problems, and his doctors admit him for a second surgery. Despite the patient's bad reaction to his first surgery—a likely indication of deficient B$_{12}$ stores—his doctors again use N$_2$O. After the surgery, he becomes confused, and the numbness in his legs grows worse. Within four months, he's paralyzed from the waist down and can barely use his arms. He becomes incontinent, and he suffers from memory loss, disorientation, and other symptoms resembling senile dementia.

It takes three months for the man's doctors to diagnose the cause of his paralysis and mental deterioration: severe vitamin B$_{12}$ deficiency, exacerbated by the use of N$_2$O. He starts B$_{12}$ therapy, but it's too late to reverse his symptoms fully, and even after an entire year of treatment and physical therapy, he can walk unaided only for short distances.[3]

This patient suffered terribly when doctors exposed him to N$_2$O without discovering his preexisting B$_{12}$ deficiency. Yet his doctors did everything "by the book"—because "the book" doesn't say anything about testing patients for B$_{12}$ deficiency before they undergo surgery.

This probably surprises you if you've had surgery, because your doctor undoubtedly ordered an alphabet soup of impressive-looking tests before your operation—CBC, LYTES, BUN, CREAT, PT/PTT, etc. Look at the list, however, and you'll probably find that serum B$_{12}$, the most basic test for B$_{12}$ deficiency, isn't on it. Neither, predictably, will be the urinary MMA, which often identifies patients in the gray zone.

A small number of anesthesiologists do give patients single injections of B$_{12}$ before procedures involving N$_2$O, to reduce the risk of a dangerous reaction in anyone who might have low B$_{12}$ stores. However, this "one-shot" approach probably won't prevent complications in severely deficient patients who are exposed to N$_2$O for several hours. It also fails to identify preoperative B$_{12}$ deficiencies that will continue to cause insidious damage and may have contributed to the disorders that led to the need for surgery in the first place. (For example, B$_{12}$ deficiency can lead to neck and back pain with paresthesias, resulting in surgery.) Also, giving an undiagnosed patient a single shot of B$_{12}$ can cloud the results of future lab tests, leaving other doctors unable to identify a deficiency if one is lurking.

Why don't doctors and dentists test for B$_{12}$ deficiency before a surgery? One reason is cost, because screening could add about $90 to your insurance company's tab. Still another reason is that many doctors assume, wrongly, that the standard pre-surgical complete blood count (CBC) will turn up any B$_{12}$ problems. The primary reason, however, is that many doctors and dentists simply aren't aware of the risks of administering N$_2$O to B$_{12}$-deficient patients and don't know that it inactivates vitamin B$_{12}$. In addition, those doctors who know about N$_2$O's potential negative effects on patients with B$_{12}$ deficiency tend to think that bad reactions, as well as B$_{12}$ deficiency itself, are extremely rare. But on this point, the doctors are almost certainly wrong. This ignorance can lead to injury, disability, and poor outcomes in millions of vulnerable patients.

TIP OF THE ICEBERG?

In one small way, patients with severe reactions to N$_2$O are lucky: Because their symptoms are so drastic, many eventually do receive a diagnosis of B$_{12}$ deficiency—although in some cases it takes months, and the diagnosis often comes too late to fully restore their health.

But what about patients who suffer side effects that are dismissed as "typical" or "not unexpected" after a surgical procedure? Millions of patients deteriorate after undergoing cardiac bypass surgery, cancer surgery, neck or back surgery, neurosurgery, or other operations. Among the most common problems we see in postoperative patients are the following:

- depression
- strokes

N$_2$O: A Dangerous "High"

Not all cases of N$_2$O-related B$_{12}$ deficiency stem from surgeries or dental procedures. A significant number are self-inflicted by people using N$_2$O as a recreational drug.

One case reported in 2006 involved a thirty-three-year-old emergency room patient who exhibited delusions and bizarre behavior. The man believed he was part of an experiment for NASA and described himself as an "interface" between humans and machines. He broke a window at home, destroyed furniture, rode his bike into a moving car, and told people he was being controlled. He stated that his actions were part of his "training," but he was unable to tell the ER staff the purpose of this training.

The man stated that he'd been told he had a second wife and must therefore kill his current wife. His wife told the ER staff that he had no history of psychiatric illness or delusions, and that he had worked previously as a medical technologist. The man's blood results were reported by the lab as "normal," and a drug screen was negative. When the ER staff questioned him about recreational drug use, he reported using inhaled nitrous oxide. He had bought several cases of N$_2$O containers ("whip-its") from a cooking store, fitted an airtight facemask, and inhaled the N$_2$O to achieve a sense of euphoria. He reportedly inhaled the N$_2$O on a daily basis for about four weeks before his arrival in the ER.

The man had a normal CBC, and his B$_{12}$ was reported as "normal" at 202 pg/ml, but was clearly deficient and fell in the gray zone. The normal range for this lab for a serum B$_{12}$ was 180–900 pg/ml. Because his level was in the lower range, doctors ordered MMA and Hcy tests, which showed extreme elevations. The patient was treated with aggressive B$_{12}$ injections. Within two weeks, he improved greatly and his delusions began resolving.[4]

Whippits are a common recreational drug, and their use must be suspected in any child, teen, or young adult who presents with psychiatric or neurological manifestations. Testing these patients' serum B$_{12}$, MMA, and Hcy could save a life.

- memory loss

- fatigue

- difficulty walking

- falls

- neuropathies or unexplained pains

- confusion

- weakness

- transient ischemic attacks (TIAs)

- balance problems

- dizziness

- incontinence

The medical profession tends to assume that these are sad but common and unavoidable risks of surgery, especially in seniors or patients undergoing back surgery or neurological procedures. But what's interesting is that all of these symptoms can also be symptoms of B$_{12}$ deficiency. Of course, patients suffer postoperative problems for many reasons, and B$_{12}$ deficiency is just one of them. But consider that as many as a third of all adults are at least marginally B$_{12}$ deficient, and at least 15 percent of seniors (and up to 40 percent of seniors with significant health problems, who are the most common candidates for surgery) are seriously deficient. This adds up to millions of at-risk patients.

Now, consider that U.S. hospitals perform more than 53 million surgical procedures each year, many involving N$_2$O—yet these hospitals screen only a handful of patients for B$_{12}$ deficiency. Dentists also perform millions of in-office surgical procedures each year, many of them involving N$_2$O, and yet few if any check to determine if patients have a history of, are at risk for, or have signs and symptoms of B$_{12}$ deficiency. Some dentists even offer N$_2$O for dental cleanings.

All of this—millions of high-risk patients, millions of surgeries using N$_2$O, and a virtual lack of B$_{12}$ screening—creates a huge potential for serious, life-threatening side effects. Anesthesiologist Jonny Hobbhahn notes that when you add to this equation the fact that symptoms often take weeks to develop, it's reasonable to assume that there is "a greater incidence of neurological deficits than reflected by the published cases."[5]

Doctors Holloway and Alberico agree, saying, "It is tempting to speculate on how many unexpected new postoperative neurological deficits in surgical patients may have actually been due to B_{12} deficiency and nitrous oxide administration."[6]

But all we can do is speculate, because the issue has never been the subject of an in-depth epidemiological investigation. Logic tells us, however, that for every patient diagnosed with obvious symptoms of B_{12} depletion due to N_2O, many more are likely to suffer symptoms that are written off as coincidental. For a patient with borderline B_{12} deficiency undergoing a short surgery, these complications could be as mild as numb or tingling legs (although these symptoms will progress over weeks or months, causing injury if not diagnosed and treated). But a severely B_{12}-deficient patient who undergoes hours of surgery—say, for a heart bypass—may suffer severe problems immediately after the operation. The patient may become paralyzed, appear to have suffered a stroke, or actually suffer a stroke or heart attack due to very elevated Hcy levels caused by severe B_{12} deficiency blocking the pathway that keeps Hcy levels normal (see Chapter 5). Given that doctors generally don't evaluate patients' B_{12} status before surgery, the likelihood of an accurate diagnosis after surgery is slim, especially when catastrophic outcomes can easily be blamed on old age or frailty.

> **Nitrous oxide, a common anesthetic agent, inactivates vitamin B$_{12}$ in the body.**

One conclusion that isn't mere speculation is that most of the N_2O-caused tragedies that are reported could have been prevented. The majority of life-threatening cases described in the medical literature involved patients with known risk factors for B_{12} deficiency or clinically symptomatic patients. These patients' suffering could have been avoided if alert doctors had spotted the warning signs—slightly abnormal blood tests, preexisting neurological or gastrointestinal problems, or other signs or symptoms of B_{12} deficiency—and ordered a couple of simple tests.

A healthy, active fifty-eight-year-old woman underwent surgery for a benign abdominal mass. A month later, her feet started tingling and she began dragging her right leg when she walked. When her surgery site became infected, she underwent a second procedure, again using nitrous oxide—despite B$_{12}$ deficiency symptoms following her first surgery, which should have raised a red flag.

"In two weeks," says the physician who reported the case, "she became so unsteady on her feet that she fell backward if she closed her eyes." Within a short time, she could no longer stand without help, button her shirt, or write legibly.[7]

How can you protect yourself from N_2O-caused pain, paralysis, or dementia? The answer is simple. If you already know that you have a history of B_{12} deficiency, *refuse to allow an anesthesiologist or dentist to use N_2O, because there are safer and equally effective substitutes.* Otherwise, calculate your risk for B_{12} deficiency (see Chapter 10). If you're at elevated risk or are symptomatic for B_{12} deficiency, insist on being tested if you're scheduled for an elective surgery involving N_2O. Even if you aren't at higher-than-average risk, it's a good idea to be tested, especially if you're middle-aged or older.

Make sure your doctor orders a serum B_{12} and understands that a serum B_{12} in the gray zone is cause for concern. A urinary MMA and homocysteine test are also needed if you've experienced any post-operative neurologic symptoms. Together, these three tests will reliably rule out B_{12} deficiency. Extra caution is called for in surgeries involving patients diagnosed with multiple sclerosis, developmental disabilities, or neurological disorders.

If you're at elevated risk, be sure to insist on testing even if a doctor or dentist tells you that your surgery will be too brief to cause problems. It's true that the longer you're exposed to N_2O, the greater your risk is, but neurologist Rose-Marie Marié warns, "In patients with borderline cobalamin (B_{12}) stores, even short exposures to nitrous oxide may be sufficient to precipitate a [B_{12}] deficiency syndrome."[8] Also, be aware that repeated surgeries, even short ones, can increase your risk of developing N_2O-caused neurological problems.

Don't be surprised, however, if your doctor is reluctant to order presurgical tests for B_{12} deficiency, or even to evaluate you for it if you experience symptoms after a surgery using N_2O. An acquaintance of ours recently became quadriplegic after a seven-hour surgery for a herniated disc. When the man's son requested tests to rule out B_{12} deficiency as a possible cause of the paralysis, the neurosurgeon refused—even when the man's wife, a registered nurse, provided the doctor with articles from medical journals describing cases of paralysis in B_{12}-deficient patients exposed to N_2O. Such egotism and opposition are particularly disturbing because, unlike many postsurgical complications, symptoms of N$_2$O-caused B$_{12}$ deficiency can be partially or wholly reversed—but only if they're caught quickly. Here are some examples from the medical literature:

- A forty-seven-year-old former ballet dancer underwent eight hours of cosmetic surgery. Her recovery went well for six weeks, but then she developed balance problems, odd sensations in her arms and legs, numbness, and weakness. She began falling, and she walked with an unsteady gait. Doctors identified her N$_2$O-caused B$_{12}$ deficiency and started her immediately on B$_{12}$ injections. Within sixteen weeks, she was back to normal, except for mild fatigue.[9]

- A fifty-nine-year-old man underwent surgery for skin cancer and soon became confused and unable to stand without staggering. An alert neurologist determined the cause of his problems and started aggressive B$_{12}$ therapy. Within four weeks, the man could stand and walk again, and within eight weeks his memory and mental functions were back to normal.[10]

- A forty-six-year-old man underwent minor cyst-removal surgery involving N$_2$O. His doctors okayed this anesthetic agent even though pre-surgical tests showed that he had macrocytosis (abnormally large red blood cells)—one sign of B$_{12}$ deficiency. Within two days, the man began experiencing numbness and tingling in his fingers. Shortly afterward, he developed abnormal sensations in both feet; that slowly spread to his trunk, and he began experiencing difficulty balancing and walking. A neurologic exam, nerve conduction studies, and an EMG revealed abnormalities, and repeat blood tests showed borderline anemia, macrocytosis, a severe B$_{12}$ deficiency (118 pg/ml), and an elevated Hcy (87 µmol/L).

  A spinal cord MRI showed myelin changes consistent with B$_{12}$ deficiency, and doctors diagnosed the man with subacute combined degeneration of the spinal cord related to N$_2$O exposure. In the following months, the man slowly improved. However, six months after the onset of his symptoms, the sensory deficits in his lower legs persisted, along with abnormal deep tendon reflexes.[11]

- A sixty-five-year-old man with no history of significant medical problems underwent a hip replacement and received nitrous oxide anesthesia. Sixteen days after surgery, he started having difficulty walking and began experiencing memory loss. An exam revealed paraplegia and subacute combined degeneration of the spinal cord. His mini mental status (MMS) exam score was 18/30—indicating cognitive impairment or dementia—and a brain MRI showed moderate cerebral atrophy. Blood work revealed that he had severe B$_{12}$ deficiency. After B$_{12}$ therapy, the man's memory improved and his MMS exam score increased to 25/30—a score considered normal. His doctors reported, "Our patient had a dementia diagnosed on the basis of DSM IV criteria including memory disorders, disturbance of executive functioning and significant impairment in social and occupational functioning, associated with a combined degeneration of the spinal cord, common in vitamin B$_{12}$ deficiency."[12] Prior to this man's hip surgery, his lab tests revealed macrocytic anemia. This sign of B$_{12}$ deficiency before his surgery was ignored, and his doctors evaluated his B$_{12}$ status only later, when his severe neurologic symptoms appeared.

N$_2$O AND CHILDREN

N$_2$O is being used increasingly often for a variety of diagnostic procedures, especially in children. Here is an advertisement from a hospital using N$_2$O. You'll notice that there is no mention of screening for B$_{12}$ deficiency and no mention of the potential dangers of using this anesthetic agent:

"The group introduced nitrous oxide at Children's in 2004. This innovation makes Children's the only nurse-administered nitrous oxide program in the United States. Nitrous oxide is now used for some procedures at Children's St. Paul and Minneapolis hospitals and at Children's West in Minnetonka. Many children receive it when they undergo a radiological test of the urinary system. For this test, a catheter is inserted into the child's bladder, the bladder is filled, and the child urinates into pads on the X-ray table while images are taken. Other children receive nitrous oxide when they need a needle inserted for an intravenous line or for nuclear medicine procedures involving a catheter and fluids."[13] (More on this in Chapter 12: The Austism-B$_{12}$ Connection).

Unlike the surgeon I mentioned earlier, who refused to evaluate our acquaintance for B$_{12}$ deficiency even after he learned about the effects of N$_2$O, most doctors are too ethical to knowingly put their patients' lives in jeopardy. From a patient's point of view, however, it doesn't matter if a missed diagnosis of N$_2$O-caused damage stems from arrogance or ignorance, because the outcome is the same: pain, debility, paralysis, dementia, or even death.

The risks of GI surgery

We've described how surgeries involving N$_2$O can worsen an existing B$_{12}$ deficiency. Certain surgeries, however, can actually *create* a lifelong B$_{12}$ deficiency. This has nothing to do with anesthesia; instead,

---

An Unheard Cry for Help?

How many patients suffer devastating symptoms of B$_{12}$ deficiency after surgery because doctors either expose them to N$_2$O when they're already B$_{12}$-deficient, or fail to recognize and treat B$_{12}$-deficiency symptoms stemming from GI surgeries? Nobody knows. However, as an informal experiment, we asked a friend who does online research to quickly skim the Internet discussion groups and see if any possible cases turned up. Within fifteen minutes, she found a dozen cases that clearly sounded suspicious. Among the desperate comments of these patients are the following:

- "My surgeon never gave me B$_{12}$ after [gastric bypass] surgery. Eventually, after getting so sick that I could not walk any longer (and calling the doctor several times asking for help, but being told that I'll 'get through it' and that it's 'just natural to feel this way'), I was admitted to the hospital where they gave me what the doctor said was 'triple the normal dose' of B$_{12}$." Sadly, this patient noted that he received no additional B$_{12}$ after this one dose, and he continues to suffer from worsening symptoms. He adds, "Now with a heavy mixture of Neurontin and Lortab from a neurologist who says that I have experienced nerve damage, I am barely able to go back to work or actually do anything besides sit there in tears."

- "I had general anesthesia during cataract surgery.... After the second eye was done, I became completely unable to get in and out

---

of bed by myself. I was told it was due to general anesthesia and would go away in a few days. [But months later there is] no change, except maybe to get worse."

- "My husband has had an ileostomy for twelve years. Just within the past three years, he has begun experiencing some serious problems related to the nervous system. He now has a condition called trigeminal neuralgia, which is a dysfunction of the cranial nerve, causing excruciating pain in his face. In the last several months, he has been losing his grip in his hands and having difficulty with speech. Because of our limited insurance plan, he has been only able to see doctors who don't really know much about this and are just medicating him and pretty much telling him he'll have to live with these things."

- "Eight weeks ago I had a gallbladder attack and a few days later had laparoscopic surgery... within a day after the surgery, I started suffering from a persistent dizziness.... I've also had blurry vision, tingling and 'pins and needles' feelings in my extremities, chest pain [and] a 'wired but tired' feeling.... I've had an MRI, which came back normal. A blood panel showed no sign of anemia." (Authors' note: As we explained earlier, a blood count alone cannot diagnose B$_{12}$ deficiency, and the serum B$_{12}$ test is not included in routine blood panels. An MRI will not detect early damage.) "...I've had many friends tell me that the anesthesia from the surgery could be the culprit. But both my doctor and the surgeon dismiss the notion."

- "I've had Crohn's [an inflammatory intestinal disease] for over twenty-five years; last four years have had increasing symptoms first in feet, now also in my hands. Had back surgery twice for stenosis of lumbar spine, then was re-diagnosed with peripheral neuropathy. Surgery once for Crohn's, removing terminal ileum. Have been tested a few times for B$_{12}$ deficiency, am told it reads normal. I take over-the-counter B$_{12}$ tablets, though I understand that's mainly a futile gesture. My neurologist wants to work me up to determine what kind of neuropathy, perhaps it's a type which is treatable, but my primary care doc won't even return my phone calls, is too busy defending the insurance company's bottom line."

Do any of these patients have B_{12} deficiency resulting from their surgeries? It's very likely, given their symptom patterns. All are in desperate need of testing, and their cases suggest that victims of post-surgery B_{12} deficiency aren't rare—just rarely identified.

it happens because some operations can impair your digestive system's ability to absorb B_{12}. These include operations that involve removing part of the stomach or small intestine (and particularly a segment of the intestine called the terminal ileum), or gastric bypass surgeries to aid in weight loss.

If you undergo a gastrointestinal (GI) surgery, you don't need to worry, as long as your physician measures your B_{12} and urinary MMA levels regularly and ensures that you receive B_{12} injections or high-dose oral/sublingual B_{12} for life. But doctors often fail to do this, even in very high-risk patients. And many other doctors do test, but again make the mistake of defining a B_{12} deficiency as a serum B_{12} less than 200 pg/ml or even less than 180 pg/ml. Still others fail to test their patients' B_{12} level if no anemia and or macrocytosis are present.

Thus, if you've had any type of gastrointestinal surgery, you'll need to take the initiative in protecting your health. If you aren't being monitored for B_{12} problems, insist on testing, even if you have no symptoms. If your doctor says you've been tested, ask which tests were done. Find out what your serum B_{12} level was and see if it fell in the gray zone.

If the tests come back normal, have them repeated yearly to ensure that a B_{12} deficiency doesn't develop over time, and always insist on screening if any B_{12} symptoms develop. If your serum B_{12} test is normal (and not in the gray zone) and you are symptomatic, urinary MMA and Hcy tests should be included. Don't assume that your doctor is looking out for you, because it's not always the case (see sidebar). We strongly advise that a therapeutic trial of high-dose B_{12} be initiated on symptomatic patients, even when test results come back normal (see Chapter 11).

All patients who have gastric bypass or have Crohn's disease with or without surgery should prophylactically be placed on high-dose B_{12} before they become symptomatic, because, in time, they will eventually become B_{12} deficient.

CHAPTER 8 NOTES:

1. McNeely, James K., Buczulinski, Bogdan, and Rosner, Diane R. Severe neurological impairment in an infant after nitrous oxide anesthesia. *Anesthesiology* (2000), 93:1549–50.

2. Holloway, Kathryn, and Alberico, Anthony. Postoperative myeloneuropathy:A preventable complication in patients with B$_{12}$ deficiency. *Journal of Neurosurgery* (May 1990), 72:732–6.

3. Marié, Rose-Marie, Le Biez, Eric, Busson, Philippe, Schaeffer, Stéphane, Boiteau, Lydia, Dupuy, Benoit, and Viader, Fausto. Nitrous oxide anesthesia-associated myelopathy. *Archives of Neurology* (March 2000), 57:380–2.

4. Sethi, N. K., et al. Nitrous oxide "whippit" abuse presenting with cobalamin responsive psychosis. *J Med Toxicol*, 2006 Jun;2(2):71–4.

5. Hobbhahn, J. Are inhaled anaesthetics still toxic? Educational paper, provided by the European Society of Anaesthesiologists (ESA), April 2000 http://www.euroanesthesia.org/pages/education/rc_Vienna/03rc1.HTM.

6. Holloway, Kathryn, and Alberico, Anthony. Postoperative myeloneuropathy:A preventable complication in patients with B$_{12}$ deficiency. *Journal of Neurosurgery* (May 1990), 72:732–6.

7. Schilling, Robert. Is nitrous oxide a dangerous anesthetic for vitamin B$_{12}$-deficient subjects? *Journal of the American Medical Association* March 28, 1986, 255:1605–6.

8. Marié, Rose-Marie, Le Biez, Eric, Busson, Philippe, Schaeffer, Stéphane, Boiteau, Lydia, Dupuy, Benoit, and Viader, Fausto. Nitrous oxide anesthesia-associated myelopathy. *Archives of Neurology* March 2000, 57:380–2.

9. Hadzic, A., Glab, K., Sanborn, K., and Thys, D. Severe neurologic deficit after nitrous oxide anesthesia. *Anesthesiology* 1995, 83:863–6.

10. Flippo, Teresa, and Holder, Walter. Neurologic degeneration associated with nitrous oxide anesthesia in patients with vitamin B$_{12}$ deficiency. *Archives of Surgery* December 1993, 128:1391–1395.

11. Renard D. et al. Subacute combined degeneration of the spinal cord caused by nitrous oxide anesthesia. *Neurol Sci* (2009) 30:75–76.

12. El Otmani H, et al. Postoperative dementia: toxicity of nitrous oxide. *Encephale* 2007 Jan-Feb;33(1):95–7.

13. www.childrensmn.org/web/whatsnew/097261.asp.

9

Can't Conceive? How B₁₂ Deficiency Contributes to Male and Female Infertility

"Vitamin B_{12} deficiency is associated with infertility.... Pregnancy may occur in the presence of B_{12} deficiency, but may be associated with recurrent early fetal loss."
—hematologist Michael Bennett, M.D.[1]

"A deficiency of B_{12} leads to reduced sperm counts and sperm motility."
—Joseph Pizzorno, M.D., and Michael Murray, M.D.[2]

Millions of couples each year are thrilled to learn that their dream of starting a family is becoming a reality. But for one in eight couples who want children, the dream becomes a nightmare of sadness and frustration as months or even years pass, and the pregnancy tests keep saying "negative." For others, there is the terrible tragedy of miscarrying a baby—and the even greater tragedy of miscarrying time after time.

For infertile couples, life often becomes an endless round of expensive (and often unsuccessful) fertility treatments. For couples who conceive babies but suffer miscarriages, trying again to become pregnant can be frightening, turning what should be a happy life experience into an anxiety-ridden ordeal that often ends, once again, in failure.

There are dozens of common causes of male and female infertility, ranging from endometriosis, pelvic inflammatory disease, and polycystic ovary disease in women to structural or hormonal problems in males, and to anti-sperm antibodies in either partner. But there is another risk factor for both male and female infertility that is often overlooked, even by infertility specialists. That problem is vitamin B_{12} deficiency.

One miscarriage is sad enough, but the woman described by physician Michael Bennett had lost seven babies before birth. After years of suffering, she was lucky to find Dr. Bennett, a hematologist (a doctor specializing in blood abnormalities), who identified her severe B_{12} deficiency. He treated her with injected B_{12}, and nine months later she delivered a healthy baby. Since then, she's given birth to two more children.[3]

The woman whose case Dr. Bennett reported was one of fourteen women he's seen over eleven years who suffered from infertility or recurrent miscarriages because of B$_{12}$ deficiency. Of these women, ten conceived successfully after receiving vitamin B$_{12}$ treatment, most within a matter of weeks. (Three women were no longer trying to conceive at the time their deficiency was diagnosed.)

> An often overlooked risk factor for both male and female infertility is vitamin B$_{12}$ deficiency.

Bennett notes that many of these women had been evaluated by obstetricians and had undergone hormonal treatments, "but the vitamin B$_{12}$ deficiency was not recognized, and only much later were they sent for a hematologic consultation."

Married for seven years, the thirty-three-year-old woman kept hoping for a baby and wondering why she couldn't conceive. She also felt increasingly weak, had trouble walking, and noticed that she didn't remember things well.

Her doctors drew a blank, until one spotted signs of macrocytic anemia and referred her to a hematology clinic. There, doctors diagnosed her with B$_{12}$ deficiency and started her on injections of the vitamin.

Within three months, she felt vastly better mentally and she could walk normally again. Within six months, she became pregnant. Her long years of waiting for a child ended when she delivered a healthy baby girl.[4]

Other doctors have also reported successful pregnancies in once-infertile women following therapy for B$_{12}$ deficiency. Yet often, sadly, this deficiency is overlooked even by infertility specialists until women have undergone months or even years of unsuccessful treatment. As a result, many couples spend tens of thousands of dollars, and they experience disappointment after disappointment, when treatment with proper B$_{12}$ replacement and high dose B$_{12}$ therapy might have solved their problem.

One group of London doctors, for instance, reported the case of a thirty-year-old woman with a history of infertility due in part to tubal disease. She underwent two attempts at *in vitro* fertilization, an expensive and time-consuming procedure, which both failed, with the second attempt producing far fewer oocytes (eggs) than the first. At a later visit to her doctor's office, where she complained about abnormal sensations in her hands, the doctor ordered a blood test that revealed low vitamin B$_{12}$ levels. The diagnosis: pernicious anemia. After treatment with injected B$_{12}$, she underwent another round of *in vitro* fertilization, this time producing a healthy number of eleven oocytes. However, she did not become pregnant, and the doctors say, "In retrospect, it may have been prudent to have waited for vitamin B_{12} treatment to restore the endometrial function, before starting a further IVF cycle."

The doctors who report this case note that anovulation (a failure to release an egg during the monthly cycle) occurs in some women with B_{12} deficiency due to pernicious anemia, and that B_{12} deficiency also causes abnormalities of the cells of the reproductive tract (see Chapter 7) which may extend to the lining of the uterus. In addition, they note, B_{12} deficiency is associated with abnormal estrogen levels that interfere with implantation of the fertilized egg.

Surprisingly, the doctors conclude, "We believe that the relation between vitamin B_{12} deficiency and infertility needs more study before serum B_{12} assays are to be included as a routine procedure in investigation of all infertile female patients to detect early cases of vitamin B_{12} deficiency."[5] We disagree, because a serum B_{12} test costs approximately ninety dollars, and a urinary MMA test (if needed) costs one hundred and fifty dollars. Either expense pales in comparison to the tens of thousands of dollars that couples spend on *in vitro* fertilization, a procedure which can fail if B_{12} deficiency exists—and which might not even be necessary when patients with such a deficiency are properly treated.

Another thirty-two-year-old infertile woman whose case is reported in the medical literature underwent four rounds of artificial insemination without success before her doctors detected both iron deficiency and vitamin B_{12} deficiency. They began treatment with oral iron and injected vitamin B_{12}, and within two months the woman became pregnant. She now has two healthy children, the second conceived without any need for fertility treatments.[6]

Researchers aren't yet sure why B_{12} deficiency makes it difficult to conceive a baby or to carry a baby to term. Dr. Bennett and his colleagues suggest that deficient B_{12} levels interfere with ovulation or normal cell division in the fertilized ovum, and that changes in the uterine lining due to B_{12} deficiency prevent implantation. The high homocysteine levels that can result from poor B_{12} status, they say, could cause fetal death by contributing to thrombosis (abnormal blood clotting), inadequate blood supply to the placenta, preeclampsia (which can lead to convulsions), premature separation of the placenta, or fetal growth retardation.

Whatever the reasons for the link between B_{12} and infertility or miscarriage, Dr. Bennett and colleagues say the number of cases they've identified in their own practice "illustrates the importance of measuring B_{12}

> ## B$_{12}$ DEFICIENCY AND MISCARRIAGE: FAR MORE COMMON THAN DOCTORS THINK
>
> A recurring theme in the medical literature is that B$_{12}$ deficiency is a fairly rare cause of miscarriage or stillbirth. The evidence, however, suggests otherwise.
>
> One recent study, for instance, compared thirty-six women who'd suffered recurrent fetal loss to forty women who'd carried healthy babies to term. The researchers found that 31 percent of the women who'd lost several babies had high homocysteine levels. (Elevated homocysteine, as we noted in Chapter 5, is caused by low levels of folic acid, B$_{12}$, and/or vitamin B$_6$, and is easily treated with these vitamins.) Sixteen percent of the women who'd suffered recurrent fetal loss carried two copies of the MTHFR gene that causes abnormally high homocysteine levels, and three of the women had overt B$_{12}$ deficiency.[7]

levels…in every patient investigated for infertility or recurrent abortion." This is particularly critical, they say, now that women of childbearing age receive large amounts of folic acid from supplements or fortified foods, because high folic acid levels can mask B$_{12}$ deficiency.

Such testing will help many women to become pregnant, and in addition, it will protect many children against the devastating effects of B$_{12}$ deficiency in utero. As we've noted elsewhere, insufficient B$_{12}$ in the developing infant is linked to serious and potentially fatal problems, including neural tube defects (see Chapter 6) and neurological abnormalities that can lead to mental retardation or autism (see chapters 6 and 12).

In 2010, we heard from a woman who underwent gastric bypass surgery for weight loss in March 2003. She became pregnant in July 2004 but suffered a miscarriage. This woman was symptomatic for B$_{12}$ deficiency and was at great risk for low B$_{12}$ because of her gastric surgery. Over the next two years, her signs and symptoms of B$_{12}$ deficiency worsened, but no connection was made by her doctors.

Two years later, this woman has a permanent neurologic injury. Her diagnosis is "subacute combined degeneration of the spinal cord—secondary to severe vitamin B$_{12}$ deficiency." Vitamin B$_{12}$ therapy following her gastric surgery would have prevented this tragedy—and it may have saved her baby's life as well.

MALE INFERTILITY AND B$_{12}$ DEFICIENCY

In about 40 percent of cases, a couple's inability to conceive is due to male infertility. Here again, vitamin B$_{12}$ plays a significant role—and, again, that role is generally overlooked by doctors.

The link between male infertility and insufficient B$_{12}$ levels first became commonly known in the 1980s, when researchers reported a study in which 27 percent of men with sperm counts less than 20 million were able to increase these counts to more than 100 million after receiving 1,000 mcg per day of vitamin B$_{12}$.[8] This research was pursued by scientists in Japan, who published a series of clinical and laboratory studies showing B$_{12}$'s beneficial effects on sperm counts. Here's what they found:

- One research group administered high-dose oral B$_{12}$ to mice previously given a drug that lowered sperm counts. After ten weeks, they say, sperm count, sperm motility, motile sperm count, and percentage of "good" sperm were all increased in B$_{12}$-treated mice as compared to controls. "These results suggest that [B$_{12}$] enhanced the testicular function," they concluded, "resulting in an increased output of mature sperm."[9]

- In another study, 57 percent of men with low sperm counts showed increases in sperm number after receiving 6,000 mcg of B$_{12}$ per day.[10]

- A different research group tested the effects of B$_{12}$, Clomid (a fertility drug generally used to treat women, but also used in some cases to treat men), and B$_{12}$ plus Clomid on infertile men. They found that for infertile men with sperm counts higher than 10 million/ml, the combination of B$_{12}$ and Clomid increased sperm count in 80 percent of cases (and B$_{12}$ alone increased sperm count in more than 60 percent).[11] In another study, this group reported that when twenty-six infertile men were treated with B$_{12}$ at a fertility clinic, sperm concentration increased in 38 percent of the men, total sperm counts increased in nearly 54 percent, sperm motility increased in 50 percent, and total motile sperm count increased in 50 percent.[12]

A newer study sheds light on the connection between B$_{12}$ and male fertility by showing that low B$_{12}$ levels affect both gonadal and sperm health. Researchers who deprived rats of B$_{12}$ found that the rats exhibited atrophy of the seminiferous tubules (where sperm are produced), as well as poor development of sperm.[13]

There's evidence, too, that supplemental B$_{12}$ may also help men whose infertility stems from causes other than deficient B$_{12}$. Studies of rodents with testicular dysfunction induced by X-ray irradiation reveal that high-dose vitamin B$_{12}$ can increase the diameter of the seminiferous tubules and increase sperm counts.[14]

INFERTILITY TREATMENT: FIRST THINGS FIRST

Americans spend millions of dollars each year on fertility drugs, artificial insemination, and *in vitro* fertilization. There is a place for these drugs and interventions, but only when simple, safe, inexpensive measures are exhausted.

High on the list of such measures is getting tested for B$_{12}$ status. This testing must include a serum B$_{12}$ level, a urinary MMA test, and a homocysteine test (see chapters 1, 10, and 11). These simple tests, if provided routinely to infertile couples, might spare thousands of men and women the suffering caused by infertility, miscarriages, and stillbirths.

Professor Ralph Gräsbeck and Olga Imerslund (noted discoverers of hereditary cubilin failure with cobalamin deficiency) have written about how vitamin B$_{12}$ and folate deficiencies can cause infertility. Gräsbeck suggests, "Every case of infertility in primary health care should initially be managed by test treatment with micronutrients, before reproduction specialists are consulted."[15]

BLADDER PROBLEMS AND MALE SEXUALITY

Are you always worrying about whether you'll make it to the bathroom on time? Or are you a man taking Viagra or Cialis? If so, you need to be screened for vitamin B$_{12}$ deficiency. Why? Because B$_{12}$ deficiency strikes one part of the nervous system called the *autonomic nervous system*. If untreated, the damage that low B$_{12}$ does to this system can result in impotence in men, hyperactive bladder in men or women, and urinary or fecal incontinence in both sexes.

The nerves in the autonomic nervous system are not under our control. These nerves are found in the stomach, bladder, intestinal tract, and genitals, and B$_{12}$ deficiency can affect any or all of these regions.

For example, B$_{12}$ deficiency can result in nerve damage in the stomach called *gastroparesis*. This damage prevents the stomach from emptying properly, resulting in symptoms such as bloating, heartburn, gastroesophageal reflux, nausea, vomiting, and constipation.

Untreated B$_{12}$ deficiency also causes bladder problems if the bladder nerves become damaged. As a result, people can't tell if their bladders are full or not. This leads to frequent bladder infections and a constant pool of unvoided urine, a problem referred to as *urinary retention.*

In addition, B$_{12}$ deficiency may also cause impotence in men. B$_{12}$ deficiency can result in erectile dysfunction (ED) because the nerves in the penis can become damaged, making it difficult or impossible to achieve or maintain an erection.

We routinely see general practitioners, internists, and urologists prescribing medications for patients with ED. We also see them blaming other disease processes, such as diabetes, for ED, impotence, or incontinence. Typically, they fail to contemplate that B$_{12}$ deficiency may be causing or contributing to these problems. This is a huge and tragic mistake, because B$_{12}$ deficiency is more common as we age, especially in older adults who suffer from ED.

> **B$_{12}$ deficiency may cause impotence and erectile dysfunction in men.**

Diabetics are particularly likely to fall victim to this type of misdiagnosis, because doctors automatically assume their ED is due to peripheral neuropathy caused by diabetes. (Peripheral neuropathy, a common problem in diabetics, is the result of problems with the nerves that carry information to and from the brain and spinal cord. Symptoms of peripheral neuropathy include pain, loss of sensation, and an inability to control muscles.)

Physicians who dismiss diabetic patients' peripheral neuropathy as a side effect of diabetes, without investigating other potential causes, fail to remember that B$_{12}$ deficiency is another common cause of autonomic nerve damage. Physicians can't tell if the nerve damage causing ED stems from diabetes or from B$_{12}$ deficiency, but only if they test their patients. Simply put, diabetic neuropathy mimics B$_{12}$ deficiency neuropathy.

The same is true for patients with alcoholism, AIDS, cancer, and other disorders that can cause damage to the autonomic nervous system. Blaming peripheral neuropathy on these conditions, without investigating the possibility of B$_{12}$ deficiency, is negligence.

When symptoms such as ED or incontinence involve B$_{12}$ deficiency, early treatment is crucial. The longer the problem continues, the more difficult treatment will be—and eventually, the damage will be irreversible. However, even at late stages, treatment can cause remarkable results.

A PRIMER ON PERIPHERAL NEUROPATHY

Peripheral neuropathy is very common, and there are numerous types and causes of this disorder. Peripheral neuropathy affects around 20 million people in the United States, and nearly 60 percent of diabetics suffer from the condition. Symptoms of neuropathy depend on which type of nerve is affected.

The three main types of nerves are sensory (those that carry sensations), motor (those that control muscles), and autonomic (those that carry information to organs and glands). Neuropathy can affect any one or a combination of these nerves. Symptoms also depend on whether the condition affects the entire body or just one nerve (as from an injury).

The autonomic nerves control involuntary or semi-voluntary functions, such as control of internal organs and blood pressure. Damage to autonomic nerves affects the urinary and reproductive organs, causing a wide range of problems including:

- Difficulty beginning to urinate (urinary hesitancy)
- A feeling of incomplete bladder emptying
- Impotence
- Urinary incontinence
- Bowel incontinence
- Slowed stomach emptying, leading to nausea, bloating, vomiting, and constipation

As you learned in Chapter 3, untreated B$_{12}$ deficiency causes subacute combined degeneration of the spinal cord (SACD). In 2008, a group of researchers investigated urination problems in eight patients—six men and two women—with SACD. All of the patients had difficulty walking, two were in wheelchairs, and four were bedridden. The researchers reported, "Urinary symptoms included retention in four, hesitancy in two, urgency in four, urge incontinence in two, frequency in three, poor stream in four, and sensation of incomplete voiding in three patients…Two patients had both urinary and fecal incontinence, five constipation, six erectile dysfunction, and one had atrophic changes in the legs."

Patients were treated with daily intramuscular injections of vitamin B$_{12}$ and followed for six months. At the end of this time, three patients' urinary issues had resolved, four had partial recoveries, and only one patient showed minimal improvement.

The researchers concluded that SACD is associated with bladder dysfunction in about one-third of patients with moderate to severe clinical symptoms and can improve on vitamin B$_{12}$ therapy.[16]

Obviously, not all people with erectile dysfunction or bladder and bowel problems have a B$_{12}$ deficiency. However, we don't know the true incidence of B$_{12}$ deficiency in these conditions, and research is sorely needed.

What we *do* know is that B$_{12}$ is a common and easily treated cause of these disorders. Testing all patients with these problems for low B$_{12}$ could save tens of thousands of patients from debility and a poor quality of life. It could also spare many people from the common and sometimes serious side effects of drugs like Viagra and Cialis.

In addition, identifying and treating peripheral neuropathy caused by low B$_{12}$ could save insurers, the government, and medical consumers huge amounts of money. In 2010, for example, a thirty-day supply of Cialis (5mg per day) sold for $137 per month, or $1,644 per year—and a single Viagra pill cost $20.92. Doctors who prescribe drugs like these without ruling out B$_{12}$ deficiency aren't just hurting many patients— they're contributing to skyrocketing medical care costs as well.

CHAPTER 9 NOTES:

1. Bennett, M. Vitamin B$_{12}$ deficiency, infertility and recurrent fetal loss. *Journal of Reproductive Medicine* 2001, 46(3):209–12.

2. Pizzorno, J. and Murray, M. "Male Infertility," in *Textbook of Natural Medicine*, Bastyr University, 1993 (online) http://www.healthy.net/library/books/textbook/Section6/MALEIN.PDF.

3. Bennett, M. Vitamin B$_{12}$ deficiency, infertility and recurrent fetal loss. *Journal of Reproductive Medicine* 2001, 46(3):209–12.

4. Menachem, Y., Cohen, A. M., and Mittelman, M. Cobalamin deficiency and infertility. *American Journal of Hematology* 1994, 46(2):152.

5. El-Nemr, A., Sabatini, L., Wilson, C., Lower, A. M., Al-Shawaf, T., and Grudzinska, J. G. Vitamin B$_{12}$ deficiency and IVF. *Journal of Obstetrics and Gynecology* 1998, 18(2):192–3.

6. Sanfilippo, J,. and Liu, Y. Vitamin B$_{12}$ deficiency and infertility: Report of a case. *International Journal of Fertility* 1991, 36(1):36–8.

7. Raziel, A., Kornberg, Y., Friedler, S., Schachter, M., Sela, B. A., and Ron-El, R. Hypercoagulable thrombophilic defects and hyperhomocysteinemia in patients with recurrent pregnancy loss. *American Journal of Reproductive Immunology* 2001, 45(2):65–71.

8. Sandler, B., and Faragher, B. Treatment of oligospermia with vitamin B$_{12}$. Infertility 1984, 7:133–8; cited in Pizzorno and Murray, "Male Infertility," in *Textbook of Natural Medicine*, Bastyr University, 1993 (online) http://www.healthy.net/library/books/textbook/Section6/MALEIN.PDF.

9. Oshio, S., Ozaki, S., Ohkawa, I., Tajima, T., Kaneko, S., and Mohri, H. Mecobalamin promotes mouse sperm maturation. *Andrologia* 1989, 21(2):167–73.

10. Kumamoto, Y., et al. Clinical efficacy of mecobalamin in treatment of oligospermia. Results of a double-blind comparative clinical study. Acta Urologica Japan 1988, 34:1109–32; cited in Pizzorno and Murray, "Male Infertility," in *Textbook of Natural Medicine*, Bastyr University, 1993 (online) http://www.healthy.net/library/books/textbook/Section6/MALEIN.PDF.

11. Isoyama, R., Baba, Y., Harada, H., Kawai, S., Shimizu, Y., Fujii, M., Fujisawa, S., Takihara, H., Koshido, Y., and Sakatoku, J. Clinical experience of methylcobalamin (CH3-B$_{12}$)/clomiphene citrate combined treatment in male infertility. *Hinyokika Kiyo* 1986, 32(8):1177–83.

12. Isoyama, R., Kawai, S., Shimizu, Y., Harada, H., Takihara, H., Baba, Y., and Sakatoku, J. Clinical experience with methylcobalamin (CH3-B$_{12}$) for male infertility. *Hinyokika Kiyo* 1984, 30(4):581–6.

13. Kawata, T., Tamiki, A., Tashiro, A., Suga, K., Kamioka, S., Yamada, K., Wada, M., Tanaka, N., Tadokoro, T., and Maekawa, A. Effect of vitamin B$_{12}$ deficiency on testicular tissue in rats fed by pair-feeding. *International Journal of Vitamin and Nutrition Research* 1997, 67(1):17–21.

14. Oshio, S., Yazaki, T., Umeda, T., Ozaki, S., Ohkawa, I., Tajima, T., Yamada, T., and Mohri, H. Effects of mecobalamin on testicular dysfunction induced by X ray irradiation in mice. *Nippon Yakurigaku Zasshi* 1991, 98(6):483–90.

15. Gräsbeck, R. Infertility—folate, cobalamin and other micronutrients [evaluation]. Rondel 2002; 10. URL: www.rondellen.net.

16. Misra, U.K., et al. Bladder dysfunction in subacute combined degeneration: a clinical, MRI and urodynamic study. *J Neurol.* 2008 Dec;255(12): 1881–8.

10

Protecting Yourself: Are You at Risk for Vitamin B₁₂ Deficiency?

"I have been convinced all of my life that an informed patient is the best patient. My advice to people has always been, 'Take charge of your health.' Now it's more important than ever because, with managed care, no one else is."
—C. Everett Koop, M.D., former surgeon general of the United States[1]

If you've read to this point, you're probably asking yourself: "Should I be worried?"

It's a smart question, because millions of people suffer from B_{12} deficiency, and far too few ever get an accurate diagnosis. That's why you need to take matters into your own hands, in order to protect your health and your life. In this chapter, we'll tell you how to determine if you're one of the victims of this silent epidemic—and, if so, what you need to do.

Remember, as you read through this chapter, that B_{12} deficiency can be a "good news" diagnosis. That's because it's simple to treat, and if it's caught in time, your symptoms will vanish. Moreover the treatment for this disorder typically costs under fifty dollars per year, making it easy on your pocketbook. And what if you receive a late diagnosis, after suffering neurological damage? Then it's even more important for you to receive aggressive methyl-B_{12} injectable therapy (see Chapter 11). Some patients with late-stage B_{12} deficiency see improvements within weeks or months, and some may even experience complete reversal of their severe neurologic manifestations.

For instance, John, a forty-seven-year-old engineer, had a severe misdiagnosed B_{12} deficiency that went undetected for years and slowly began to cripple him. When he finally received a diagnosis and his primary neurologist began treating him with daily injectable cyanocobalamin, he improved slightly but still had fine and gross motor problems. After reading the first edition of this book, he asked his neurologist if the doctor would be willing to prescribe methyl-B$_{12}$ injections instead of cyanocobalamin. His neurologist was unaware of the different forms of B$_{12}$ and told John that he would investigate it. He did, and agreed to try it.

John began receiving methyl-B$_{12}$ injections daily, and within five days of starting treatment he began to notice major improvements. He continued to improve over the next three weeks, and after three months of treatment his neurologic symptoms were completely reversed.

John's case shows that there is no way of knowing who will improve and who will not. When John initially shared his story with us, we doubted that he would be able to reverse all of his symptoms, but he did. So if you receive a late-stage diagnosis, insist on aggressive treatment.

Of course, the earlier a diagnosis of B$_{12}$ deficiency is made, the better the chances for a total recovery are. Some cases of B$_{12}$ deficiency are diagnosed too late, and these stories don't have a happy ending. So if you suspect after reading this chapter that deficient B$_{12}$ levels could be playing a role in your medical problems, don't hesitate—find out!

CALCULATING YOUR ODDS

B$_{12}$ deficiency isn't like the measles or a sprained ankle. There's not one obvious symptom, like a red rash or a swollen joint, which allows you (or your doctor) to make an instant diagnosis. Instead, there are signs and symptoms that can strongly implicate deficient B$_{12}$ as a culprit and risk factors that make a deficiency more likely. To know if you're at risk for B$_{12}$ deficiency, you need to recognize these signs, symptoms, and risk factors. If you spot them, your next step should be to call your doctor.

> The earlier a diagnosis of B$_{12}$ deficiency is made, the better the chances are for a full recovery.

How can you tell if you're at risk? On the following pages, you'll find a checklist of the risk factors and symptoms most often associated with B$_{12}$ deficiency, along with a point score to assign to each of these. To make the checklist easier to use, we've divided it into categories. To determine your risk, add up your point score for all of the categories and check it against the scoring chart at the end. If you are filling in the questionnaire for a loved one, simply answer as that person would.

ARE YOU AT RISK?

1. NEUROLOGICAL SYMPTOMS

If you have any of the symptoms listed below, give yourself two points. If you have more than one of the symptoms listed below, give yourself another point for each additional symptom.

- Do you experience a "pins and needles" feeling or suffer from numbness or burning in your feet, hands, legs, and/or arms?

- Have you been diagnosed with diabetic or peripheral neuropathy?

- Do you suffer from weakness in your arms and/or legs?

- Do you experience light-headedness or dizziness?

- Are you prone to falling or do you fall frequently?

- Have you or others noticed any unusual changes in your ability to move? For instance, do you walk clumsily or with your feet wide apart, or have difficulty writing legibly?

- Have you noticed problems with your memory or thinking: for instance, increased difficulty in remembering names or dates, or more trouble in adding numbers, balancing your checkbook, or making change? Do you sometimes become confused or disoriented? Do you suffer from memory problems or other symptoms of dementia?

- Do you have trouble knowing where various parts of your body are, if you aren't looking? (For instance, do you have trouble walking in the dark, when you can't see your feet?)

- Does your sense of touch, or your perception of pain, appear distorted?

- Has a doctor ever told you that you have muscular spasticity (lack of coordination and excessive muscle contraction)?

- Do you have a tremor?

- Do you suffer from urinary or fecal incontinence?

- Do you suffer from impotence?

- Do you have visual impairment, visual loss, or abnormal visual evoked potential tests?

2. Psychiatric Symptoms

If you have any of the symptoms listed below, give yourself two points. If you have more than one of the symptoms listed below, give yourself another point for each additional symptom.

- Have you undergone any unusual personality changes? For instance, do your friends say that you're "not acting like yourself," or do you find that you are more irritable than usual?

- Are you unusually apathetic or depressed, or have you ever been diagnosed with depression (including postpartum depression)? Have you ever had suicidal thoughts?

- Do you ever experience hallucinations or delusions?

- Do you ever exhibit violent behavior?

- Have you been diagnosed with any other form of psychosis or mental illness, including schizophrenia or bipolar disorder?

- Do you find yourself becoming more paranoid about other people's actions or intentions?

3. Hematologic Signs (Abnormalities of the blood cells)

If you have any of the signs listed below, give yourself two points. If you have more than one of the signs listed below, give yourself another point for each additional symptom.

- Has a doctor ever told you that your red blood cells are abnormally large (macrocytosis)?

- Has a doctor ever told you that you have abnormally small red blood cells, an iron deficiency, or iron deficiency anemia?

- Has a doctor ever told you that you are anemic (low blood count or low hemoglobin)? Do you have low platelets, or a low white blood cell count?

4. Gastrointestinal Risk Factors

If you have any of the risk factors listed below, give yourself two points. If you have more than one of the risk factors listed below, give yourself another point for each additional symptom.

- Have you been diagnosed with inflammation and/or wasting of the stomach lining (gastric atrophy)?

- Have you been diagnosed as having low stomach acid?

- Do you suffer from gastritis?

- Do you suffer from ulcers?

- Have you been diagnosed with gastroesophageal reflux disease (GERD)?

- Do you have diverticulosis?

- Have you been diagnosed with precancerous gastrointestinal growths or gastrointestinal cancer?

- Have you undergone a gastrointestinal resection (partial or complete gastrectomy), undergone a gastric bypass surgery for weight loss, or had either partial or complete removal of your ileum (last part of the small intestine)?

- Have you been diagnosed with a malabsorption syndrome (Crohn's disease, inflammatory bowel disease, irritable bowel syndrome, or celiac disease [gluten enteropathy])?

- Do you have a family history of pernicious anemia (an autoimmune disease)?

- Have you been diagnosed with small bowel overgrowth?

- Have you been diagnosed with a tapeworm or other gastrointestinal parasite?

5. GENERAL RISK FACTORS

If you have any of the risk factors listed below, give yourself one point.

- Are you age sixty or over?

- Do you have a thyroid disorder, or do you have an autoimmune disorder: for instance, lupus, insulin-dependent diabetes, rheumatoid arthritis, Hashimoto's thyroiditis, Graves' disease, Addison's disease, vitiligo, hypogammaglobulinemia, or agammaglobulinemia?

- Have you ever had cancer? Have you undergone chemotherapy, or undergone radiation therapy?

- Have you ever undergone surgery (including dental surgery) in which nitrous oxide was used?

- Do you abuse nitrous oxide as a recreational drug?

- Are you a vegan or vegetarian, or do you follow a macrobiotic or raw food diet?

- Are you an alcoholic?

- Are you taking any of the following medications: proton pump inhibitors (omeprazole [*Prilosec*], Nexium, Prevacid, Protonix), H2-blockers (ranitidine [*Zantac*], Pepcid, Tagamet, Axid), metformin (*Glucophage*), anticonvulsants (phenytoin [*Dilantin*], phenobarbital, Mysoline), potassium supplements, birth control pills, colchicine, neomycin, methotrexate, cholestyramine (*Questran*), colestipol (*Colestid*), or aminosalicylic acid?

6. OTHER SIGNS/SYMPTOMS OFTEN ASSOCIATED WITH B$_{12}$ DEFICIENCY

If you have any of the signs or symptoms listed below, give yourself one point.

- Do you suffer from fatigue, lack of energy, or weakness?

- Do you suffer from generalized weakness?

- Have you experienced a loss of weight or loss of appetite?

- Do you suffer from chest pain, or from shortness of breath with exertion (e.g., walking from your bed to the toilet or to your kitchen)?

- Are you unusually pale, does your skin have a grayish cast, or do you have a lemon-yellow skin color?

- Do you have a sore, inflamed, or "beefy red" tongue?

- Do you suffer from tinnitus (ringing in the ears)?

- If you are female, has a doctor ever told you that your Pap smear showed abnormal cells (cervical dysplasia)?

- Do you suffer from infertility?

> **TO CALCULATE YOUR SCORE:**
>
> Add the points in every category. Your score is:
>
> **Low Risk:**   with less than 3 points
>
> **Moderate Risk:** with 3 to 6 points
>
> **High Risk:**   if your points are 7 or greater

WHAT SHOULD YOU DO NOW?

- **If you scored in the low-risk range,** and you do not have any of the medical conditions listed in the section following this one, your B$_{12}$ levels are probably fine. Remember, however, that as you age, your B$_{12}$ levels may drop—meaning that a healthy level today won't guarantee that you're safe a year from now—so be aware of the symptoms and risk factors we've described, and have your B$_{12}$ levels checked yearly or sooner if you develop any of them.

- **If you scored in the moderate-risk range,** you need B$_{12}$ screening. Make an appointment with your doctor and get tested. If B$_{12}$ deficiency is indeed the culprit, catching it early may lead to a complete remission of symptoms.

- **If you scored in the high-risk range,** there is no time to waste: Call your doctor, and get the earliest appointment possible and get tested. If your doctor is skeptical or resistant, be assertive—and, if necessary, find another doctor. Your physician must also rule out other disease processes that mimic B$_{12}$ deficiency, such as an underactive thyroid.

ARE THERE SPECIFIC MEDICAL CONDITIONS THAT PUT YOU AT RISK?

Regardless of your score on this questionnaire, we believe that if you currently suffer from, or have suffered from, any of the following conditions, you need to be tested for B$_{12}$ deficiency as soon as possible:

- dementia/Alzheimer's disease
- multiple sclerosis

- autism
- any neurologic disorder
- any psychiatric disorder
- peripheral neuropathy (related to diabetes, CIDP or other disorders)
- any form of anemia
- acquired immune deficiency syndrome (AIDS)
- optic neuritis or optic atrophy
- macular degeneration
- congestive heart failure (CHF)
- hyperhomocystinemia
- insulin-dependent diabetes mellitus (IDDM) (also known as Type I diabetes)
- vertigo
- fibromyalgia
- chronic fatigue syndrome
- cervical spondylosis
- impotence

You also need to be tested if you suffer from chronic pain, have an occlusive vascular disorder (transient ischemic attacks—TIAs or mini-strokes), or have a history of cerebrovascular accident (CVA or stroke), pulmonary embolism (blood clot in the lung), myocardial infarction (heart attack), coronary artery disease, or deep vein thrombosis (DVT). People with iron deficiency anemia, radiculopathy (nerve irritation in an arm or leg, from a back or neck disorder or from surgery), a history of alcoholism, or the blood disorders polycythemia or thrombocytopenia should also be tested. Vitamin B₁₂ deficiency can cause signs and symptoms that mimic or hide behind many of these diseases. People with kidney problems, patients on dialysis, and people with liver disorders (e.g., hepatitis or alcoholic liver disease) need to have

> **If your doctor is skeptical or resistant, be assertive—and, if necessary, find another doctor.**

AVOID SELF-TREATING!

We can't stress enough that you should avoid the temptation to self-treat possible symptoms of B$_{12}$ deficiency. Taking B$_{12}$ before undergoing tests will skew your lab results, making it difficult to diagnose or rule out B$_{12}$ deficiency, which can prevent you from getting a proper diagnosis and treatment. Therefore, if you have signs and symptoms of B$_{12}$ deficiency, get tested before taking any over-the-counter B$_{12}$ supplements (pills, lozenges, spray, nasal-B$_{12}$ or creams). After screening, your doctor can determine if you have a B$_{12}$ deficiency and begin treatment.

People often think they can take high-dose B$_{12}$ for a few days or weeks and then stop for a month to get tested. This will alter test results and confuse physicians, making it appear as though the people never had a B$_{12}$ deficiency. Once tested, you can begin over-the-counter (OTC) high-dose B$_{12}$ lozenges while waiting for your test results—but not before! Depending on your symptoms and results, your physician will prescribe OTC lozenges or injections.

However, if you've already been taking a multi-vitamin or another product that has B$_{12}$ in it and are having symptoms, you still need to be tested. Just don't start taking any new B$_{12}$ before the tests, and do inform your doctor that you've been taking B$_{12}$ supplements.

If you've already been on high dose B$_{12}$ and have noticed an improvement, continue to take it. Your physician may want to do further tests on you, or may want to tweak your treatment (for instance, by switching you to B$_{12}$ injections), depending on your physical exam and symptoms.

the urinary MMA test along with the serum B$_{12}$, because these disorders often give falsely elevated serum B$_{12}$ results.

WHAT ABOUT TREATMENT?

In our opinion, B$_{12}$ injections are preferable to oral B$_{12}$ in many cases, and *they are absolutely necessary when neurological symptoms are present.* This is an area of controversy, but we've personally seen cases in which high-dose oral B$_{12}$ and lozenges simply didn't work, and such cases are reported in the literature as well.

What Tests Should I Have?

Your health care provider may choose one of the following five methods for determining if you have a B_{12} deficiency. In chapters 1 and 11, we explain these tests. In Chapter 11, we advise clinicians on how to proceed with testing and treatment.

1. B_{12} (using updated range B_{12} > 450 pg/ml or 332 pmol/L)

2. B_{12} and the urinary MMA (see Chapter 11 for detailed discussion)

3. B_{12} and HoloTC (see chapters 1 and 11)

4. B_{12}, MMA, and homocysteine (see Chapter 11)

5. B_{12}, MMA, HoloTC, homocysteine (see Chapter 11)

Many doctors will argue that the literature indicates—although it does not prove—that oral B_{12} is adequate in most cases (see Chapter 11 for an extensive discussion of this topic). Doctors may also consider rising serum B_{12} levels or normalization of blood cells as evidence that oral treatment is effective, not taking into account the physical exam or how a patient feels subjectively. Our philosophy is simply this: Given that bimonthly shots of B_{12} are virtually painless thanks to microfine needles, and given the multiple ways (see Chapter 1) in which the B_{12} pathway can be disrupted between your mouth and your bloodstream, why take a chance? The bonus is that injectable B_{12} therapy is cheap.

Moreover, while there are many over-the-counter B_{12} lozenges, pills, drops, nasal gels, skin patches, gums and drinks, it's not possible to know the efficacy of each of these products or to predict each individual's response. What studies were done to test them, and how many people were involved? Were these studies done on healthy people or B_{12}-deficient patients? What was the cause of the patients' B_{12} deficiency? Did any of the studies include patients with severe neurologic symptoms? All of these factors—as well as the form of B_{12} in a product and the shelf life of the product—must be considered when selecting a B_{12} therapy.

Thus, we advise caution. If a patient responds to oral B_{12} or B_{12} lozenges—great! But if not, injections are always indicated as a trial.

Here's a case in point. A forty-eight-year-old female diagnosed with pernicious anemia ten years earlier was switched from B_{12} injections to oral B$_{12}$ pills for two years. She took 2,000 mcg of cyanocobalamin daily. For the last six months of this time, she complained of foggy thinking, paresthesias, depression, and severe fatigue. This led us to recheck her serum B$_{12}$, which was found to be 216 pg/ml. Switching her to B$_{12}$ injections (hydroxocobalamin) corrected her symptoms.

And here's another good reason to opt for injections: if you're counting pennies, the shots are cheaper than the pills if you inject yourself or have a family member administer the injections for you. Shots are also the safest route if you're dealing with a B$_{12}$-deficient loved one who is forgetful or non-compliant, and thus likely to skip oral doses. Hundreds of thousands of diabetics can testify—as can one of the coauthors of this book, who self-administers her B$_{12}$ shots twice a month—that shots take only seconds to prepare and are simple to administer after the first time or two.

If you aren't sure if you can handle self-administering monthly shots, ask your doctor for a prescription and a little training, and give it a try for a month or two. We can just about guarantee that you'll find self-injections easy—and if not, you can always have your doctor's staff administer the shots, or have a family member trained to give them to you.

Don't quit!

A few causes of B$_{12}$ deficiency are temporary. Many, however, are permanent, and taking extra B$_{12}$ for only a few weeks or months won't solve the problem. If you have one of these conditions, you'll need to take supplemental B$_{12}$ for life, and it's both your responsibility and your doctor's to make sure that there's no break in your treatment.

Sometimes doctors order serum B$_{12}$ tests for patients who've undergone long-term B$_{12}$ treatment, in order to demonstrate to these patients that

---

A Final Word about Oral B$_{12}$

We don't dismiss the use of oral B$_{12}$ supplements entirely. If you and your doctor agree on oral B$_{12}$, we recommend a high dose (2,000 mcg per day) in lozenge or sublingual (under the tongue) form, and prefer methyl-B$_{12}$. You should switch to an oral formula only after you've received initial shots to get your B$_{12}$ stores back to normal, and you should have at least yearly B$_{12}$ tests to make sure the oral formula is working for you. We review all the different forms and routes in Chapter 11.

they're not deficient—or even to convince them that they never suffered from a deficiency in the first place. This is misguided, because people who've been correctly treated for B_{12} deficiency will have adequate serum B_{12} levels, and these levels will stay adequate for months or years when treatment is stopped. Eventually, however, the deficiency will return, and with it the risk of debilitating symptoms, or even death.

In other cases, problems arise when patients switch to new doctors who aren't knowledgeable about B_{12} deficiency. We recommend that patients who receive a diagnosis of B_{12} deficiency obtain their test results and medical records and give copies of these papers to any new doctors. A physician who's skeptical about your assertion that you're B_{12}-deficient is likely to be more accepting if you have the documentation to prove it. Again, however, this is a time to be assertive. If you know you're B_{12}-deficient, and a doctor says, "You don't need treatment for that any more," don't be afraid to speak up. Insist on treatment, and if you don't get it, find a more knowledgeable doctor.

Of course, as medical professionals, we're all too aware that this is easier said than done. As physician Charles Inlander points out in *Medicine on Trial*, "Doctors over recent generations have established the ground rules for patient behavior, especially regarding the patient's relationship to (and critique of) the doctor. Many of us are taught (or intuit) that it is not good form to play too active a role, never mind a contentious one. Questions to doctors should be polite and deferential, acknowledging their superior knowledge and the wisdom of experience. If we are irritated with the doctor's demeanor in any way or left with any uneasy feeling that something is not right in the care being given, we might save our gripes for relatives or friends."

Unfortunately, when it comes to B_{12} deficiency, this politeness can be fatal. In our own practices, we've seen dozens of people who were diagnosed as B_{12}-deficient at some point in their lives but later allowed doctors to discontinue their treatment. Several paid a high price for this lack of assertiveness, because they now have permanent neurological damage or dementia.

Conversely, we know of patients with B_{12} deficiency who are alive and well today only because they, or an assertive family member, insisted—sometimes in the face of significant resistance—on proper diagnosis and treatment.

A MEDICAL MIRACLE—OR JUST ANOTHER CASE OF UNTREATED AND MISDIAGNOSED B$_{12}$ DEFICIENCY?

Bill, an active seventy-seven-year-old retired engineer, had a history of pernicious anemia, diagnosed fifteen years earlier. Not long ago, Bill suffered a heart attack, and tests indicated that he needed a heart valve replacement. At the time, he was also suffering from severe iron-deficiency anemia. Bill's doctors suspected that the anemia stemmed from occult gastrointestinal bleeding, but they could find no evidence of this, so they simply gave him two units of blood to improve his anemia.

A few months later, Bill underwent successful surgery. After the operation, however, he began experiencing hand tremors, light-headedness, extreme weakness, and fatigue. As the weeks passed, he became increasingly weak and eventually could no longer walk. He became very anemic again, and required multiple blood transfusions. His surgeon, diagnosing Bill as iron-deficient because his red blood cells were very small, told Bill to take iron supplements.

The iron supplements didn't help, and Bill's condition continued to worsen. Bill's cardiologist, informed of his patient's decline, had him admitted to the emergency department, and Bill's nephew Michael, who happens to be a nurse at the same hospital, accompanied him there. Michael informed the emergency department (ED) doctor that Bill had pernicious anemia, and that he hadn't received a B$_{12}$ injection for at least four months. (Bill had been told by his family doctor prior to surgery that he didn't need the B$_{12}$ shots, and that they would interfere with his new heart medications—both untrue statements.)

Despite Michael's input, the ED doctor, and the other admitting physicians who cared for Bill during his hospital stay, did not order any B$_{12}$ testing or provide any treatment for Bill's symptoms. Michael called Bill's cardiologist, cardiovascular surgeon, internist, and general practitioner, but none would agree to investigate Bill for B$_{12}$ deficiency. In the course of his calls, Michael learned that the general practitioner treating Bill's pernicious anemia had been administering B$_{12}$ shots only every three to four months, rather than monthly, thus setting the stage for Bill's postsurgical B$_{12}$ crisis.

When transfusions failed to help Bill, the cardiothoracic surgeon— persuaded in large part by Michael's determined advocacy—called in a hematologist (a specialist in blood disorders). While Bill's recent blood transfusions skewed his test results, as did his earlier pre-surgery transfusions, the doctor recognized Bill's clear-cut symptoms of deficiency and immediately began B₁₂ injections. By the third injection, Bill was remarkably improved, and he was soon discharged home. He could stand again, and his tremor, weakness, fatigue, and unsteadiness were dramatically reduced. The expensive wheelchair, hospital bed and other medical equipment needed to care for Bill were not needed.

It took weeks, and a series of B₁₂ shots, for Bill to completely regain his strength, but his story has a happy ending: He's now fully recovered and back to enjoying life. The credit for his recovery belongs in large part to his nephew, who became educated about B₁₂ deficiency and refused to take "no" for an answer when it came to his uncle's need for proper treatment.

Bill, now eighty-five, is an active senior who lives half the year in Florida and the other half in Michigan. He drives, golfs, and fishes. His lifestyle is vastly different from the grim prognosis and nursing home sentence his doctors gave him eight years ago.

SPREAD THE WORD!

It's not unusual for B₁₂ deficiency to run in families, so if you're diagnosed with this disorder, let your relatives know. When the authors of this book urged other family members to have their B₁₂ levels checked, they uncovered several cases of B₁₂ deficiency which were causing symptoms ranging from dizziness, to tremor, to autistic behavior.

At first, your family members may tease you about your "over-zealousness" in educating them about the dangers of B₁₂ deficiency. (We can sympathize, because it's happened to us!) But if your generosity in sharing your new knowledge leads to a diagnosis for another family member, that teasing will quickly turn to gratitude. It may also lead to a cure for your relatives' troubling or life-threatening medical symptoms, and that's one of the greatest gifts you can give your loved ones.

CHAPTER 10 NOTES:

1. Dr. Koop's remarks were made in an interview in the *Reformed Quarterly* (newsletter of the Reformed Theological Seminary), Winter 1998.

11

Information for Physicians

"Vitamin B$_{12}$ (cobalamin) deficiency should be on your radar screen for several reasons. Prevention, early detection, and treatment of vitamin B$_{12}$ deficiency are important public health issues, because they are essential to prevent development of irreversible neurologic damage which can impact quality of life."
—Centers for Disease Control and Prevention, June 29, 2009.[1]

"Vitamin B$_{12}$ deficiency affects about one quarter of the U.S. population and is more common in the elderly and in adults with several predisposing conditions.... Health-care professionals need to recognize that vitamin B$_{12}$ deficiency is often undetected and can lead to devastating and irreversible complications. Early treatment is effective and prevents disability from hematologic or neuropsychiatric complications, or both."
—T. S. Dharmarajan, M.D., and Edward P. Norkus, Ph.D., in *Postgraduate Medicine.*[2]

In the emergency department (ED), we never know who will come through our doors next. On a typical shift our patients could include a confused elderly woman, a man complaining of chest pains, a young woman with puzzling neurological symptoms, an elderly man with a hip fracture, a pregnant woman suffering a miscarriage, a young man in the grip of an acute episode of paranoia, a depressed and suicidal patient, a stroke victim, a gastric bypass patient with weakness, an AIDS patient or diabetic crippled by neuropathy, or a child whose diagnosis is listed as "autistic spectrum disorder."

As we look over these patients' records, we see the obvious battery of tests: X-rays, blood tests, psychiatric evaluations, EKGs, MRIs, CT scans. What we don't see, however, is evidence that a significant percentage of the patients who present with signs and symptoms of B$_{12}$ deficiency—including all of the patients we just described above—have been tested for this common, simple-to-treat, and potentially deadly problem.

In the ED, we have the greatest opportunity to witness the frequent misdiagnosis of B$_{12}$ deficiency, because we are caring for many other physicians' patients. We see a greater volume and wider variety of patients than other doctors and nurses. We are not limited to a specific group of patients in regard to disease, body system, age, or sex, as are other health care professionals. We care for whoever comes in, from infants to the elderly, insured or uninsured. We treat psychiatric patients, the homeless, drug abusers, and chronic pain patients. We frequently find B$_{12}$ deficiency because we know the signs, symptoms, and risk factors, and are actively looking for it, where other clinicians are not.

> In our experience, there are eight reasons why physicians often miss a diagnosis of B$_{12}$ deficiency.

Obviously, only a fraction of the patients we treat have symptoms caused by B$_{12}$ deficiency. This problem, however, affects as much as 25 percent of the population,[3] causing a remarkable array of debilitating and dangerous medical problems. Yet many physicians, including those who primarily treat older patients, will rarely or never diagnose a case of B$_{12}$ deficiency.

Why? In our experience, there are eight reasons why physicians often miss a diagnosis of B$_{12}$ deficiency:

PROBLEM 1: FAILURE TO RECOGNIZE THE NEUROLOGICAL AND PSYCHIATRIC SYMPTOMS OF B$_{12}$ DEFICIENCY

The number one reason for the high rate of missed diagnoses is that physicians fail to recognize the neuropsychiatric signs and symptoms of B$_{12}$ deficiency. It is well known and has been well documented that B$_{12}$ deficiency damages the brain, spinal cord, peripheral nerves, and the nerves of the eye, often well before blood abnormalities appear. Thus, doctors who think of B$_{12}$ deficiency only in the context of anemia will miss the majority of cases that pass through their offices and hospitals. Physicians must become aware that *macrocytic anemia is a late sign of vitamin B$_{12}$ deficiency, frequently occurring long after potentially irreversible neurological damage has taken place.*

The common and striking neuropsychiatric manifestations of B$_{12}$ deficiency, including depression, altered mental status, dementia, psychosis, vertigo, tremor, neuropathy, visual problems, extremity weakness, dizziness, balance problems, and gait disorders, have been long forgotten by physicians. This is perplexing, because physicians as far back as 190 years ago—Combes (1820), Addison (1855), and Biermer (1872)—documented that "pernicious anemia" caused severe neurologic complications. Later, physicians Osler (1877), Lichtheim (1887), and Cabot (1908) reported on post-mortem exams of pernicious anemia patients revealing subacute combined degeneration of the spinal cord. An array of published medical articles exist describing neurologic symptomatology preceding the classic blood signs, yet clinicians ignore or have forgotten this and, rather than testing for B_{12} deficiency, simply prescribe other medications in an attempt to alleviate their patients' symptoms.

In 1988, Lindenbaum et al. reported in the *New England Journal of Medicine* that neurologic manifestations associated with B_{12} deficiency occurred in the absence of anemia or macrocytosis. This article generated a great deal of interest and was interpreted as new information, which it clearly was not. It is evident that the knowledge of B_{12} deficiency as a cause of neurologic and/or psychiatric disease has been lost.

IDENTIFYING THE SYMPTOMS OF B_{12} DEFICIENCY

B_{12} deficiency affects all body systems, is a master mimic, and can masquerade as a wide variety of medical problems. In addition to neuropsychiatric manifestations, it can cause shortness of breath, fatigue, generalized weakness, anemia, poor digestion, GERD-like symptoms, constipation, diarrhea, weight loss, recurrent miscarriage, abnormal pap smears, infertility, osteoporosis, poor wound healing, and poor immune response. Patients with B_{12} deficiency may have few or subtle signs, or present with a wide variety of overt signs and symptoms that are easy to blame on other disorders, preexisting diseases and comorbid conditions.

PROBLEM 2: THE NAME "PERNICIOUS ANEMIA"

Many physicians fail to diagnose B_{12} deficiency because the name "pernicious anemia" is misleading. Physicians believe that to have B_{12} deficiency, a patient must have a macrocytic anemia. The name "pernicious anemia" was coined in 1872 by German physician Anton Biermer, over fifty years before vitamin B_{12} was discovered. The medical community has kept the name for historical purposes, adding to the confusion for today's practicing physician.

PROBLEM 3: PRACTICE MISTAKES OF THE PAST

There are other historical reasons, too, for doctors' failure to diagnose B$_{12}$ deficiency. Many physicians remember the days when thousands of patients got B$_{12}$ shots whether they needed them or not. Their justified scorn for this practice leads them to overreact now by making the opposite mistake: failing to realize that B$_{12}$ deficiency is, indeed, a real, common, and serious medical disorder.

When diagnosis-related groups (DRGs) came about in the early 1980s, physicians who billed for B$_{12}$ shots had to prove that their patients had "pernicious anemia" or another medical reason for their malabsorption syndrome, or the doctors could be accused of fraud. Because many physicians weren't testing their patients for B$_{12}$ deficiency to begin with, they discontinued using B$_{12}$ injections for fear of legal consequences.

Some of these doctors had created more revenue for their practice by administering cheap B$_{12}$ shots and then billing patients' insurance. Many of them stopped B$_{12}$ treatment because they equated B$_{12}$ therapy with placebo, having only given the shots to make money. Unknowingly, these physicians had been doing many patients some good (those with a true B$_{12}$ deficiency), while the others were not harmed. But the practice has unfortunately given vitamin B$_{12}$ a bad name within medical circles.

PROBLEM 4: DANGEROUSLY LOW VALUES FOR THE SERUM B$_{12}$ TEST

Another problem is the serum B$_{12}$ test itself. Even when physicians do consider B$_{12}$ deficiency as a diagnostic possibility, they tend to treat only when a patient's serum B$_{12}$ is under 200 pg/ml—and often they wait for it to drop below 180 pg/ml, the lower limit of some B$_{12}$ assays.

These "normal" lower limits are considered by many experts to be far too low. Setting the "normal" cutoff for serum B$_{12}$ at less than 200 pg/ml translates into poor patient health, neurological changes, and possibly injury or disability. It also increases costs by forcing clinicians to order more expensive tests to "prove" a patient's deficiency. These additional tests (MMA, Hcy, holo-TC), however, are not "gold standard" tests. What we see in our own practices, and what the medical literature shows, is that the MMA, Hcy, and even the holo-TC have their own limitations. They not only increase costs but can actually confuse the diagnosis, delaying treatment and possibly causing physicians to stop treatment that has already been started.

INTERPRETING B$_{12}$ VALUES

Physicians need to be aware that in some research studies, B$_{12}$ values are measured in picomoles per liter (pmol/L)*, while clinical laboratories express values in picograms per milliliter (pg/ml) or nanograms per liter (ng/L). The conversions are as follows:

pmol/L = pg/ml x 0.738 -> 200 pg/ml = 148 pmol/L

pg/ml = pmol/L ÷ 0.738 -> 450 pg/ml = 332 pmol/L

ng/L = pg/ml = 200 ng/L -> 200 pg/ml

*Some other countries use pmol/L versus pg/ml for the serum B$_{12}$ test depending on the assay used.

PROBLEM 5: CONFUSION REGARDING *SUBCLINICAL* VERSUS *CLINICAL* B$_{12}$ DEFICIENCY

Reviewing the medical literature, we observe "experts" in B$_{12}$ deficiency, as well as officials at the CDC, describing *subclinical* and *clinical* vitamin B$_{12}$ deficiency. The problem is that these "experts"[4] are not following the proper definitions of *subclinical* and *clinical*, which is causing confusion, late diagnosis, and misdiagnosis of vitamin B$_{12}$ deficiency.

The definition of subclinical disease is: *"An illness that stays below the surface of clinical detection. A subclinical disease has no recognizable clinical findings. It is distinct from a clinical disease, which has signs and symptoms that can be recognized."*[5] The CDC report confuses this issue, writing, "Although most health care providers already recognize the occasional person who presents with obvious signs and symptoms, they are far less likely to screen and diagnose the majority of patients who have a subclinical or mildly symptomatic vitamin B$_{12}$ deficiency."[6]

This quote contains several errors. First, overt B$_{12}$ deficiency is not an "occasional" problem. Second, we commonly see physicians failing to diagnose patients with obvious clinical signs and symptoms. And the CDC refers to "subclinical or mildly symptomatic vitamin B$_{12}$ deficiency," but it can't be both—subclinical is *without* symptoms. Therefore, mildly symptomatic patients have clinical disease, no matter how the medical community tries to minimize their symptoms.

In the ED, we test patients who are symptomatic. This is the way most clinicians practice. Of course, there will be patients who need to be screened if they are at risk (due to gastric bypass, Crohn's disease, or a vegetarian diet, for example), but often even these "at risk" patients have signs and symptoms of B$_{12}$ deficiency when a complete history and physical is obtained. It is a mistake for the clinician to fail to recognize the neuropsychiatric signs and symptoms of B$_{12}$ deficiency, and then label patients as *subclinical* and withhold treatment, when the serum B$_{12}$ is found to be low or in the gray zone. Simply put, if patients have signs and symptoms of B$_{12}$ deficiency, they have clinical, not subclinical disease.

Hematologist Asok Antony, an authority on B$_{12}$ deficiency, notes, "What has been termed a subclinical state of vitamin B$_{12}$ deficiency should be revisited in the light of the availability of far more sophisticated questionnaires, instruments, and other methods use to test brain function. Investigators have consistently found abnormalities in electroencephalography, evoked potentials, and P300 event-related potentials (electric signals from the brain that are found during the performance of various cognitive tasks and measured as an electrophysiologic marker of cognitive ability) in one-half or more of those with metabolically defined mild preclinical cobalamin deficiency. In most cases these abnormalities were reversed with cobalamin therapy, which supported the hypothesis of a causal relation."[7]

PROBLEM 6: POTENTIALLY HARMFUL GUIDELINES FROM LEADING MEDICAL AUTHORITIES

The CDC's report on B$_{12}$ contains some additional errors that can easily misguide the clinician. It states, "…all patients with *unexplained* hematologic or neurologic signs or symptoms should be evaluated for a vitamin B$_{12}$ deficiency." Many clinicians will interpret this statement to mean that patients with "explained" signs or symptoms—for example, neuropathy attributed to diabetes, anemia related to iron deficiency, or dementia related to Alzheimer's disease—don't need to be tested. This is harmful advice, because it doesn't take into account the fact that B$_{12}$ deficiency may be the actual cause of the signs and symptoms, but can also coexist with other conditions and will only worsen if left undiscovered.

The CDC report also states, "The Hcy and MMA can be used to confirm B$_{12}$ deficiency in cases with ambiguous initial results because metabolic changes often precede low cobalamin levels." Again, based on this statement, many physicians may assume that a patient does not need to be treated if these tests are normal. The MMA and Hcy, however, are not gold standard tests (see pages 216–217). Patients who are symptomatic and have serum B_{12} levels that are low or in the gray zone need to be treated, regardless of the MMA and Hcy results.[8,9,10]

The CDC report goes on to say, "Vitamin B_{12} deficiency is simple to prevent and simple to treat, but the diagnosis is easy to miss and is often overlooked in the outpatient setting."[11] This is true, but we would counter that B_{12} deficiency is easy to recognize when clinicians are educated about the signs and symptoms. Additionally, the CDC forgot to note the fact that B_{12} deficiency is often overlooked in inpatient settings as well.

Lastly, the report claims, "Clinical vitamin B_{12} deficiencies are relatively rare."[12] We couldn't disagree with this statement more. We do wonder if the CDC, along with many B_{12} experts and everyday clinicians, thinks of "clinical B_{12} deficiency" only in terms of subacute combined degeneration of the spinal cord or severe macrocytic anemia requiring blood transfusions—both severe complications due to chronic misdiagnosis—rather than thinking of B_{12} deficiency in its earlier stages, when symptoms are potentially reversible.

PROBLEM 7: LACK OF A UNIVERSALLY ACCEPTED SCREENING PROTOCOL FOR VITAMIN B_{12} DEFICIENCY

Can you imagine what it would be like if we didn't have an accepted protocol for chest pain? If clinicians only contemplated cardiac complaints in men with "crushing" chest pain radiating down the left arm? Many patients with indigestion or women with vague upper abdominal pain would be missed.

Today, our treatment of chest pain has evolved to the point where we appreciate the wide variety of symptoms that can occur in acute coronary syndrome and acute myocardial infarction. What is long overdue is a similar protocol for recognizing and treating B_{12} deficiency.

Physicians and other health care professionals are failing to address B_{12} deficiency, ignoring patients' symptoms, and discharging these patients without diagnosing the cause of their symptoms. This is dangerous, especially for elderly patients who are at high risk for fall-related trauma when discharged home with B_{12} deficiency.

For example, one elderly woman broke her leg and was sent to rehabilitation. She returned to the ED two weeks later after

> Can you imagine what it would be like if we didn't have an accepted protocol for chest pain? What is long overdue is a similar protocol for recognizing and treating B_{12} deficiency.

she suffered another fall and broke her other leg. At this point, she was found to be severely B_{12} deficient. Clearly, this woman hadn't suddenly developed severe B_{12} deficiency. Instead, her condition had been worsening over an extended period of time. If she had been worked up by her internist or other specialists as an outpatient (or even during her last hospitalization), her injuries could have been prevented.

Orthopedic surgeons must also get involved, because not only does B_{12} deficiency cause falls, but fractured bones will not mend properly when B_{12} deficiency is present (see Chapter 2). Doctors may assume that their patients' poor outcomes, including an inability to stand, balance themselves, or walk, are due to age, debility, or other conditions. Many times, however, these problems simply stem from chronically untreated B_{12} deficiency. We need to address B_{12} deficiency in healthcare using a team approach.

PROBLEM 8: OUTDATED TREATMENT PROTOCOLS

The last problem we need to address is that B_{12} treatment has been miserly. Treatment protocols were developed more than fifty years ago, establishing which form of B_{12} to use, the frequency at which to treat, and which route to select. However, researchers at that time were more focused on resolving the hematologic picture than the neuropsychiatric symptoms. This is why treatment with injections is performed monthly.

Patients often complain that monthly injections are not enough, but clinicians typically disregard their reports and complaints, believing their problems are "all in their heads." Instead, we need to approach B_{12} treatment using a collaborative approach with our patients. This is no different than a patient being placed on a psychotropic medication. The patient is started on the lowest dose, and the dose is then titrated over time based on the patient's progress. The titration of dose and frequency continues until an optimal level is reached.

B_{12} therapy should be approached in the same manner. Some patients will require more frequent dosing, while others may do fine with monthly shots. We often find that bi-monthly subcutaneous injections or even weekly injections are better tolerated as maintenance therapy. These injections can be self-administered by patients themselves or by a reliable family member.

Unfortunately, many physicians prescribe B_{12} even more cautiously than they prescribe narcotics or controlled substances, hesitating to give

B_{12}-deficient patients more than a minimal dosage. Ironically, we see clinicians prescribe narcotics without hesitation for patients who are highly symptomatic for B_{12} deficiency. Unlike narcotics, B_{12} is not addictive, does not impair patients when they are driving, working or operating machinery, and does not cause social or other health problems.

The combined result of the eight factors we've discussed here is that millions of patients, both young and old, suffer because their physicians miss an easy diagnosis or prescribe incorrect treatment. Patients with symptoms, no matter how slight, need to be tested. Early and aggressive treatment is key to preventing devastating neurologic injury. We encourage physicians to become educated on the neurologic presentation of B_{12} deficiency and actively use the Cobalamin Deficiency Criteria List (see Appendix M) to evaluate patients.

B_{12}'S CRUCIAL ROLES

Very few doctors are aware of the full range of problems that can stem from B_{12} deficiency, and we frequently encounter skepticism when we tell physicians that their patients' low B_{12} levels could be responsible for symptoms as diverse as dementia, heart disease, muscle weakness, radiculopathy, and infertility. But deficient B_{12} levels can indeed affect almost every system of the body, because cobalamin plays an integral role in a wide range of neurologic, hematologic, immunologic, metabolic, vascular, and reproductive functions, including the following:

- the division of all cells.

- numerous enzymatic reactions.

- the synthesis of nucleic acids, the transmethylation of amino acids, and the metabolism of carbohydrates and fatty acids.

- maintenance of a healthy nervous system (peripheral nerves, spinal cord, and brain).

- maintenance of a healthy immune system.

- the proper function of folic acid, because B_{12} allows folic acid to assist in the conversion of the amino acid homocysteine (Hcy) into the essential amino acid methionine. Elevated Hcy is both vasculotoxic and neurotoxic.

Because B$_{12}$ deficiency severely impairs many systems in the body, and because it is so easily treated, doctors should make it a point to routinely identify and treat its victims. This is particularly crucial now, as the "Baby Boomer" generation ages into its senior years—the years of highest risk for B$_{12}$-deficiency-related problems.

B$_{12}$ METABOLISM: A COMPLEX PATHWAY

In its natural state, cobalamin occurs only in animal products. Unlike other vitamins, this large molecule must undergo several major steps in the digestion process in order to be properly absorbed, and a breakdown can occur at any of the following stages:

- In the stomach, vitamin B$_{12}$ is released from its protein-bound state by pepsin. This step requires the acidic environment of a healthy stomach producing hydrochloric acid.

- The stomach's parietal cells also secrete intrinsic factor, which is required for B$_{12}$ absorption.

- Once vitamin B$_{12}$ is freed from its protein-bound state, it connects to salivary vitamin B$_{12}$ receptors, called cobalophilins, or R-binders.

- These complexes are further broken down in the duodenum by pancreatic proteases, which allow the released vitamin B$_{12}$ to attach to intrinsic factor.

- The vitamin B$_{12}$-intrinsic factor complex is then transported to the ileum (requiring the participation of free calcium). This complex adheres to receptors on the ileal cells and penetrates the mucosal wall.

- Free B$_{12}$ attaches to a plasma protein called transcobalamin II (TC II), which then is able to transport B$_{12}$ into the blood stream where it can be taken up by organs, bone marrow, and various cells of the body. Any excess is transported to the liver for storage.

The metabolism of B$_{12}$ is a complex and easily disrupted process, and a variety of problems—genetic, digestive, metabolic, surgical, dietary, pharmaceutical, autoimmune—can stop it in its tracks. This explains why cobalamin deficiency is so widespread, despite the ready availability of this vitamin in a typical diet.

How Common Is B$_{12}$ Deficiency?

In 2000, coauthor Jeffrey Stuart, D.O., conducted a retrospective study of all emergency department patients for whom he personally had ordered B$_{12}$ levels after observing possible risk factors for B$_{12}$ deficiency (see appendices O and P).

Dr. Stuart calculated the number of patients found to be B$_{12}$ deficient (Cbl level<180pg/ml), as well as those with levels between 180 and 211 pg/ml., and those termed in the "indeterminate range" of 212–350pg/ml. (He included the last range because hematology experts report that a significant number of patients in this range are deficient.[13] Some experts even advocate screening patients whose cobalamin levels are below 400pg/ml.[14])

The analysis included 302 patients. Of these, twenty-four (7.9 percent) were found to be overtly deficient, with levels of less than 180pg/ml. An additional sixteen (5.3 percent) patients were in the range of 180–211pg/ml and were also deficient. Finally, the 212–350 pg/ml range included ninety-one (30.1 percent) patients who warranted treatment. Thus, a total of 131 patients, or 43.3 percent of the total, had B$_{12}$ levels less than 350pg/ml. Notably, of this group, 30 percent were less than sixty years of age.

These findings are consistent with other studies showing that 15 to 20 percent of seniors are B$_{12}$-deficient, and that as many as 40 percent of hospitalized elderly patients have low or borderline serum B$_{12}$ levels.[15] Additionally, as we note in Chapter 1, more than 80 percent of long-term vegans who do not supplement their diets correctly, and over 50 percent of long-term vegetarians, show clear evidence of B$_{12}$ deficiency.[16,17] Additional evidence comes from the large-scale Framingham study, which found that nearly 40 percent of participants between the ages of twenty-six and eighty-three had plasma B$_{12}$ levels in the low-normal range—a level at which some people begin experiencing neurological symptoms.[18]

In Dr. Stuart's study, 13 percent of the symptomatic ED patients tested were under 200 pg/ml, which the CDC currently defines as a B$_{12}$ deficiency. More alarmingly, over 43 percent of symptomatic patients presenting to the ED were found to be under 350 pg/ml, which in our opinion (as well as that of many other experts) constitutes B$_{12}$ deficiency and warrants subsequent treatment.

WHO IS AT HIGHEST RISK?

If you're a physician who treats adult patients—no matter what your specialty is—odds are at least one of the patients you see this week will be at least moderately (and possibly severely) B$_{12}$-deficient. Even if you treat children or teens, your patient population almost undoubtedly includes some people at risk for B$_{12}$ deficiency.

B$_{12}$ deficiency can strike anyone, at any age, but some patients are at far greater risk than others. The majority of cases of B$_{12}$ deficiency stem from malabsorption disorders (see Chapter 2), and seniors are at highest risk because 30 to 40 percent of them have atrophic gastritis. This condition (as well as chronic proton pump inhibitor use) drastically reduces levels of stomach acid needed to free B$_{12}$ from animal proteins.

In addition, seniors often have unrecognized small intestinal bacterial overgrowth (SIBO), resulting in malabsorption and subsequent B$_{12}$ deficiency. SIBO has been reported to affect 15 to 50 percent of older adults. B$_{12}$ deficiency in this disorder is caused by the uptake of B$_{12}$ by microorganisms in the small intestine.[19]

However, malabsorption problems are also common in people of any age who have the following medical conditions (see Appendix A for a more complete list):

- Crohn's disease, blind loop syndrome, celiac disease, helicobacter pylori, or other digestive disorders
- a history of gastrointestinal surgeries, including surgery for weight loss, such as gastric bypass (see Chapter 10)
- a history of radiation treatment for GI, breast, or pelvic cancers

Another cause of B$_{12}$ deficiency is pernicious anemia (PA), in which an autoimmune process destroys the cells that produce intrinsic factor. PA can occur at any stage of life (one of the authors of this book was in her early twenties when she was diagnosed), but it is typically thought to develop in middle age or later. Although many doctors think of PA as a "northern European disease," recent studies show that it affects all ethnic groups. Genes play a strong role in PA, and immediate relatives of people with pernicious anemia have nearly twenty times the normal risk of developing the condition.[20]

A diet low in B_{12} can also cause deficiency, and it frequently does so even in people with no other risk factors. In fact, one at-risk group largely overlooked by doctors consists of health-conscious vegans, vegetarians, and followers of macrobiotic diets. Many of these people fail to take the proper amount of supplemental B_{12}; a number of others take spirulina or tempeh, supplements that are touted as being high in B_{12} but actually contain B_{12} analogues that block the absorption of cobalamin and cause falsely normal serum

> **If you're a physician who treats adult patients, odds are at least one of the patients you see this week will be B_{12} deficient.**

B_{12} levels on testing. Unless they are knowledgeable about B_{12} nutrition, vegans and vegetarians can easily become deficient, as can infants who are nursed by B_{12}-deficient vegan or vegetarian mothers. In these infants, B_{12} deficiency can manifest as developmental delay, autistic-like symptoms, motor problems, loss of language and social skills, or failure to thrive.

Infants also can develop B_{12} deficiency if their mothers have undiagnosed pernicious anemia, particularly if the mothers breast-feed. Children of mothers who have undergone gastric bypass are also high risk for a deficiency. But it is important to note that mothers who are B_{12}-deficient for *any* reason may produce B_{12}-deficient children.

In addition, some children suffer from inherited forms of B_{12} deficiency, which often manifest early in life and can rapidly become fatal (see Chapter 12). In these cases, it is important to determine which genetic error is present in order to treat patients properly. (For instance, orotic aciduria is a genetic disorder of pyrimidine metabolism and patients present with megaloblastic anemia. This disorder does not respond to treatment with B_{12} or folic acid, but is treated with oral uridine). Immediate treatment for any inborn error needs to be started to prevent permanent mental retardation or death.

Inherited defects are usually, but not always, obvious during infancy. Some are not apparent until early childhood, when they can take the form of developmental delays and can be mistaken for autism (see chapter 12).

Surgical patients are another group at high risk of suffering debility due to B_{12} deficiency. Nitrous oxide, a commonly used anesthetic, inactivates methylcobalamin by inducing irreversible oxidation on the cobalt atom of vitamin B_{12}. This can cripple or kill patients who go into the operating room with low B_{12} stores—particularly if they undergo surgical procedures requiring several hours of nitrous oxide exposure. In one report, researchers found that the urinary MMA in one patient rose to 314 mcg/ml creatinine (normal is less than 3.8) after nitrous oxide exposure for eighty minutes.[21]

Due to the absence of preoperative B$_{12}$ testing and the high prevalence of B$_{12}$ deficiency, this problem is far more common than physicians realize. Doctors often fail to diagnose postsurgical B$_{12}$ deficiency, assuming that patients' weakness, paralysis, or other neuropsychiatric symptoms are unfortunate but unavoidable side effects of their surgeries. When patients are elderly, surgeons may tend to blame these symptoms on age rather than considering B$_{12}$ deficiency. A few physicians, aware of the harmful effects of nitrous oxide, have published their accounts in medical journals and have suggested administering B$_{12}$ shots prior to operations. This may protect patients in the short term, but it does not adequately protect at-risk patients who should be screened prior to surgery so they can receive appropriate long-term care if they prove to be B$_{12}$-deficient.

Dental patients can also become B$_{12}$-deficient after long procedures using nitrous oxide, and several cases involving dentists and dental assistants exposed to N$_2$O have been reported in the medical literature.[22] Physicians often forget to ask their patients about recent dental procedures (dental cleaning or surgeries) where N$_2$O could have been administered, causing or contributing to their patient's symptoms. Recreational users of nitrous oxide, a popular drug of abuse called "whip-its," can develop neurological problems and florid mental symptoms due to B$_{12}$ depletion, and physicians should suspect this problem in any teen or young adult patient who develops MS-like symptoms, numbness, weakness, visual disturbance, depression, psychosis, or other mental or neurological problems. Physicians need to ask about nitrous oxide use or abuse (whippets) as part of their routine history, especially when patients present with new psychiatric symptoms.

A number of prescription drugs, too, can deplete B$_{12}$ stores, particularly in older patients. Among the most common are proton pump inhibitors, metformin (Glucophage), H-2 blockers, antacids, anticonvulsants, some antibiotics, and colchicine. Nitric oxide and other nitrates (nitroprusside) oxidize B$_{12}$ and may also induce deficiency. In young and middle-aged women, birth control pills are a common culprit. (See Appendix A for a more complete list.)

B$_{12}$ DEFICIENCY AND VISION PROBLEMS

Research is desperately needed to document the incidence of B$_{12}$ deficiency in patients with visual defects. Visual field loss is often the initial manifestation of disorders involving the optic chiasm. There are multiple etiologies of chiasmal lesions (traumatic, congenital, iatrogenic, intrinsic, and extrinsic), but cases have been published in medical journals documenting B$_{12}$ deficiency as the cause of some of these chiasmal visual field defects (bitemporal hemianopsia or junction scotoma).[23]

For example, a twenty-nine-year-old female presented with bitemporal hemianopsia. She had normal MRI and CT scans and normal visual evoked potentials (VEP). B$_{12}$ deficiency was found to be the cause of her visual impairment.[24]

Some patients have experienced improvement and partial recovery of vision after B$_{12}$ therapy. John, a fifty-four-year-old male, was diagnosed with cortical basal ganglionic degeneration and had visual field loss. After B$_{12}$ treatment, his visual acuity improved by 80 percent.

In another case, Mary, an eighty-five-year-old female who had macular degeneration, was being followed due to worsening vision in her left eye. She was scheduled to have surgery, and came to have her vision rechecked before the operation. Mary's doctor was surprised. When she examined Mary's left eye, it had dramatically improved. What had changed Mary's condition? Four months previously, her underlying B$_{12}$ deficiency was finally diagnosed and treated. It wasn't her diabetes and old age causing the problem; it was an unidentified B$_{12}$ deficiency. How many more people like Mary are out there?

Most nutritional supplements prescribed to treat or prevent macular degeneration do not contain vitamin B$_{12}$, which many macular degeneration patients may actually need. Typical vitamins and other nutrients found in suggested retinal supplements are vitamins A, C, and E, zinc, copper and lutein.

SENSITIVE ADJUNCTIVE TESTS THAT AID IN DIAGNOSIS

As we noted earlier, the standard serum B$_{12}$ test may fail to identify some patients with low cobalamin levels. For example, patients with underlying liver disease, alcoholism, myeloproliferative disorders, lymphoma, or intestinal bacterial overgrowth often have falsely elevated serum B$_{12}$ levels. Also, as we've discussed, the lower limit for this test currently is far too low.

There are adjunctive tests that can aid in the diagnosis of B$_{12}$ deficiency. These include tests for urine and serum methylmalonic acid (MMA) and plasma homocysteine (Hcy), two metabolites that are biochemical markers of B$_{12}$-dependent enzyme activity. Because high levels of MMA and Hcy may indicate B$_{12}$ deficiency, these tests can sometimes help identify patients with a deficiency when serum B$_{12}$ levels fall within the "normal" range. Another test, the serum holotranscobalamin II (holo-TC), measures one of the binding proteins used to transport B$_{12}$ throughout the body. See Chapter 1, which details the pros and cons of each test.

In 2005, research began emerging that questioned the reliability of the serum MMA and plasma Hcy assays. In one paper, Ralph Green, M.D., Ph.D., reported, "The startling and disturbing findings in this study are that all assays showed considerable variability before any treatment was initiated and that the results of these assays taken singly or in combination often did not reliably predict or preclude a response to specific treatment with vitamin B$_{12}$. Taken at face value and given the general reliance placed on the clinical reliability of these tests for identification of cobalamin deficiency, these findings are extremely troubling." Over-diagnosis of B$_{12}$ deficiency is essentially innocuous; but as this report notes, "missed diagnosis is quite clearly, a matter of greater gravity, particularly since the risk of formidable devastation from neurologic damage that results from uncorrected cobalamin deficiency is preventable."[25] Green went on to say, "Many have come to accept at face value the glib messages and mantras conveyed by assay kit manufacturers and the enshrined dogmas that permeate the literature that the laboratory identification of clinically significant cobalamin deficiency is a 'cake walk.' Indeed, it may be time to carefully reassess a field that is perhaps in a state of confusion and disarray not dissimilar to what existed when radioassays were introduced to replace microbiologic assays for measuring B$_{12}$."[26]

Green suggested, "At this stage, it would be prudent to conclude that the currently available assays for identifying or excluding cobalamin deficiency, though potentially useful, should be used with full awareness of their possible limitations, at least until unresolved issues have been settled."[27] We couldn't agree more, and this is exactly why detailed histories, clinical exams, and ongoing research in B_{12} deficiency are critical.

One problem is that there is limited information on patients with clinical findings of B_{12} deficiency but normal serum B_{12} and metabolite levels. Lawrence Solomon, M.D., of Yale University Health Services, evaluated thirty-seven patients who responded to vitamin B_{12} therapy and found that pretreatment values of serum B_{12} and Hcy were normal in about 50 percent of the subjects and MMA values were normal in 25 percent.[28] Over the past several years, we have encountered similar patients, and have talked with other colleagues who express the same concerns.

"Moreover," Solomon said, "because studies from academic centers usually employed special diagnostic or research laboratory facilities, their findings may not be representative of those obtainable in other ambulatory care settings."[29]

Solomon performed a retrospective review of patients evaluated for B_{12} deficiency during a ten-year period at a staff model HMO using a national commercial laboratory. Initially, only patients with low serum B_{12} levels or elevated MMA/Hcy levels received therapeutic trials of B_{12}. "However," he reported, "in the seventh year of the study period, one patient with total absence of vibratory sensation in the ileac crest, knees, and ankles had complete recovery following two months of Cbl therapy despite normal Cbl, MMA and HCy levels. Thereafter, therapy was offered to all patients with hematologic or neurologic abnormalities consistent with Cbl deficiency, regardless of the results of screening studies."[30]

The results of this revised treatment approach were eye-opening. "If therapy had been restricted to symptomatic patients with *both* low or intermediate Cbl levels *and* increased metabolite values, 63 percent of responders would not have been treated," Solomon reported. "Twenty-five patients did not respond to treatment, including 5 of 11 patients (45 percent) with low Cbl, 22 of 49 patients (45 percent) with high MMA, and 13 of 30 patients (43 percent) with high HCys values. It is concluded that Cbl, MMA, and HCys levels fluctuate with time and neither predict nor preclude the presence of Cbl-responsive hematologic or neurologic disorders."[31]

This study illustrates why clinicians must take into account patients' subjective symptoms and clinical signs when forming a treatment plan. At this point, we believe the first step in diagnosing B$_{12}$ deficiency is to take a complete history and perform a thorough neurologic exam along with obtaining a serum B$_{12}$ level. The clinician should keep in mind the gray zone when interpreting the serum B$_{12}$ results. If patients are symptomatic and their serum B$_{12}$ is <200 pg/ml or falls in the gray zone (200–450pg/ml), treatment must be initiated.

We must point out that the Solomon study used the serum MMA rather than the urinary MMA. The urinary MMA is preferred, but it still has limitations. We have seen patients with normal urinary MMAs who nonetheless had dramatic responses to injectable B$_{12}$ therapy. (Interestingly, these adult patients' serum B$_{12}$ levels were low or in the gray zone.) We have also seen symptomatic children with elevated urinary MMAs, but normal or even high serum B$_{12}$ levels, who had a significant response to B$_{12}$ therapy. This suggests that "normal" serum B$_{12}$ for children may need to be even higher than for adults because of critical brain growth and development. Van Tiggelen found in adults that serum B$_{12}$ levels below 550 pg/ml were associated with low B$_{12}$ in cerebral spinal fluid (CSF). Repeated larger studies need to be done comparing serum B$_{12}$ with CSF B$_{12}$ to determine the optimal serum B$_{12}$ range.[32] (After a thorough review of the medical literature pertaining to the serum MMA and the urinary MMA/creatinine ratio tests, and after using both tests for more than ten years, we firmly believe that the urinary MMA is preferable, particularly for elderly patients or those with renal disease. The urinary MMA, unlike the serum MMA, is validated for screening senior populations, and clinicians can be confident that the results are not skewed due to hydration or renal status.)

At this time, because the lower limit for the serum B$_{12}$ test is too low, we recommend two options for clinicians: 1) clinical exam and use of the serum B$_{12}$ (treating symptomatic patients in the gray zone—B$_{12}$ < 450 pg/ml); or 2) clinical exam and use of both the serum B$_{12}$ and urinary MMA for patients who present with symptoms consistent with B$_{12}$ deficiency. If either test is abnormal (or the serum B$_{12}$ is in the gray zone), treatment needs to be initiated. Research is needed to determine if raising the lower limit of the serum B$_{12}$ test to 450 pg/ml or even 550pg/ml in adults would eliminate the need for these adjunctive tests.

Is the holotranscobalamin test better than the serum B_{12} or urinary MMA? A study from 2006 concluded that "HoloTC and total vitamin B_{12} have equal diagnostic accuracy in screening for metabolic vitamin B_{12} deficiency. Measurement of both holoTC and total vitamin B_{12} provides a better screen for vitamin B_{12} deficiency than either assay alone."[33] This is similar to what we have found with the urinary MMA and serum B_{12}.

According to John Dommisse, M.D., "The one major step that would bring B_{12} deficiency back into the mainstream of medicine and psychiatry would be the general recognition that the normal range should be regarded as 600 to 2000 pg/ml. Below 550 to 600pg/ml, deficiencies start to appear in the CSF, as shown by several papers over the past 20 to 30 years. Humans and other mammals are all born with serum levels of about 2000 pg/ml, which decline gradually throughout life." Dommisse further states, "In severe deficiencies (less than 300 or 400 pg/ml), it is best to start with B_{12} injections, which get the largest amount of B_{12} to the deficient tissues in the shortest time." Dommisse believes that once six to twelve weekly-to-twice-weekly 1,000 mcg injections are given, the route can be changed to high-dose oral tablets (2,000 to 2,500 mcg) twice daily, providing the patient has an intact terminal ileum (not resected, or damaged by Crohn's disease/terminal ileitis).[34] Dommisse states that older adults ought to have a level of at least 600 to 2,000 pg/ml. For children, he recommends a level of 1,000 to 2,000 pg/ml.

Dr. Joseph Chandy, a general practitioner from the U.K., has been researching and treating vitamin B_{12} deficiency since 1981. He recommends that B_{12} deficiency be diagnosed on the basis of signs and symptoms, clinical features, and family history, and we fully agree. He defines subtle deficiency as a serum B_{12} level between 300 and 450 pg/ml, intermediate deficiency as a level between 200 and 300 pg/ml, and severe deficiency as a level below 200 pg/ml. (Visit www.B12d.org to review "The Chandy Diagnostic Criteria.")

Which of your patients should receive screening for B_{12} deficiency? After years of clinical experience and research, as well as an extensive review of the literature, we developed the Cobalamin Deficiency Criteria List (CDCL) in 1999 as a screening tool for doctors and other health-care providers. We have updated it in 2010 (see Appendix M). The CDCL's point system allows physicians to estimate a patient's relative risk of B_{12} deficiency, defined as the Cobalamin Deficiency Risk (CDR) Score.

SERUM VITAMIN B$_{12}$

1. Cost-effective

2. New parameters are needed for accepted lower-limit

3. Clinicians need to treat symptomatic patients < 450 pg/ml

4. Can give false-negative results (elevated serum B$_{12}$ levels in the presence of deficiency) in patients with the following conditions:

   - active liver disease (hepatitis, alcoholism)

   - transcobalamin II deficiency

   - intestinal bacterial overgrowth

   - myeloproliferative disorders:

     - polycythemia vera

     - chronic myelogenous leukemia

     - acute promyelocytic leukemia

     - chloral hydrate medication

     - lymphoma

5. Can give false-positive results (low serum B$_{12}$ levels in the absence of deficiency) in patients with the following conditions:

   - folate deficiency

   - pregnancy (although we question the validity of this finding, because it is possible that B$_{12}$ deficiency is under-recognized in pregnancy)

   - multiple myeloma

   - excessive vitamin C intake

   - transcobalamin I deficiency

URINARY MMA/CREATININE RATIO TEST

1. Typically elevated in vitamin B$_{12}$ deficiency

2. Elevated in some inborn errors of B$_{12}$ metabolism

3. Adjusts for poor renal function

4. Adjusts for hypovolemia/dehydration

5. Non-invasive

6. No fasting required (spot urine)
7. Cost-effective

SERUM MMA

1. Sometimes elevated in vitamin B_{12} deficiency
2. Elevated in certain inborn errors of B_{12} metabolism
3. Falsely high in renal insufficiency
4. Falsely high in intravascular volume depletion
5. Twelve-hour fasting required
6. Invasive
7. Less sensitive and specific than urinary MMA

PLASMA HOMOCYSTEINE

1. Sometimes elevated in vitamin B_{12} deficiency
2. Elevated in folate deficiency
3. Elevated in vitamin B_6 deficiency
4. Elevated in renal insufficiency
5. Elevated in intravascular volume depletion
6. Elevated in chronic diseases (hypothyroidism, systemic lupus erythematosus, severe psoriasis, some cancers, renal failure)
7. Elevated with the use of specific medications (Dilantin, Tegretol, nitrous oxide, methotrexate, lipid-lowering drugs [colestipol and niacin in combination with thiazide diuretics], estrogen-containing oral contraceptives)
8. Elevated in inherited errors of methionine metabolism:
   - cystathionine ß-synthase deficiency
   - methionine synthase deficiency
   - methylenetetrahydrofolate reductase deficiency
9. Elevated in certain inborn errors of B_{12} metabolism
10. Twelve-hour fasting required
11. Invasive

The History of the Urinary MMA

By 1967, researchers knew that elevated urinary MMA revealed B$_{12}$ deficiency. However, because testing for urinary MMA was laborious and time-consuming at that time, urinary MMA was not adopted as a clinical procedure.

What clinicians needed was a sensitive and rapid test measuring MMA in the urine—a test that was developed in 1982 by researcher Eric J. Norman, Ph.D., in collaboration with the late Dr. M. Drue Denton and coworkers at the Hematology Division of the University of Cincinnati College of Medicine. Dr. Norman's laboratory team developed an assay for urinary MMA using a gas chromatography/mass spectrometric (GC/MS) method that was fast, sensitive, and reproducible. In tests involving nearly 2,000 subjects with megaloblastic anemia, other anemias, elevated red cell mean corpuscular volume, or unexplained neurologic disorders, the researchers found that the urinary MMA test was a better indicator of B$_{12}$ deficiency than the serum B$_{12}$, the Schilling test, and other basic hematologic tests. They also found that many patients without anemia had already suffered permanent neurologic disability due to a delay in diagnosis, stemming, in a number of cases, from the lack of accurate tests.

By 1985, the urinary MMA/creatinine ratio test was perfected, and Dr. Norman and his wife Claudia opened their own laboratory (Norman Clinical Laboratory) to provide B$_{12}$ screening. Around this time a separate research group, studying Dr. Norman's data and research, analyzed stored blood samples from patients with pernicious anemia and other types of B$_{12}$ deficiency and concluded that MMA testing was superior to serum B$_{12}$ tests. The results of this study (using blood rather than urine) were published in the *New England Journal of Medicine* in 1988.[35] This study's conclusions began to dominate medical practice, even though the serum MMA was actually inferior. Dr. Norman explains, "MMA is concentrated about 40-fold in the urine over serum, therefore temporary fluctuations may affect the serum test more." Despite this early confirmation of the value of the urinary MMA, the medical community has made only minimal use of this screening tool—but interestingly endorses the less accurate serum MMA and Hcy tests. In 1993, an 809-patient study funded by the NIH documented the usefulness of the urinary MMA, yet it is ignored.[36]

RECOMMENDED B$_{12}$ DEFICIENCY TREATMENT PROTOCOL

There are three forms of supplemental vitamin B$_{12}$: cyanocobalamin, hydroxocobalamin, and methylcobalamin. (We will review the advantages and disadvantages of the different forms later in this chapter.) Different recommendations exist for initial and maintenance vitamin B$_{12}$ therapy. Here is the most commonly used protocol, but one that we feel should be updated to reflect current knowledge:

OLD TREATMENT PROTOCOL:

- Initial intramuscular injections of vitamin B$_{12}$, 1,000 mcg daily or every other day for five to seven days, followed by

- Intramuscular injections of 1,000 mcg weekly for four weeks, followed by

- Maintenance intramuscular injections of 1,000 mcg every month. This maintenance therapy must be life-long.

Under the regimen outlined above, hematologic improvements typically commence within five to seven days, and the deficiency should resolve after three to four weeks of therapy. If the B$_{12}$ deficiency has been long-standing, and neurological manifestations are present, it can take six months or longer before signs of improvement appear. In cases where neurologic signs and symptoms have been present for a year or longer, or where impairment is severe, neurologic damage may be permanent. Overall, neurological symptoms are completely resolved in about half of cases, while residual deficits remain in the other half; however, nearly all patients improve to some degree.

NEWER TREATMENT PROTOCOL:

Today, maintenance therapy should be titrated based on a patient's response to treatment. It is important to remember that 80 percent of the injected cyanocobalamin dose is excreted within the first twenty-four hours. G. Richard Lee, M.D., notes in *Wintrobe's Clinical Hematology* that a single injection, even of massive amounts of B$_{12}$, is not sufficient to replenish body stores. This is because the body's ability to retain the injected B$_{12}$ is limited. Thus, he writes, "If greater than 1 mg of B$_{12}$ is to be stored, several injections separated by at least twenty-four hours need to be administered, rather than a single dose." Lee also notes that some people are "short responders" whose serum B$_{12}$ concentrations may drop to dangerously low levels within two weeks of an injection.[37]

Therefore, B$_{12}$ injections need to be individualized. Some patients do well on monthly injections; however, many will do better with bi-monthly or even weekly injections. There is no harm in giving B$_{12}$ more frequently. Actually, it makes more sense to maintain a steady state, rather than waiting thirty days between injections, creating periods of relative deficiency. We recommend teaching patients, or willing family members, to administer subcutaneous injections (similar to diabetics administering insulin). This will save time for the patient and physician, as well as money for the patient. Most patients will be able to tell how long a B$_{12}$ injection is effective and, along with their physician, can adjust the interval accordingly. The old protocol of monthly injections is simply out of date and does not sufficiently benefit patients.

It is important to note that the toxicity of vitamin B$_{12}$ is nil, except for extremely rare allergic reactions. The only exception, discussed later in this chapter, involves patients with Leber's hereditary optic neuropathy, a very uncommon disease in which the use of cyanocobalamin is contraindicated.

B$_{12}$ is safe, water-soluble, and non-toxic. To further illustrate its safety, examine the treatment for cyanide poisoning, which uses hydroxocobalamin. The protocol calls for five grams of hydroxocobalamin (five thousand times the amount of a single 1,000 mcg B$_{12}$ shot) diluted in 150ml of normal saline and infused intravenously over 15 minutes. The dose can be repeated in thirty minutes if needed.

WHICH FORM OF COBALAMIN IS BEST?

Current evidence indicates that hydroxocobalamin is superior to cyanocobalamin, and methylcobalamin may be superior to hydroxocobalamin for neurologic disease. Lee notes in *Wintrobe's Clinical Hematology*, "The initial retention of hydroxocobalamin is better than that of cyanocobalamin; twenty-eight days after injection, retention still is nearly three times greater. In addition, hydroxocobalamin is more available to cells and is processed more efficiently by them."[38]

Methylcobalamin (available at compound pharmacies, with or without preservatives) is not widely used in the United States, but Japanese studies indicate that it is even more effective in treating the neurological sequelae of B_{12} deficiency. Its greater efficacy presumably stems, at least in part, from the fact that, like hydroxocobalamin, it does not need to be decyanated. In addition, unlike either hydroxocobalamin or cyanocobalamin, it does not need to be reduced to the (+1) state (the only form that can cross the blood-brain barrier).* Thus, it bypasses several potentially problematic steps in B_{12} metabolism. Furthermore, methylcobalamin provides the body with methyl groups essential for various biological oxidation-reduction reactions. Studies show that a small oral dose of methylcobalamin results in a greater accumulation of cobalamin in the liver than an oral dose of cyanocobalamin, and that methylcobalamin is retained approximately three times longer in tissues than cyanocobalamin.

Some concerns have been raised about using a cyanide-based vitamin B_{12} derivative. Patients with Leber's hereditary optic neuropathy (LHON) should *never* receive cyanocobalamin; LHON is associated with an inability to properly clear cyanide from the body, and there is evidence that the optic atrophy associated with LHON can be exacerbated by the administration of cyanocobalamin. (Hydroxocobalamin and methylcobalamin can, of course, be used to treat LHON patients, as they do not contain the cyano-group [cyanide]. In fact, there is evidence that some cases of optic neuropathy respond dramatically to hydroxocobalamin, which acts as a cyanide antagonist.)

People with hepatic dysfunction can also have elevated cyanide levels, and children with inborn errors of B_{12} metabolism may have a metabolic defect involving cyanide metabolism. Smokers, too, have elevated cyanide levels, and research shows that hydroxocobalamin injections can decrease smokers' blood cyanide levels by 59 percent; conversely, administration of cyanocobalamin could potentially raise the cyanide levels of smokers.[39]

Given the greater safety of hydroxocobalamin and methylcobalamin (both available in the U.S.) as well as their greater effectiveness, we agree with physician Steve Roach, who says, "I would not expect any adverse effects in most patients with either preparation [cyanocobalamin or

---

* Researchers have proposed that there are approximately four steps required to convert cyanocobalamin to the active coenzyme forms (methylcobalamin and adenosylcobalamin).[40] Methylcobalamin is found in blood plasma, cerebral spinal fluid, and the cytosol of cells. Adenosylcobalamin predominates in cellular tissues, where it is retained in the mitochondria. If there is a defect not allowing the conversion of cyanocobalamin to methylcobalamin, B_{12} is not in its usable form, and is limited or unusable in the blood plasma, cerebral spinal fluid, and the cytosol of cells.

225

hydroxocobalamin]. However, it seems wise to avoid a potentially harmful form of a drug when the more physiologic variety is available and is excreted at a more desirable rate."[41]

More importantly, studies have demonstrated that hydroxocobalamin is superior to cyanocobalamin. One study concluded, "After intramuscular injection of about 1 mg CN-B$_{12}$ and OH-B$_{12}$, normal subjects excreted within 24 hours about 80 per cent and about 25 per cent, respectively, in the urine. This corresponds to a retention of about 20 per cent CN-B$_{12}$ compared with about 75 per cent OH-B$_{12}$. These two factors—greater binding to the serum proteins and slower diffusion of non-bound OH-B$_{12}$—reduce glomerular filtration and must be considered the main explanation why far less of injected OH-B$_{12}$ than of injected CN-B$_{12}$ is lost in the urine."[42]

In light of the current evidence, we recommend hydroxocobalamin over cyanocobalamin for the treatment of typical pernicious anemia patients, as well as patients with neurologic symptoms resulting from delayed diagnosis. Recent research has found that patients with neurologic involvement may benefit even more from high-dose methylcobalamin[43] (see Chapter 3).

No matter which form of cobalamin is used, it is crucial to inform any of your patients who need long-term treatment, such as those with autoimmune pernicious anemia or a history of gastric or ileal surgery, about the need to continue treatment for life. It is important, too, to provide them with documentation that will make it easier for them to obtain treatment in the future, if they need to switch doctors. Also, encourage the hospitals with which you are affiliated to develop protocols for effective B$_{12}$ screening and treatment (using hydroxocobalamin and methylcobalamin). B$_{12}$ deficiency is a public health crisis, and it is crucial, particularly as the huge Baby Boomer generation ages, that we develop appropriate standards of care in order to acknowledge, address, and handle this crisis.

> We recommend hydroxocobalamin over cyanocobalamin for the treatment of B$_{12}$ deficiency.

THE ORAL VERSUS INJECTED ISSUE

There are studies noting that high-dose oral cyanocobalamin (1,000–2,000 mcg daily) is equivalent to cyanocobalamin injections. A recent U.S. study, for example, demonstrated that daily high-dose oral B$_{12}$ (2,000 mcg) was as effective in producing hematologic and neurologic responses as a standard injectable regimen in patients with B_{12} deficiency. This study strongly supports the view that oral B_{12} at doses of 2,000 mcg can replace injection therapy in *some* situations. Although this was a very small study with only thirty-three patients, it used serum MMA and Hcy markers, demonstrating a reduction in these metabolites.[44]

This study is consistent with findings from the 1950s and 1960s, which showed that 1 percent of the oral B_{12} dose consumed is absorbed by an alternate pathway, via passive diffusion throughout the small intestine, in the presence of intrinsic factor or a functioning terminal ileum. It also is consistent with clinical practice in Sweden, where oral B_{12} maintenance therapy has been used for more than twenty-five years.

We believe, however, that additional research is needed to confirm the efficacy and safety of oral B_{12} for patients whose deficiencies stem from a variety of etiologies. Studies need to be conducted comparing oral methylcobalamin to oral cyanocobalamin, and comparing injectable hydroxocobalamin and methylcobalamin to oral and injectable cyanocobalamin. It is also important to note that oral and sublingual B_{12} formulations are not regulated by the Food and Drug Administration.

Emmanuel Andres, M.D., noted recently in the *Annals of Pharmacotherapy*, "As Lane and Rojas-Fernandez demonstrated, to date only case reports or small studies have focused on oral vitamin B_{12} therapy for the treatment of cobalamin deficiencies. Thus, the ideal doses of oral cobalamin and treatment duration remain to be determined.... In several studies, cobalamin deficiency is not well established, be it low serum vitamin B_{12} concentrations or true cobalamin deficiency with biological or clinical features; nor is the etiology known, be it nutritional deficiency, pernicious anemia, or food-cobalamin malabsorption. To our knowledge, these limitations involve major difficulties with interpretation of the data."[45] Lane and Rojas-Fernandez concluded in their summary, "There are inadequate data at the present time to support the use of oral cyanocobalamin replacement in patients with severe neurologic involvement."[46] We ourselves have seen cases in which injected B_{12} resulted in far greater benefits than oral supplementation.

It may be true that some cases of B_{12} deficiency caused by malabsorption can be treated with high-dose oral B_{12} (2,000 mcg daily). Unfortunately, doctors may fail to accurately determine which patients fall into this category, and the assumption that all elderly patients have B_{12}

deficiency caused by malabsorption will endanger those with other conditions. In addition, physicians prescribing oral B$_{12}$ must be aware that while the bottle label on B$_{50}$ complex says it contains 833 percent of the recommended daily intake, it contains only 50 mcg of B$_{12}$. Common "senior" multivitamins contain only 25 mcg of B$_{12}$, and typical adult multivitamins contain only 6 mcg. These amounts are grossly inadequate for patients who have malabsorption problems and need to ingest at least 2,000 mcg of oral B$_{12}$ daily.

Moreover, even in cases of malabsorption, some patients, especially those with neurologic symptoms, would benefit from having their stores rapidly replenished. Further, in cases involving patients who are non-compliant or suffer from memory problems or mental illness, injections administered in the office or by a family member are far more reliable than oral supplements which patients may forget to take. Also, some patients object to taking an increased number of pills, while others have problems swallowing tablets, or have sensitive stomachs and can easily be nauseated by oral supplements. (High-dose sublingual B$_{12}$ may be an option for these patients.)

With the development of virtually painless microfine needles, the only significant problem associated with injected B$_{12}$—injection pain—has been greatly reduced. Moreover, patients can easily learn to inject themselves, making injected B$_{12}$ much less expensive than other formulations (oral, nasal, transdermal patches, and creams—see Chapter 13). And the efficacy of injections has been well studied, which is not the case for many over-the-counter B$_{12}$ products.

The argument for injections is simple: Given that injectable B$_{12}$ is safe, effective, inexpensive, and virtually painless, why take a chance on oral formulations that may not be as effective? In cases of B$_{12}$ deficiency due solely to an inadequate diet, however, oral supplementation is, of course, effective, once normal B$_{12}$ levels have been reestablished and any other reasons for the deficiency have been carefully ruled out.

One final note: It's important to remember that patients prescribed *any* form of B$_{12}$ treatment must be monitored for efficacy, symptom resolution, or failed treatment response.

AN OBLIGATION FOR ALL SPECIALTIES

We're often told, as emergency department (ED) staff, that B_{12} testing is inappropriate in our setting. Yet a significant percentage of our "repeaters"—the patients who come in month after month suffering from mental status changes, syncope, chest pain, anemia, weakness, dizziness, or fractures caused by falls—have been found to be grossly B_{12} deficient. Health care providers need to realize that their patients may indeed be suffering from a B_{12} deficiency which is causing or exacerbating their health problems.

We believe that the ED is an appropriate place for B_{12} testing. We have an ethical obligation to rule out B_{12} deficiency in ED patients who present with signs and symptoms, or are at high risk. We and our colleagues have saved the health and lives of many patients by doing this, so we encourage ED staff to order tests when indicated.

Ideally, however, this diagnosis should occur in the office of a primary care physician or specialist who can provide long-term follow-up. B_{12} deficiency is a problem that should be identified and treated long before it causes symptoms serious enough to require emergency care. In the great majority of cases, B_{12} deficiency develops slowly and can easily be diagnosed months or even years before it causes painful or dangerous symptoms. But until primary care doctors, internists, and other specialists become reeducated and change their practice, emergency medicine physicians must step up and assist in combating this epidemic.

Early diagnosis and treatment can become the norm if doctors in every specialty take responsibility for identifying patients deficient in B_{12}. The neurologist or neurosurgeon whose patient complains of dizziness or neuropathy or pain; the psychiatrist whose patient is depressed or paranoid or psychotic; the gynecologist whose patient continues to have abnormal Pap smears or infertility; the gastroenterologist caring for patients with Crohn's disease, celiac disease, GERD, or other GI disorders; the cardiologist treating patients with heart attacks, congestive heart failure, and hyperhomocystinemia; the endocrinologist who sees patients with thyroid and other autoimmune disorders, and patients with neuropathy seemingly related to diabetes; the orthopedic surgeon who treats patients with fall-related fractures; the anesthesiologist treating chronic pain and fibromyalgia, or administering nitrous oxide to at-risk patients; the pediatrician or pediatric neurologist treating children with mental retardation, cerebral palsy, developmental delay, or symptoms resembling autism—all must realize that B$_{12}$ testing is a crucial part of a thorough workup.

Very rarely in medicine can such a severely debilitating and potentially life-threatening disorder be so easily diagnosed, and so easily and inexpensively treated. The doctor who fails to screen patients with suspicious symptoms or histories consistent with B$_{12}$ deficiency will indeed save a few minutes, and one to two hundred dollars worth of tests in the short run, but he or she will almost certainly be condemning some of these patients to severe, life-long debility—and condemning the health-care system to the financial burden of caring for them. Conversely, the wise doctor who remembers to include B$_{12}$ deficiency in a differential diagnosis whenever symptoms warrant will save both health-care dollars and patients' lives.

Moreover, doctors who look diligently for B$_{12}$ deficiency often save the lives of their own loved ones. One of us (J. S.), initially skeptical about routinely testing for B$_{12}$ deficiency, changed his mind when he discovered that it affected not just many of his patients but four members of his own family as well. Luckily, he diagnosed them in time to protect their health. Since then, we've convinced a number of colleagues to have relatives tested, and many have come back to us saying, "You were right, the tests showed B$_{12}$ deficiency—thank you!"

A thoracic surgeon, writing in the *Journal of the American Medical Association*, wasn't as lucky. His wife suffered severe and probably irreversible neurological symptoms, because a number of specialists missed her B$_{12}$ deficiency. "Her experiences with competent physicians at a major medical center convinced me that vitamin B$_{12}$ deficiency is not a benign condition, and it is not diagnosed easily by general physicians," he wrote.[47] But it *is* easy to diagnose. Unfortunately, it's also easily overlooked. Many physicians are failing not only their patients, *but even their own family members, friends, and colleagues.*

> Very rarely in medicine can such a severely debilitating and potentially life-threatening disorder be so easily diagnosed, and so easily and inexpensively treated.

In contrast, physicians willing to learn about this widespread problem and share their knowledge with others are our best hope for confronting the growing problem of B$_{12}$ deficiency. One of these doctors is David

QUESTIONS THAT NEED ANSWERS:

According to Asok C. Antony, M.D. of the Indiana University School of Medicine, who has published numerous articles regarding B_{12} deficiency, as well as authored chapters in hematology textbooks: "We still lack prospective trials to define the optimum diet for various at-risk populations.... The international nutrition community must take up the challenge posed by this body of evidence and enact practical steps to ensure parity in the vitamin B_{12} status of vegetarians and omnivores.... Clearly, recommendations for supplementation of vitamin B_{12} are not that easily implemented." Antony poses these questions for researchers:

"How can the conversion of vitamin B_{12} to inactive analogues as a result of multivitamin-mineral chemical interaction or interaction with foods and other nutrients be avoided?"

"Does the cooking of certain 'ethnic-specific' foods containing vitamin B_{12} lead to conversion to vitamin B_{12} analogues?"

"What is the influence of large-scale processing on the shelf life and subsequent bioavailability of foods fortified with vitamin B_{12}?"

"Worldwide, vegetarians number in the hundreds of millions," he states, "so public health initiatives that seek to improve the health of this population will have a global effect."[49]

Spence, M.D., who wrote in *The Lancet* [48] about his own misdiagnosis when he developed B_{12} deficiency. His neurologist, interpreting his B_{12} level as "normal" (his level was 200 pmol/L = 271 pg/ml; reference range 150–800 pmol/L), concluded that Spence's neuropathy and other marked neurological abnormalities stemmed from an old neck injury. Spence himself concluded that his troubling, unexplained neuropathy and myelopathy probably were due to an occult malignancy, and he spent six months worrying about this possibility.

By luck, however, Spence's personal interest and study regarding homocysteine and vascular disease led him to begin taking high-dose B vitamins, including 500 mcg of B_{12} daily, around this time. His lab results revealed that he had a high homocysteine level (a natural consequence of his undiagnosed B_{12} deficiency), and he was aware of the vitamin's effects in lowering homocysteine. When his neuropathy began improving, and when a follow-up test showed that his serum B_{12} level was still in the low normal range—at a time when it should have been very high due to the fairly high dose of oral B_{12} he was taking—the correct diagnosis dawned on him: "It was clear that I was malabsorbing vitamin B_{12}." As it turned out, his problem involved a defect of transcobalamin II, a protein needed to transport B_{12} once it crosses the ileal mucosa.

Spence now makes every effort to inform physicians about the widespread phenomenon of B_{12} deficiency and its consequences. "I am working on reducing the prevalence of this knowledge gap," he says, citing a quotation from Sir William Osler: "It is the obligation and the joy of the physician to be a perpetual student."

GENE MUTATIONS MAY CAUSE B₁₂ DEFICIENCY IN SOME PATIENTS

In addition to the many common causes of B_{12} deficiency, some patients may have mutations in genes encoding important proteins of the B_{12} metabolic pathway. These defects can be complete, causing death in infancy, or partial, with a delayed onset. N. Dali-Youcef and Emmanuel Andres wrote in the *Quarterly Journal of Medicine* 2009, "Mutations in genes encoding the intrinsic factor (GIF), cubilin, amnionless, transcobalamin II or its receptor provoke defects in cobalamin absorption and/or cellular uptake which translates into functional cobalamin deficiency and its clinical manifestations."[50]

Endocytic receptors and proteins are responsible for vitamin B_{12} intestinal absorption and transportation to the various cells of the body. Partial B_{12} errors and defects may not express themselves until young adulthood (similar to partial errors in Hcy metabolism causing early vascular disease). Partial gene defects in B_{12} metabolism may be the actual cause of many chronic debilitating neurologic disorders such as multiple sclerosis. This could explain why some patients clinically diagnosed with B_{12} deficiency have normal tests, yet respond greatly to B_{12} therapy.

We fully agree with Dali-Youcef and Andres, who concluded, "Many clinically diagnosed cobalamin deficiencies remain unexplained and molecular tools aimed at targeting genes involved in vitamin B_{12} absorption and cellular uptake signaling pathways will pave the way for new therapeutic approaches to efficiently treat functional cobalamin deficiency."[51]

Osler's quote is indeed apt, because the current epidemic of B_{12} deficiency presents physicians with both a tremendous obligation—the obligation to combat this epidemic—and a tremendous opportunity to conduct exciting research in an area of medicine that is in desperate need of more study. Indeed, it is remarkable, given the destruction that B_{12} deficiency wreaks on so many body systems (hematologic, neurologic, psychiatric, cardiovascular, reproductive, gastrointestinal, musculoskeletal) that so many questions about the disorder remain unanswered. Medical professionals interested in clinical or laboratory research would be well advised to aid in bridging this knowledge gap by making research on B_{12} deficiency a top priority.

Among the issues that researchers need to address are the following:

- What percentage of older adults who suffer fall-related trauma are B_{12} deficient?

- What percentage of elderly patients who fall and sustain fractures are B_{12} deficient?

- Should emergency departments and trauma centers include serum B_{12} testing for trauma patients (i.e., fall-related trauma, motor vehicle crashes) who are symptomatic or at risk for B_{12} deficiency? (We know first-hand the answer is yes!)

- What percentage of diabetics have peripheral neuropathy caused in part by B_{12} deficiency?

- What percentage of patients who experience transient ischemic attacks, strokes, chest pain, or congestive heart failure have underlying B_{12} deficiency?

- What percentage of patients diagnosed with dementia or Alzheimer's are actually deficient in B_{12}?

- What percentage of patients institutionalized or admitted to outpatient psychiatric facilities have B_{12} deficiency?

- Postoperative patients often suffer complications, ranging from weakness, paresthesias, or paralysis to depression and memory loss. How often are these symptoms due to untreated B_{12} deficiency which was exacerbated by exposure to nitrous oxide during surgery and/or increased metabolic demands and tissue repair after surgery?

- What is the rate of B$_{12}$ deficiency among infertile men and women? What percentage of women with abnormal Pap smears are B$_{12}$-deficient?

- What percent of AIDS patients with neuropathy or dementia actually have neurological symptoms due to untreated B$_{12}$ deficiency, a common condition in AIDS patients?

- How many motor vehicle accidents (particularly among the elderly) involve B$_{12}$ deficiency, which often causes confusion, dizziness, slowed reflexes, and neuropathy that can leave sufferers unable to control a vehicle's gas and brake pedals, or cause poor judgment behind the wheel?

- How many dialysis patients have B$_{12}$ deficiency? Does giving hydroxocobalamin or methylcobalamin (IM or IV) decrease these patients' elevated MMA and Hcy levels and aid in treating uremic neuropathy? (Recent studies indicate the answer is "yes."[52]) Early treatment in this group could be preventive as well as curative, because dialysis patients are at high risk for thrombotic events.

- How many children diagnosed with "autism" actually have an acquired B$_{12}$ deficiency, a defect in the transport of B$_{12}$, or an undiagnosed inborn error of B$_{12}$ metabolism?

We strongly encourage teaching hospitals and other medical facilities to put research into these issues at the very top of their "to do" lists. Answers to these critical questions will aid us in bringing the hidden epidemic of B$_{12}$ deficiency out into the open, identifying its victims, and offering them the help they so desperately need.

A QUIZ FOR PHYSICIANS: DID YOU KNOW THESE FACTS ABOUT VITAMIN B$_{12}$ DEFICIENCY?

1. Vitamin B$_{12}$ deficiency and/or pernicious anemia may be present without anemia or macrocytosis.

2. Vitamin B$_{12}$ deficiency and/or pernicious anemia may be present in patients with a normal CBC or a microcytic anemia.

3. Patients with B$_{12}$ deficiency have been misdiagnosed as having anemia of chronic disease and internal bleeding. After extensive testing

proves no bleeding has occurred, patients are given the diagnosis of "unexplained anemia."

4. In the past, by the time anemia was symptomatic, more than 80 percent of patients had neurologic manifestations, and in 50 percent this led to some permanent incapacity.

5. Patients have acquired permanent neurological damage because of delayed diagnosis or misdiagnosis of B_{12} deficiency.

6. Patients with B_{12} deficiency have been confined to wheelchairs or bedridden because of chronic misdiagnosis.

7. Permanent spastic gait or paralysis can result from misdiagnosed B_{12} deficiency.

8. Peripheral neuropathy occurs in about 25 percent of untreated patients.

9. Subtle changes in mental status are present in as many as two-thirds of patients before treatment is started.

10. Patients with vitamin B_{12} deficiency have been misdiagnosed with diabetic neuropathy.

11. Patients with B_{12} deficiency/pernicious anemia have been misdiagnosed with multiple sclerosis.

12. Patients with B_{12} deficiency have been misdiagnosed with dementia, requiring nursing home placement.

13. Patients with B_{12} deficiency have been misdiagnosed with psychiatric disorders.

14. Vitamin B_{12} deficiency is found in all ages, from infants to geriatrics, and in all ethnic groups.

15. Research indicates that B_{12} deficiency affects one of every seven seniors. Some studies indicate that the number is even higher, with up to 25 percent of the elderly suffering from undiagnosed B_{12} deficiency.

16. Emergency medicine physicians encounter undiagnosed or misdiagnosed B_{12}-deficient patients during nearly every shift in their current practice.

17. Vitamin B_{12} deficiency causes hyperhomocystinemia, which leads to an increased risk of strokes, MIs, DVTs, and PEs.

18. B_{12} deficiency causes dizziness, imbalance, and orthostatic hypotension.

19. Many elderly patients who have fallen and sustained fractures have been found to be B_{12}-deficient.

20. Patients administered nitrous oxide during surgery or dental procedures can have poor outcomes or even die if they have undiagnosed B_{12} deficiency preoperatively.

21. Patients two to six weeks post-op who complain of paresthesias, TIA symptoms, frequent falls, and/or mental status changes could have nitrous oxide-induced myelopathy due to undiagnosed B_{12} deficiency.

22. Vitamin B_{12} deficiency is easy to diagnose and inexpensive to treat, and testing is reimbursable.

23. Costly malpractice suits have resulted from failure to diagnose B_{12} deficiency.

24. Early diagnosis of B_{12} deficiency would save healthcare dollars by dramatically reducing ED, hospital, rehabilitation, home care, and nursing home usage.

25. Billions of dollars could be saved with early diagnosis.

26. There is a critical window of opportunity for treating B_{12} deficiency before irreversible neurological damage results.

27. The CDC reports that 1 out of every 31 Americans over age fifty has B_{12} deficiency. This report underestimates the incidence by using a serum B_{12} cut-off that is far too low.

28. The incidence of B_{12} deficiency in infants and young children is unknown, but the medical literature clearly shows that pediatric B_{12} deficiency is under-diagnosed.

CHAPTER 11 NOTES:

1. http://www.cdc.gov/ncbddd/b12/intro.html.

2. Dharmarajan, T. S., and Norkus, E. P. Approaches to vitamin B_{12} deficiency: Early treatment may prevent devastating complications. *Postgraduate Medicine* 2001;110(1); 99–105.

3. Ibid.

4. http://www.cdc.gov/ncbddd/b12/history.html.

5. MedicineNet.com.

6. http://www.cdc.gov/ncbddd/b12/intro.html.

7. Antony, A. C. Vegetarianism and vitamin B_{12} (cobalamin) deficiency. *American Journal of Clinical Nutrition*, Vol. 78, No. 1, 3–6, July 2003.

8. Green, R. Unreliability of current assays to detect cobalamin deficiency: "nothing gold can stay." *Blood*, 2005;105: 910–911.

9. Solomon, L. R. Cobalamin-responsive disorders in the ambulatory care setting: unreliability of cobalamin, methylmalonic acid, and homocysteine testing. *Blood* 2005;105:978–985.

10. Solomon, L. R. Disorders of cobalamin (Vitamin B_{12}) metabolism: emerging concepts in pathophysiology, diagnosis and treatment. *Blood* 2007;21:113–130.

11. http://www.cdc.gov/ncbddd/b12/summary.html.

12. http://www.cdc.gov/ncbddd/b12/history.html.

13. Antony, A. C. Megaloblastic anemias. In R. Hoffman et al. (3rd Ed.), *Hematology: Basic Principles and Practice* (pp. 457–467). 2000, Philadelphia: Churchill, Livingstone; and Savage, D. G., Lindenbaum, J., Stabler, S. P., and Allen, R. H. Sensitivity of serum methylmalonic acid and total homocysteine determinations for diagnosing cobalamin and folate deficiencies. *American Journal of Medicine* 1994, 96:239–246; and Norman, E. J., and Morrison, J. A. Screening elderly populations for cobalamin (vitamin B_{12}) deficiency using the urinary methylmalonic acid assay by gas chromatography mass spectrometry. *American Journal of Medicine* 1993, 94:589–594; and Stabler, S. P., Lindenbaum, J., and Allen, R. H. The use of homocysteine and other metabolites in the specific diagnosis of vitamin B_{12} deficiency. *Journal of Nutrition* 1996, 126:1266S–1272S.

14. Dharmarajan, T. S., Norkus, E. P. Approaches to vitamin B_{12} deficiency: Early treatment may prevent devastating complications. *Postgraduate Medicine* 2001;110(1); 99–105; and Snow, C. F. Laboratory diagnosis of vitamin B_{12} and folate deficiency. *Archives of Internal Medicine* 1999;159:1289–98.

15. Shahar, A., Feiglin, L., Shahar, D. R., Levy, S., and Seligsohn, U. High prevalence and impact of subnormal serum vitamin B_{12} levels in Israeli elders admitted to a geriatric hospital. *Journal of Nutrition, Health and Aging* 2001, 5(2):124–7.

16. Crane, M. G., Register, U. D., Lukens, R. H., and Gregory, R. Cobalamin (CBL) studies on two total vegetarian (vegan) families. *Vegetarian Nutrition: An International Journal* 1998, 2(3):87–92.

17. Bissoli, L., Di Francesco, V., Ballarin, A., Mandragona, R., Trespidi, R., Brocco, G., Caruso, B., Bosello, O., and Zamboni. Effect of vegetarian diet on homocysteine levels. *Annals of Nutrition and Metabolism* 2002, 46(2):73–9.

18. "B$_{12}$ deficiency may be more widespread than thought," USDA Agricultural Research Service, August 2, 2000.

19. Dharmarajan, T. S, Adiga, G. U, Norkus, E. P. Vitamin B$_{12}$ deficiency. Recognizing subtle symptoms in older adults. *Geriatrics* 2003;58:30–8.

20. Lee, G. R. Pernicious anemia and other causes of vitamin B$_{12}$ (cobalamin) deficiency. In G. R. Lee (10th Ed.), *Wintrobe's Clinical Hematology*, (pp. 941–958). 1999, Baltimore: Williams & Wilkins.

21. Kalikiri, P. C., and Sachan, R. S. G. S. Nitrous oxide induced elevation of plasma homocysteine and methylmalonic acid levels and their implications. *The International Journal of Anesthesiology* 2004, 8(2).

22. Ostreicher, D. S. Vitamin B$_{12}$ supplements as protection against nitrous oxide inhalation: *New York State Dental Journal* 1994, 60(3):47–9; and Quarnstrom, F. Nitrous oxide analgesia. What is a safe level of exposure for the dental staff? *Dentistry Today* 2002, 21(4):104–9.

23. Kowing, D., Kesler, E. Patient's B$_{12}$ deficiency causes chiasmal lesion. *Review of Optometry*, February 15, 2007.

24. Wilhelm, H., et al. Uncommon chiasmal lesions: demyelinating disease, vasculitis, and cobalamin deficiency. *German J Ophthalmol* (1993) 2:234–240.

25. Green, R. Unreliability of current assays to detect cobalamin deficiency: "nothing gold can stay." *Blood*, 2005;105: 910–911.

26. Ibid.

27. Ibid.

28. Solomon, L. R. Cobalamin-responsive disorders in the ambulatory care setting: unreliability of cobalamin, methylmalonic acid, and homocysteine testing. *Blood* 2005;105:978–985.

29. Ibid.

30. Ibid.

31. Ibid.

32. VanTiggelen, C. J. M. et al. Assessment of vitamin-B$_{12}$ status in CSF. *American Journal of Psychiatry* 141, 1:136–7, 1984.

33. Miller, J. W. Measurement of total vitamin B_{12} and holotranscobalamin, singly and in combination, in screening for metabolic vitamin B_{12} deficiency. *Clinical Chemistry* (2006) 52:2;278–285.

34. Dommisse, J. Subtle vitamin-B_{12} deficiency and psychiatry: a largely unnoticed but devastating relationship? *Medical Hypotheses* (1991) 34,131–140.

35. Lindenbaum, J., et al. Neuropsychiatric disorders caused by cobalamin deficiency in the absence of anemia or macrocytosis. *New England Journal of Medicine* 1988, 318:1720–8.

36. Norman, E. J., Morrison, J. A. Screening elderly populations for cobalamin (vitamin B_{12}) deficiency using the urinary methylmalonic acid assay by gas chromatography mass spectrometry. *The American Journal of Medicine* (1993) 94,589–594.

37. Lee, G. R. Pernicious anemia and other causes of vitamin B_{12} (cobalamin) deficiency. In G. R. Lee (10th Ed.), *Wintrobe's Clinical Hematology*, (pp. 941–958). 1999, Baltimore: Williams & Wilkins.

38. Ibid.

39. Forsyth, J. C., et al. Hydroxocobalamin as a cyanide antidote: Safety, efficacy and pharmacokinetics in heavily smoking normal volunteers. *Journal of Toxicology and Clinical Toxicology* 1993, 31(2):277–94.

40. Pezacka, E., Green, R., and Jacobsen, D. W. Glutathionylcobalamin as an intermediate in the formation of cobalamin coenzymes. *Biochem Biophys Res Comm* 1990, 2:443–50.)

41. Roach, E. S., and McLean, W. T. Neurologic disorders of vitamin B_{12} deficiency. *American Family Physician* 1982, 25(1):111–5.

42. Hertz, H., Kristensen, H. P. Ø. and Hoff-Jørgensen, E. (1964), Studies on Vitamin B_{12} Retention Comparison of Retention Following Intramuscular Injection of Cyanocobalamin and Hydroxocobalamin. *Scandinavian Journal of Haematology*, 1: 5–15. doi: 10.1111/j.1600–0609.1964.tb00001.x.

43. Kira, J., Tobimatsu, S., and Goto, I. Vitamin B_{12} metabolism and massive-dose methyl vitamin B_{12} therapy in Japanese patients with multiple sclerosis. *Internal Medicine* 1994, 33(2):82–6.

44. Kuzminski, A. M., et al. Effective treatment of cobalamin deficiency with oral cobalamin. *Blood* 1998, 92(4):1191–8.

45. Andrès, E. Comment: Treatment of vitamin B₁₂ deficiency anemia: Oral versus parenteral therapy. *Annals of Pharmacotherapy* 2002, 36:1268–72.

46. Lane, L. A., and Rojas-Fernandez, C. Treatment of vitamin B₁₂-deficiency anemia: oral versus parenteral therapy. *Annals of Pharmacotherapy* 2002, 36:1268–71.

47. Brantigan, C. O. Folate supplementation and the risk of masking vitamin B₁₂ deficiency. *Journal of the American Medical Association* 1997, 277(11):884–5.

48. Spence, D. Uses of error: Knowledge gaps. *The Lancet* 2001, 358(9297):1934.

49. Antony, A. C. Vegetarianism and vitamin B₁₂ (cobalamin) deficiency. *American Journal of Clinical Nutrition*, Vol. 78, No. 1, 3–6, July 2003.

50. Dali-Youcef, N., Andrés, E. An update on cobalamin deficiency in adults. *QJM* 2009 102(1):17–28.

51. Ibid.

52. Kuwabara, S. et al. Intravenous methylcobalamin treatment for uremic and diabetic neuropathy in chronic hemodialysis patients. *Internal Medicine* 1999, 38(6):472–5; and Koyama, K., Usami, T., Takeuchi, O., Morozumi, K., and Kimura, G. Efficacy of methylcobalamin on lowering total homocysteine plasma concentrations in haemodialysis patients receiving high-dose folic acid supplementation. *Nephrology, Dialysis, Transplantation* 2002, 17(5):916–922; and Rostand, S. G. Vitamin B₁₂ levels and nerve conduction velocities in patients undergoing maintenance hemodialysis. *American Journal of Clinical Nutrition* 1976, 29(7): 691–7.

12

The Autism-B_{12} Connection: When Low B_{12} Causes Pediatric Brain Injury

What every parent, pediatrician, obstetrician, and health care provider caring for children must know.

Over the years, as we've heard the stories of people whose lives were altered by undiagnosed B_{12} deficiency, the cases that have affected us most are those of infants and children. Many of these children were diagnosed too late and will spend their entire lives crippled both mentally and physically by this devastating—and entirely preventable—disorder.

In an effort to increase awareness of this horrific problem, we recently prepared a concise summary detailing the signs, symptoms, and consequences of pediatric B_{12} deficiency. We are making this document available as a chapter in this book in the hope that we can save the lives of many at-risk children and spare their families from tragedy as well as bankrupty.

We believe that B_{12} Deficiency Acquired Brain Injury (BABI) is an unrecognized epidemic of the twenty-first century that deserves serious research and attention. We encourage physicians treating developmentally delayed children to remember the ABCs –an acronym standing for the Autism B_{12} Connection. In the following chapter, we describe this connection.

If you are a lay reader, you may find some of this information a bit technical. However, if you are a parent, we hope that you will read this chapter and share it with your child's physicians.

Problem Statement:

Cobalamin (vitamin B_{12}) deficiency is an easily treated disease that often goes undiagnosed in infants and young children, placing them at high risk for permanent brain injury. It is well documented that B_{12} deficiency causes developmental delay, hypotonia, failure to thrive, reduced IQ, and mental retardation. Children with B$_{12}$ deficiency exhibit speech, language, and social delays, as well as problems with fine and gross motor movement. Magnetic resonance imaging (MRI) scans reveal brain atrophy and structural abnormalities, which often times reverse after B$_{12}$ therapy. However, if the deficiency is diagnosed late, permanent impairment of intellectual functioning typically occurs even after treatment, and cognitive and language development often remain seriously retarded.

The signs and symptoms of pediatric B$_{12}$ deficiency frequently mimic those of autism spectrum disorders (ASDs). However, very few children presenting with autistic symptoms receive adequate testing for B$_{12}$ deficiency. While the medical literature is replete with cases of developmental disability and mental retardation stemming from B$_{12}$ deficiency, we do not know how many children diagnosed on the autism spectrum actually have an undiagnosed cobalamin (B$_{12}$) deficiency. It is imperative that health care professionals screen at-risk and symptomatic children to prevent misdiagnosis, permanent brain injury, and life-long disability.

> B$_{12}$ Deficiency Acquired Brain Injury is an unrecognized epidemic of the 21st century.

Limited information about the prevalence of B$_{12}$ deficiency in older children in the U.S. is available. A study of 3,766 children aged 4 to 19 years (using data from the second phase of NHANES III 1991–1994) found that 1 in 200 children had serum B$_{12}$ levels less than 200pg/ml. This clearly indicates that B$_{12}$ deficiency is more common than previously recognized.[1] It is alarming that the prevalence of B$_{12}$ deficiency in infants and young children has not been studied or documented, because these are the most crucial times for brain growth and development.

ONSET AND PROGRESSION OF B$_{12}$ DEFICIENCY IN INFANTS AND YOUNG CHILDREN

In adults, symptoms of B$_{12}$ deficiency often develop slowly over several months or years. If B$_{12}$ stores initially are adequate, it can take two to six years for deficiency to develop. An adult's normal storage of vitamin B$_{12}$ in the liver is approximately 2,500 mcg. Newborns of mothers with normal B$_{12}$ stores have body stores of only 25 mcg, which is *thought to be* enough to cover all of their metabolic needs in their first year of life.

However, infants who are born to mothers with B$_{12}$ deficiency due to nutritional preferences (e.g., vegetarianism), disease states (e.g., pernicious anemia, short-gut syndrome, celiac disease), or surgical states (e.g., gastric bypass, partial ileectomy) and who are exclusively breast-fed may have significantly less stored B$_{12}$ and can develop a deficiency within the first year of life. Even infants who are formula-fed by these mothers may still have suboptimal B$_{12}$ levels, because the amount of B$_{12}$ in their formula may not be enough to correct their deficiency.

Compared to adults, infants with B$_{12}$ deficiency typically have a much more rapid onset of symptoms. Many children are deficient even before birth, either because their mothers have an unidentified B$_{12}$ deficiency or because the children have an inborn error of B$_{12}$ metabolism. The existing deficiency is worsened when an infant or young child is breast-fed by a mother with unidentified B$_{12}$ deficiency.

The symptoms of B$_{12}$ deficiency in infants and young children are often misdiagnosed. For example, irritability or gastric symptoms of B$_{12}$ deficiency can be easily mistaken for colic or gastroenteritis. The apathetic or dull infant can be mistaken for an "easy" or "good" baby. Additional symptoms of infant B$_{12}$ deficiency include poor head growth, insufficient weight gain, repetitive vomiting, drowsiness, swallowing problems, constipation, and tremors. Over time, B$_{12}$ deficiency causes failure to thrive and if not promptly corrected may lead to coma or death. Infants are also more vulnerable than adults to permanent brain injury because their central nervous systems are still developing.

> **Children with B$_{12}$ deficiency exhibit speech, language, and social delays.**

If B$_{12}$ deficiency goes unrecognized in infancy, treating the disorder later at the toddler stage can result in rapid improvement but some areas of the brain may be permanently injured, giving rise to fine motor difficulties, lower IQ, speech and language deficits, developmental delay, and behavioral problems. "Infantile vitamin B$_{12}$ deficiency may cause lasting neurodisability even though vitamin B$_{12}$ supplementation leads to rapid resolution of cerebral atrophy and EEG abnormality" (*Arch Dis Child* Aug 1997;77: 133–139). The extent of recovery and level of post-treatment functioning depend on the age at which the B$_{12}$ deficiency began, the severity of the deficiency, how long it was present, and at what age treatment was instituted.

A SAMPLING OF CASES OF B$_{12}$ DEFICIENCY IN INFANTS AND CHILDREN REPORTED IN THE MEDICAL LITERATURE:

A 15-month-old boy diagnosed with B$_{12}$ deficiency. He had normal development until 8 months of age. He was irritable and apathetic, had poor food intake, and exhibited drowsiness before arrival in the ER. He had marked hypotonia, hepatomegaly, slight anemia and macrocytosis when diagnosed. Psychometric testing when he was 5 years old revealed him to be functioning in the borderline range of intellectual ability.

—Graham, S. M., et al. Long-term neurologic consequences of nutritional vitamin B$_{12}$ deficiency in infants (*J Pediatr.* 1992 Nov;121:710–4).

§

An 8-month-old boy diagnosed with B$_{12}$ deficiency. EEG showed diffuse slow-wave activity. His eyes did not fix or follow, and he had an exaggerated startle response. His head circumference and weight were below the 3rd percentile. The child's response to B$_{12}$ was remarkable, with an improvement in head growth up to the 90th percentile, disappearance of choreoathetoid movements, and improved development. At 2.5 years he had language delay, and at 5 years mild to borderline intellectual retardation.

—Graham, S. M., et al. Long-term neurologic consequences of nutritional vitamin B$_{12}$ deficiency in infants (*J Pediatr.* 1992 Nov;121:710–4).

§

A 15-month-old boy diagnosed with B$_{12}$ deficiency (failure to thrive, hypotonia, and developmental delay). Brain CT showed widened subarachnoid spaces that suggested cerebral atrophy. Follow-up at 21 months showed sustained improvement: he was walking with a hand held and said approximately ten words.

—Graham, S.M., et al. Long-term neurologic consequences of nutritional vitamin B$_{12}$ deficiency in infants (*J Pediatr.* 1992 Nov;121:710–4).

§

A 9-month-old girl presenting with developmental delay, weakness, anorexia, tremor, and myoclonic jerks of the extremities. EEG was abnormal and brain CT showed marked dilation of the cerebral ventricles and brain atrophy.

—Avinoam, R. et al. Cobalamin deficiency in a breast-fed infant of a vegetarian mother (*IMAJ* 2003;5:534–536).

§

A 14-month-old boy whose MRI showed severe frontal and frontoparietal cranial atrophy due to B_{12} deficiency. After six weeks of treatment the child's EEG was normal, and cranial MRI after 10 weeks showed complete disappearance of all structural abnormalities. "Cognitive and language development remained seriously retarded at the age of 2 years."

—von Schenck, U. et al. Persistence of neurological damage induced by dietary vitamin B_{12} deficiency in infancy (*Arch Dis Child* 1997;77:137–139).

§

A 30-month-old boy presenting with developmental delay and failure to thrive. At 9 months of age his parents and physician were concerned regarding his growth and development. He had abnormal tongue movements. Poor motor skills and speech were documented at 11 months. At the age of 30 months he was diagnosed and treated. He experienced catch-up development in motor skills and completed physical therapy, but needed continued speech, language and occupational therapy. At 36 months (6 months after B_{12} treatment began) the child exhibited speech and fine motor delays.

—Muhammad, R. et al. Neurologic impairment in children associated with maternal dietary deficiency of cobalalmin Georgia, 2001 (*MMWR Weekly*, January 31, 2003;52(04);61–64).

§

A 9-year-old female, 8-year-old boy, and 6-year-old boy, all diagnosed with B_{12} deficiency and all treated before 15 months of age. All three children have IQs around 70. The researchers believed the first two patients were spared serious effects of developmental delay/mental retardation due to the occasional 1mg doses of B_{12} given in the early stages as part of the treatment for their suspected celiac disease and for the Schilling tests. "However, the fact that their IQs are at the borderline of subnormality (about 70) suggests that at some stage minor cerebral damage may have occurred."

—McNicholl, B. and Egan, B. Congenital pernicious anemia: effects on growth, brain, and absorption of B_{12} (*Pediatrics*, Vol. 42, No. 1, July 1968).

An 8-month-old boy who became fretful and apathetic, and stopped smiling and socializing, when he was between 3 and 6 months of age. At 6 months of age he had a dull, vacant stare, had poor head control, and made no attempt to play with his hands and feet. He showed occasional involuntary chewing movement of the mouth and rolling movements of the arms. Brain CT at 8 months showed marked cerebral atrophy and moderate ventricular enlargement. EEG showed an excess of slow rhythms. At 8 months he was diagnosed with B$_{12}$ deficiency and treated.

Over the following months, sustained improvement occurred. At 10 months of age he sat, socialized, babbled and grasped at toys. He crawled at 12 months and at 14 months he pulled himself up and cruised around holding on to furniture. By 17 months his EEG was normal but he could not walk alone. His neurological and psychometric assessment revealed his development was that of a child of 11 months of age.

—Wighton, M. C. et al. Brain Damage in infancy and dietary vitamin B$_{12}$ deficiency (*Med. J. Aust.* 1979, 2: 1–3).

When breastfeeding mothers deficient in B$_{12}$ switch their infants to formula or table foods, the children may obtain sufficient B$_{12}$ from these foods, but not enough to correct the existing deficiency. The minute amounts of B$_{12}$ in formula or table foods will protect a child from failure to thrive or death, but are sub-optimal for restoring the additional B$_{12}$ needed for critical brain growth and development.

EVIDENCE LINKING B$_{12}$ DEFICIENCY AND AUTISM

Autism is currently reaching epidemic proportions. In 2007, the Centers for Disease Control and Prevention reported, "For decades, the best estimate for the prevalence of autism was four to five per 10,000 children. More recent studies from multiple countries using current diagnostic criteria conducted with different methods have indicated that there is a range of ASD prevalence between 1 in 500 children and 1 in 166 children." Rick Rollens, cofounder of the U.C. Davis M.I.N.D. Institute, reported in 2007, "Twenty years ago in 1987 there were 2,273 persons with autism in California's system. Today, 20 years later, there are 32,809." In 2010, the prevalence is now reported to be 1 in 110 children.

EXAMPLES OF B$_{12}$ DEFICIENCY AND AUTISTIC SYMPTOMS

In 1997, a 14-month-old boy was brought to an emergency room comatose on arrival. Severe B$_{12}$ deficiency was diagnosed, with severe brain atrophy demonstrated by MRI. The boy regained consciousness within hours of treatment and by day three of B$_{12}$ injections he was able to walk, eat, and drink, and was discharged. Brain MRI 10 weeks post-treatment revealed all structural brain abnormalities had disappeared, but the patient continued to show nerve damage. At two years of age he still displayed psychomotor retardation, was agitated, and had poor concentration. He could not speak any words.

—von Schenck, U. et al. Persistence of neurological damage induced by dietary vitamin B$_{12}$ deficiency in infancy. *Arch Dis Child* 1997 Aug;77(2):137–9.

§

I recently contacted the mothers of two children whose cases were presented to me. At the time of our conversation, their children were 5 and 12 years post-treatment. Their B$_{12}$ deficiency had been detected too late to reverse all of their symptoms. While the children were reported in their medical and school evaluations to be "low IQ" and "developmentally delayed" as a result of chronic B$_{12}$ deficiency, the mothers described their children's behaviors in later childhood as strikingly similar to classical features of autism (fixation on spinning objects, obsession with particular object(s), toe-walking, flapping, social/behavioral problems, repetitive and ritualistic behavior). In addition, when the children were tested by licensed evaluators unaware of their B$_{12}$-deficiency diagnoses, they both met criteria for placement in autism classrooms and were labeled as "autistic."

There is strong evidence to indicate that B$_{12}$ deficiency plays a significant role in the epidemic of autism spectrum disorders. Among this evidence:

- The signs and symptoms of B$_{12}$ deficiency are strikingly similar to autism. B$_{12}$ deficiency in children causes developmental delay, problems with fine and gross motor skills, and lower IQ, all of which autistic children demonstrate. Both autistic and brain-injured B$_{12}$-deficient children have difficulty with speech and language. B_{12} deficiency can also cause aloofness and withdrawal.

- Many doctors report anecdotally that administration of B_{12} injections ameliorates autistic symptoms in a significant percentage of patients. One of these physicians, James Neubrander, M.D., reports that 94 percent of his autistic patients improve when they receive injected methylcobalamin (a form of B_{12}). This improvement has also been reported in children receiving hydroxocobalamin injections.

- Because doctors typically administer B_{12} treatment to autistic children without adequately testing them beforehand, we do not yet have accurate statistics on the numbers of these children who are proven to have a true B_{12} deficiency prior to treatment. However, one pilot study found that the rate of elevated urinary methylmalonic acid (MMA) levels in one group of autistic children was 19 percent. We have personally tested eight children with autistic symptoms—relatives, friends, or friends of friends—and seven had an elevated urinary MMA, proving B_{12} deficiency. Of the seven children, five received B_{12} therapy and all improved (some more than others, depending on the severity of B_{12} deficiency and the age at diagnosis).

> There is strong evidence to indicate that B_{12} deficiency plays a significant role in the epidemic of autism spectrum disorders.

- Many autistic children improve on gluten-free diets. It is well established that children with gluten intolerance or celiac disease have sub-optimal B_{12} levels or frank B_{12} deficiency, and that as the lining of the small intestine rejuvenates, B_{12} can again be absorbed. Thus, the improvement of autistic children on gluten-free diets could very well stem from enhanced B_{12} absorption.

MOUNTING RISK FACTORS FOR PEDIATRIC B_{12} DEFICIENCY

Most cases of B_{12} deficiency in infants and children stem from deficiencies occurring in their mothers during pregnancy and/or breastfeeding. Women of child-bearing age are exposed to many risk factors for B_{12} deficiency, and these risks are increasing. Among the most important factors contributing to high rates of B_{12} deficiency in pregnant and breastfeeding women:

- Increasing numbers of women are vegans or vegetarians, or follow other diets (i.e., the raw food diet, macrobiotic diets, very low-calorie diets) that drastically limit intake of vitamin B$_{12}$. Many of these women supplement their diets with foods such as tempeh and spirulina which, although purported to be rich in B$_{12}$, actually contain B$_{12}$ analogs that block the uptake of B$_{12}$. Even women who abandon low-B$_{12}$ diets and return to diets containing adequate B$_{12}$ may remain deficient for many years if their intake is not adequate to fully replenish their depleted stores.

- Many women of child-bearing age have unidentified B$_{12}$ deficiency resulting from a malabsorption problem (e.g., autoimmune pernicious anemia, celiac disease, Crohn's disease, H. pylori, bacterial overgrowth of the small intestine, gastrointestinal surgery, or gastric bypass surgery for weight loss).

- Increasing numbers of young women are taking metformin, proton-pump inhibitors, H-2 blockers, or large amounts of antacids, all of which decrease B$_{12}$ absorption.

- More women practice breast-feeding now than did 30 years ago. While this is a healthy trend, children of breast-feeding mothers are at higher risk of developing B$_{12}$ deficiency than those of mothers using formula. This risk occurs because women are not being screened for B$_{12}$ deficiency during the prenatal, post-partum, or lactating period.

- Women who become pregnant shortly after a previous delivery are at increased risk for B$_{12}$ deficiency.

- Vaccinations containing mercury as a preservative (including RhoGAM, tetanus diphtheria, the TB skin test, and flu vaccines) bind vitamin B$_{12}$, robbing it from women's body stores.

- Hydrocarbons in pollution can lower B$_{12}$ levels, as can smoking, by producing cyanide which binds to cobalamin and decreases the body's stores.

- Women are now placed on high-dose folic acid before and during pregnancy, as well as during breast-feeding. Folic acid masks the signs of anemia and macrocytosis which, while not always present in B$_{12}$ deficiency, can alert doctors to a B$_{12}$ problem. In addition, the FDA fortified all cereals and grains with folic acid in 1998 to help decrease birth defects; this fortification can also contribute to masking a B_{12} deficiency.

- B_{12} deficiencies can stem from anorexia or bulimia, which affect increasing numbers of women. Women who recover from eating disorders may remain deficient in B_{12} for months or years afterward.

- Nitrous oxide (laughing gas) administration to women of childbearing age contributes to lower B_{12} stores and can even cause a B_{12} deficiency. Nitrous oxide inactivates B_{12} and is routinely used in emergency caesarian sections. Also, some women use nitrous oxide as a recreational drug—a relatively new phenomenon—and thus put themselves at high risk for B_{12} deficiency.

Medical practitioners may mistakenly believe that the prenatal vitamins prescribed to pregnant women significantly reduce the risk of B_{12} deficiency. Prenatal vitamins, however, do not contain enough vitamin B_{12} to correct a deficiency.

CURRENT DEFICITS IN DIAGNOSIS OF PEDIATRIC B_{12} DEFICIENCY

For more than a century, the medical literature has clearly defined the effects of B_{12} deficiency on the brain and nervous system. These effects include cerebral atrophy, demyelination, degeneration of cortical neurons, and decreased production of neurotransmitters. B_{12} deficiency causes an array of neuropsychiatric manifestations including depression, apathy, paranoia, hallucinations, psychosis, self-injury, paresthesias, balance and gait problems, tremor, neuropathy, visual problems, taste, smell, and hearing problems, dizziness, and vertigo.

Unfortunately, the common diagnostic practice is to identify B_{12} deficiency only in the presence of anemia and macrocytosis. However, these symptoms often are not detectable even in people with advanced B_{12} deficiency. This is particularly true now that foods are heavily fortified with folic acid, which masks the hematologic effects of B_{12} deficiency. Moreover, many women have iron deficiency, which can mask a B_{12} deficiency, as can thalassemia and sickle cell anemia. (Note: Some of the children reported in the medical journals did have macrocytosis, which is a known sign of B_{12} deficiency, yet their physicians initially failed to diagnose it. By neglecting to perform further tests or provide treatment, these physicians allowed the deficiency to worsen until severe neurologic signs and symptoms were present as well as brain atrophy documented on CT or MRI scans.)

The prevalence of B$_{12}$ deficiency is not known for children under the age of four years. There are also no standard of care guidelines for

---

B$_{12}$ AND uMMA IN PEDIATRIC PATIENTS: SOME FINDINGS

Urinary methylmalonic acid (uMMA) testing is beneficial in children. Table 1 shows the serum B$_{12}$ and uMMA results for nine children diagnosed with varying degrees of developmental delay.

TABLE 1: URINARY MMA TESTING VERSUS SERUM B$_{12}$ IN CHILDREN.

Cases	Age	Sex	B$_{12}$ >200 pg/ml	Urine MMA <3.8 µmol/L	Serum MMA <0.4 µmol/L	Hcy <14 µMol/L
1	25 months	M	130	28.9		89.2
2	10 months	M	257	26.4	8.0	
3	3 years	M	643	4.1		9
4	3 years	F	1,894	5.5		
5	3 years	M	505	12.1	0.8	10
6	4 years	M	608	4.2		10.3
7	10 months	M	209	16.4	1.70	7.3
8	14 months	F	64	+4 significantly elevated	12.6	46.2
9	10 years	M	997	4.4		

All children had an elevated uMMA, whereas only two children had low B$_{12}$ levels. Two children had B$_{12}$ levels in the gray zone. Therefore, five children would not have been treated because their serum B$_{12}$ levels were high and even above the gray zone. All of these children were symptomatic, which is why testing was initiated. All nine children responded to B$_{12}$ therapy in varying degrees. Two children (1, 8) have severe brain injuries from late-diagnosed B$_{12}$ deficiency. Both children were proven to have B$_{12}$ deficiency because of maternal B$_{12}$ deficiency, not an inborn error of B$_{12}$ metabolism. Both mothers had prenatal care, took prenatal vitamins, and breastfed. One mother was a lacto-ovo vegetarian and the other was not a vegetarian of any kind.

This nine-patient sample reveals that urinary MMA testing must be included when B$_{12}$ deficiency is suspected in infants and children. We have not found this consistently in adults (where the serum B$_{12}$ is high or outside the gray zone and urinary MMA elevated). Research on serum B$_{12}$, urinary MMA, and holoTC must be done to determine which test, or combination of tests, can provide the most accurate and cost-effective way to diagnose B$_{12}$ deficiency in children and adults.

Norman Clinical Laboratory, Inc. reviewed its records for infants and children tested for B$_{12}$ deficiency using urinary MMA during 2006 and 2007. Results showed 17 children out of 30 screened (56 percent) had elevated urinary MMA indicating vitamin B$_{12}$ deficiency (Table 2). Children were tested for B$_{12}$ deficiency because they were symptomatic, exhibited developmental delay, or were at risk for B$_{12}$ deficiency. Below are details about the 17 children with B$_{12}$ deficiency (71 percent boys and 29 percent girls) and their uMMA results. Normal uMMA is <3.8 μmol/L.

TABLE 2: POSITIVE URINARY MMA RESULTS OF CHILDREN WITH DEVELOPMENTAL DELAY 2006–2007.

Case	Age	Sex	uMMA	Case	Age	Sex	uMMA
1	10 years	F	4.4	10	2 years	M	19.9
2	8 years	M	4.7	11	2 years	M	35.7
3	3 months	M	20.0	12	5 years	M	4.6
4	3 years	M	41.0	13	10 months	M	26.4
5	4 years	M	5.6	14	22 months	F	33.3
6	4 years	M	4.2	15	10 years	M	4.4
7	4 years	M	5.1	16	3 yr, 10 mo	M	56.0
8	4 years	F	5.3	17	10 years	F	8.3
9	9 years	F	5.2				

CONSEQUENCES OF LATE DIAGNOSIS

A B$_{12}$-deficient child reported in the medical literature presented with failure to thrive, developmental delay, grossly elevated uMMA, and low serum B$_{12}$. At the time she was diagnosed at 15 months of age, a brain MRI revealed "global cerebral atrophy." B$_{12}$ treatment began immediately with hydroxocobalamin injections. At 28 months of age, the patient's fine motor skills were at the 9-month level, and her gross motor skills were comparable to an 18-month-old's. Her expressive language was at 10 months and her receptive language was at 12 months. At 32 months, she had made developmental progress but continued to have developmental delays, especially in speech and language.

—Muhammad, R., et al. Neurologic impairment in children associated with maternal dietary deficiency of cobalamin—Georgia, 2001. *MMWR Weekly*. January 31, 2003/52(04);61–64.

screening and diagnosing B$_{12}$ deficiency in pregnant or breastfeeding women. Urinary MMA, which is non-invasive and helpful in diagnosing B$_{12}$ deficiency in infants and children, is rarely used. Complete blood counts which look for anemia and macrocytosis are inappropriate and late screening tools. The current "normal" lower limit for the serum B$_{12}$ test in all age groups is far too low, and needs to be changed. This is especially problematic for infants and young children during critical brain growth and development. Because of this, testing in infants and children needs to include the urinary MMA test. The uMMA has diagnosed many children whose serum B$_{12}$ was "normal."

Studies have revealed that adults with serum B$_{12}$ levels below 550 to 600pg/ml have early B$_{12}$ deficiency. (This was documented by comparing the patients' serum B$_{12}$ to the B$_{12}$ in their cerebral spinal fluid.) According to John Dommisse, M.D., infants' and young children's serum B$_{12}$ should be well over 1,000 pg/ml. "Humans and other mammals are all born with serum levels of about 2,000 pg/ml," he notes, "which decline gradually throughout life" (Dommisse, J. V. The Experts Speak Interviews: Psychiatry and vitamin B$_{12}$ deficiency. *Clinical Pearls News*, March 1998;51–52). Most doctors, however (including those in the U.S., United Kingdom, and Australia), typically do not contemplate a diagnosis of B$_{12}$ deficiency (regardless of a patient's age) unless serum B$_{12}$ is under 200 pg/ml in the U.S. and under 180 pg/ml in the U.K. As a result, B$_{12}$-deficient pediatric patients often go for many months or years without receiving a diagnosis. By the time diagnosis occurs, it is often too late for complete reversal of the initial brain injury.

Testing in later childhood may not reveal as dramatic a deficiency as it would if the child had been tested in early childhood, or when autism or developmental delay first presented. This is because test results may become normal if a child is currently obtaining some B$_{12}$ from food or supplements (for example, if the child's B$_{12}$-deficient mother stopped nursing him and switched him to a formula containing B$_{12}$, or started administering children's vitamins). However, the standard amount of B$_{12}$ in food or supplements, while it may result in test results that appear "normal," is not sufficient to replenish the body's stores and often is not provided soon enough during critical brain development to reverse brain injury.

RATIONALE FOR INVESTIGATION OF THE ROLE OF B$_{12}$ DEFICIENCY IN AUTISM SPECTRUM DISORDERS

The diagnosis of B$_{12}$ deficiency using urinary MMA is simple, non-invasive and relatively inexpensive (approximately $150 per test). The treatment of B$_{12}$ deficiency is even less expensive—only a few dollars per month. The estimated lifetime cost of caring for a person with autism, in contrast, is approximately $3.2 million. Clearly, if a significant percentage of cases of autism involve B$_{12}$ deficiency, the identification of this problem and the implementation of steps to prevent or treat B$_{12}$ deficiency in infants and children would result in huge financial savings for society and, more importantly, would protect the lives and health of many children.

If research shows that B$_{12}$ deficiency is a key factor in autism spectrum disorders, autism rates could be reduced through the following interventions:

1. Screening mothers and children at recommended intervals.

2. Increasing the B$_{12}$ in prenatal vitamins from 12mcg to 1,000mcg, and increasing the B$_{12}$ content of infant formulas. Methyl-B$_{12}$ formulation should be used in conjunction with prenatal vitamins, but at much higher doses (1,000 mcg versus 16mcg), and methyl-B$_{12}$ should be used rather than cyanocobalamin.

3. Educating medical professionals to use the urinary MMA test in conjunction with the serum B$_{12}$, rather than relying solely on less accurate tests such as the complete blood count (CBC). The serum B$_{12}$ test would be more accurate if the U.S. increased the adult range for "normal" to the lower cut-off of 450 pg/ml rather than 200 pg/ml. For infants and children, the lower limit may need to be raised to 1,000 pg/ml.

4. Educating clinicians regarding the effects of B$_{12}$ deficiency in women and children.

5. Paying special attention to the care and screening of high-risk mothers including vegans, vegetarians, women with eating disorders, and women with GI disorders, autoimmune diseases, or a history of gastric bypass surgery. Women who underwent emergency c-sections, and those with a history of medical or dental procedures involving nitrous oxide before or during pregnancy or while breastfeeding, should also be screened.

6. Educating mothers who breastfeed about the importance of adequate B$_{12}$, and monitoring these women's B$_{12}$ status.

7. Cautioning both breastfeeding and bottle-feeding mothers against the extensive use of microwaved milk, formula, or baby food, as microwaving partially destroys the B$_{12}$ in milk and meats (*Agricultural and Food Chemistry*, 1998).

8. Immediately screening any child for B$_{12}$ deficiency when a clinician or parent expresses concerns regarding developmental delay, failure to thrive, poor head growth, or insufficient weight gain.

9. Avoiding the use of nitrous oxide in medical or dental procedures performed on infants and children; or, if such use cannot be avoided, giving high-dose B$_{12}$ pre- and post-operatively.

> **The estimated lifetime cost of caring for a person with autism is approximately $3.2 million.**

10. Avoiding the use of pediatric immunizations/vaccinations that contain mercury. Thimerosal interferes with folate-dependent methylation by inhibiting the biosynthesis of the active form of vitamin B$_{12}$ (methylcobalamin). Using high-dose B$_{12}$ pre- and post-vaccination may be another option.

These interventions could be implemented rapidly and easily, and at a minimal cost to the health care system. The savings, both financially and in terms of human life, would be incalculable.

Autism spectrum disorders have multiple causes, and B$_{12}$ deficiency is only one piece of the puzzle. But *it is the most treatable and preventable part of the autism puzzle.* Thus, given the epidemic of autism we are facing and the devastating social and financial costs of this disorder, it is crucial that we explore the autism/B$_{12}$ link immediately.

UNANSWERED QUESTIONS INVOLVING B$_{12}$ DEFICIENCY AND AUTISM SPECTRUM DISORDERS

To fully elucidate the relationship between B$_{12}$ deficiency and autism, the following questions must be answered:

1. How many children diagnosed with autism spectrum disorders or pervasive developmental disorder actually suffer from an unidentified or misdiagnosed B$_{12}$ deficiency?

2. Can chronic sub-optimal B$_{12}$ during fetal development and/or infancy cause mild brain injury that manifests as high-functioning autism? Can overt B$_{12}$ deficiency in infancy cause moderate to low-functioning autism?

3. What impact would the universal screening of children with developmental delay for B$_{12}$ deficiency have on the identification of children with reversible symptoms that might otherwise be diagnosed as "incurable" autism?

4. Would the screening of infants and toddlers as well as women in the prenatal, post-partum, and breastfeeding period for B$_{12}$ deficiency significantly reduce the rates of autism and developmental delay?

5. Would high-dose methyl-B$_{12}$ therapy (1,000 mcg daily) taken by women before conception, during pregnancy, and during breast feeding reduce the rising rates of autism?

6. Should pregnant women also receive monthly B$_{12}$ shots during their prenatal visits? (Many women who bore children in the 1960s relate that they received B$_{12}$ injections before and during pregnancy from their obstetricians.)

7. Should the lower-end normal criterion for serum B$_{12}$ in infants and young children be raised to at least 1,000 pg/ml?

8. Are some cases of cerebral palsy caused by unknown B$_{12}$ deficiency that injures the brain during fetal growth and development? Are cerebral palsy patients having B$_{12}$ deficiency ruled out at the first opportunity?

The answers to these questions will not be found until we look for them. Currently, most medical professionals are unaware of the neuropsychiatric manifestations of B$_{12}$ deficiency and the role that this deficiency plays in developmental disorders (and, in particular, autism). The minority of doctors who *are* aware of B$_{12}$'s role in autism typically prescribe high-dose cobalamin to autistic children without first performing tests to determine these children's B$_{12}$ status. The latter physicians, while well-intentioned, are actually preventing us from obtaining crucial information about the role of B$_{12}$ deficiency in autism. The same is true of parents who "self-treat" children on the autism spectrum with B$_{12}$ without first having these children tested.

Because the medical community ignores the problem of B$_{12}$ deficiency or at best offers hit-or-miss treatments to at-risk children without testing them, thousands of B$_{12}$-deficient children are going undiagnosed, misdiagnosed, or undertreated. It is imperative that we begin to investigate, document, and report the true incidence of cobalamin deficiency in children (particular those with symptoms of autism or developmental disability) and in women of child-bearing age, so that we can determine the magnitude of this problem and take steps to address it. It is also vital that we revise our standard of care to reflect the critical role that B$_{12}$ plays in the mental and physical health of both children and their mothers.

FACTS REGARDING B$_{12}$ DEFICIENCY IN CHILDREN:

1. Inadequate B$_{12}$ during pregnancy has been associated with adverse outcomes including neural tube defects, preterm birth, intrauterine growth-retardation, and recurrent miscarriage.

2. The most common cause of B$_{12}$ deficiency in young children is maternal dietary deficiency which typically manifests in breastfed infants at four to eight months of age.

3. Vitamin B$_{12}$ is necessary for the normal growth and development of infants and children.

4. Cerebral and spinal cord lesions resulting from B$_{12}$ deficiency are well-documented.

5. B$_{12}$ deficiency can cause neurologic damage if untreated, and diagnosis must be made early to prevent permanent neurologic injury. Infants are more vulnerable to permanent damage.

6. B$_{12}$ deficiency identified late in the infant or child causes lower IQ.

7. B$_{12}$ deficiency is capable of causing mental retardation.

8. B$_{12}$ deficiency can rapidly lead to failure to thrive and if not promptly treated can lead to coma or death.

9. High-dose folic acid supplementation masks the traditional signs of B$_{12}$ deficiency in the blood count (anemia and/or macrocytosis). High-dose folic acid is prescribed to all pregnant women in prenatal vitamins.

10. Many women of child-bearing age have undiagnosed celiac disease, autoimmune pernicious anemia, or B$_{12}$ deficiency stemming from other causes (primarily dietary). These women's children are at high risk for B$_{12}$ deficiency. Their risk of brain injury is increased if the mother breastfeeds.

11. Children who were found to be B$_{12}$ deficient and then treated have lower IQs, "which suggests that at some stage minor cerebral damage may have occurred: this may have been in the latter part of their first years when they showed regression or slowing in motor development, or during their long periods without B$_{12}$" (McNicholl and Egan, *Pediatrics*, 1968, 42(1):149–156). As reported in a study of children of vegetarians, reduced IQ is common in children who have B$_{12}$ deficits during early development, even if these children receive adequate amounts of B$_{12}$ later in life.

12. There is an increased use of proton-pump inhibitor (PPI) drugs in infants and young children due to gastroesophageal reflux disease (GERD). These drugs cause B$_{12}$ deficiency with chronic use.

KEY POINTS FOR DIAGNOSTICIANS:

B$_{12}$ deficiency in infants that goes undiagnosed will lead to irreversible neurological damage. B$_{12}$ deficiency is progressive, and variable damage occurs to the brain, spinal cord, and peripheral nerves, depending on the duration of misdiagnosis. B$_{12}$ deficiency is one of the few potentially reversible causes of neurologic injury, *when promptly identified and properly treated*. Early diagnosis and treatment may prevent significant long-term sequelae.

Vitamin B$_{12}$ deficiency in infants and young children may produce the following neurologic and hematologic signs:

1. developmental delay

2. developmental regression

3. poor socialization

4. poor motor skills

5. language delay

6. speech problems

7. lower IQ

8. mental retardation

9. irritability

10. weakness

11. hypotonia

12. ataxia

13. apathy

14. tremor

15. myoclonus of the head, limbs, and tongue

16. involuntary movements

17. seizures

18. anorexia

19. failure to thrive

20. poor weight gain

> B$_{12}$ deficiency is one of the few potentially reversible causes of neurologic injury, *when promptly identified and properly treated.*

21. poor head growth (microcephaly)

22. anemia (may be present but is not a requirement)

23. pancytopenia

24. macrocytosis (may be present but is not a requirement—and may be masked)

COMMON FINDINGS:

1. abnormal brain CT: cerebral brain atrophy, enlarged ventricles

2. abnormal brain MRI: cerebral brain atrophy, enlarged ventricles

3. abnormal EEG: generalized slow activity

THE HUMAN COST OF UNDIAGNOSED PEDIATRIC B$_{12}$ DEFICIENCY

The information we've presented in this chapter outlines the medical aspects of acquired brain injury due to pediatric B$_{12}$ deficiency. To demonstrate the costs of this problem in human terms, we're concluding this chapter with the stories of two children who suffered the crippling effects of B$_{12}$ deficiency. One story has a happy ending. Sadly, the other story does not.

JACK'S STORY

In March 2006, Kelly, the mother of a ten-month-old baby named Jack, called us. Jack had spina bifida occulta and a tethered spinal cord. He was scheduled for surgery in a week at the University of Michigan. Kelly's mother-in-law read the first edition of our book, and she urged Kelly to read the children's chapter immediately.

After reading the chapter and speaking with us, Kelly decided to have Jack tested for B$_{12}$ deficiency because of his poor head growth and developmental delays. She was concerned as well about the upcoming surgery, and learned that it would involve nitrous oxide. Kelly sent Jack's urine sample to Norman Clinical Laboratory, Inc., where testing showed that his urinary MMA was grossly elevated at 26.4 µmol/L. This led Kelly to return to her pediatrician and pediatric gastroenterologist to get Jack treated.

The Chief of Neurosurgery postponed Jack's spinal surgery, stating that "B$_{12}$ deficiency can lead to neurological complications." Despite this, several specialists denied Jack B$_{12}$ treatment because it wasn't "normal" protocol, though they all acknowledged that B$_{12}$ treatment is harmless.

Kelly says, "I was told nothing was wrong with my son, and that we should take no action. I was told head measurement varies and is subjective. I was told that his level of B$_{12}$ was within the normal range, and that since he was not anemic and did not have megaloblastic cells, he did not have a B$_{12}$ deficiency. I was told his elevated MMA was only an indicator of [a metabolic condition called] methylmalonic aciduria. All of which is, unfortunately, completely wrong."

Luckily, Kelly was armed with the information in our book. She says, "I have no doubt that without this book, and the information therein, my son would now be mentally retarded, and might be suffering from neurological damage, and even autistic behaviors."

Kelly continued to take Jack to specialists, and finally a pediatric gastroenterologist determined that he did indeed have a B$_{12}$ deficiency. Upon treatment, Jack's levels of serum B$_{12}$ increased and his urine methylmalonic acid decreased to normal levels, making the B$_{12}$ deficiency diagnosis conclusive.

After Jack received treatment, his head growth accelerated and his head circumference climbed from the 8th to the 20–25th percentile (and has remained there since). Now five years old, Jack has met all his physical milestones according to his physical therapist, and his mental development is also right on track

B$_{12}$ treatment has made all the difference. Jack had been headed for microcephaly, retardation, and permanent mental disability—a tragic outcome prevented only by his mother's determination and the good fortune that put our book in her mother-in-law's hands. (Jack's results in Table 1 are listed under case #2.)

LENNON'S STORY

Lennon, a beautiful baby boy, began to fall behind developmentally at nine months of age. His head stopped growing, and his weight and growth flat-lined.

When Lennon was eleven months old, his pediatrician diagnosed anemia and started him on iron. As the months passed, Lennon continued to exhibit developmental delay. His language, speech, socialization, mobility, and eating were all abnormal.

Lennon's parents, Melinda and Greg, were extremely concerned and took Lennon to their pediatrician regularly. The doctor assured them that Lennon's weakness and developmental delays were due to his previous iron deficiency anemia. He also assured them that Lennon's development was along the lines of some of his other patients, and that there was no need to worry.

At fifteen months, Lennon was taken off the iron because the pediatrician told the parents his anemia had resolved. At twenty-one months, the pediatrician placed Lennon on a nutritional supplement called "Juice Plus." He continued to decline developmentally, and his growth was also affected. He was referred to a pediatric neurologist who specialized in developmental delay. A detailed assessment, a brain MRI, and an array of blood work were done, including testing for eleven enzyme defects. The pediatric neurologist said she was "100 percent sure" that Lennon had a form of a rare genetic disorder called mucopolysaccharide disease.

The neurologist also referred Lennon to a pediatric endocrinologist "to evaluate him for pituitary insufficiency and for nutritional issues regarding him having been breastfed by a vegetarian mother." Lennon saw the endocrinologist at twenty-three months of age, and the physician had nothing else to add to the pediatric neurologist's diagnosis but said to follow up with her again in six months.

Lennon was now twenty-four months old and growing weaker. He was approaching death, but not from some incurable disease. Melinda and Greg trusted the pediatricians' diagnosis of a rare, incurable genetic disease that was fatal. They consulted a close friend who was a medical researcher, desperately looking for anything to save their baby's life. The friend told them to gather Lennon's records, saying he would review them and find the best specialist working with mucopolysaccharide diseases.

Greg picked up the medical records from the pediatrician's office, and when Melinda began reviewing them, she realized that Lennon's blood had been abnormal for over a year and that he was severely macrocytic. She immediately called the pediatric neurologist, stating that she thought Lennon had a B$_{12}$ deficiency and asking that he be tested immediately.

Indeed, Melinda was correct. Lennon did have a severe vitamin B$_{12}$ deficiency. None of Lennon's doctors suspected or checked him for B$_{12}$

deficiency, despite clear documentation in the medical records that he had exhibited consistently abnormal blood counts, and that he was being breast fed by a lacto-ova vegetarian mother, which placed him at higher risk for this life-threatening problem.

Lennon's subjective and physical exams shouted out B$_{12}$ deficiency, but all of his doctors missed an easy diagnosis. His serum B$_{12}$ was 130 pg/ml (normal: 211–911), his urinary MMA was 28.9 (normal: < 2.4 μmol/L), and his homocysteine was 89.2 μmol/L (normal: 5–15). An even more disturbing fact emerged as Melinda reviewed Lennon's medical records: she discovered that he'd had macrocytic anemia for the past eight months. Lennon had also displayed numerous textbook signs and symptoms of B$_{12}$ deficiency, including poor eating, poor sucking, poor growth, failure to thrive, irritability, speech and language problems, socialization problems, poor gait/ataxia, poor muscle tone (hypotonia), developmental delay, macrocytosis, anemia, pallor, elevated red cell distribution width, and frequent infections.

Melinda remembers bringing up B$_{12}$ deficiency to her pediatrician on three different occasions because she had read about it in the American Medical Association *Family Medical Guide* when Lennon was first diagnosed with iron deficiency anemia. Her pediatrician repeatedly dismissed her input and reassured her that, "Nobody gets a B$_{12}$ deficiency. He is getting enough from your milk." When Lennon was twenty-one months old, the pediatrician stated that his mean corpuscular volume was elevated because he had a metabolic disease, not because of B$_{12}$ deficiency.

Melinda fully trusted her pediatrician, who was the Chief of Pediatrics with a "special interest in developmental pediatrics." How could he and all of the other medical and health care professionals the family encountered fail to make this straightforward diagnosis? Kelly, the first mother we talked about, was very fortunate that her mother-in-law had our book in hand. For Melinda, who fought just as hard to find a reason for her son's symptoms, the explanation came too late.

Lennon finally received B$_{12}$ therapy at the late age of twenty-six months. He had been symptomatic for over a year and his brain was actually starving from B$_{12}$ deficiency.

Lennon, now eleven years of age, compensates for the brain injury he suffered due to his late-diagnosed B$_{12}$ deficiency. He has a strong spirit and works hard to make up for his speech, language, and cognitive delays.

He has fine motor difficulties and is enrolled in numerous therapies to help him do things that come naturally to his peers.

Lennon's behavior resembles autism to the casual observer, as well as to trained professionals. But Lennon does not suffer from autism. He suffers from an acquired brain injury due to B$_{12}$ deficiency. Worse yet, there are many more Lennons out there, suffering silent and devastating brain injuries that are written off as incurable autism or other disorders by practitioners who fail to diagnose an easily treated condition.

How many specialists miss a diagnosis of B$_{12}$ deficiency and then compound the tragedy by dismissing the symptoms of the deficiency as autism—thus cutting off further investigation? How many of the tens of thousands of children receiving therapy for autism or other special education services could have been diagnosed early and spared from a lifetime of disability? And how many can still improve or even recover if they receive treatment immediately?

We don't know—and we won't know until doctors begin aggressively diagnosing and treating pediatric B$_{12}$ deficiency. Lennon's lifelong disability is proof that it is far past the time for doctors to stop saying—as his

INBORN ERRORS OF B$_{12}$ METABOLISM AND TRANSPORT[1]

GENETIC DISORDERS CAUSING METHYMALONIC ACIDURIA AND /OR HOMOCYSTINURIA

1. Cbl-A	increase MMA	usually responsive to B$_{12}$	no megaloblastic anemia
2. Cbl-B	increase MMA	50 percent responsive to B$_{12}$	no megaloblastic anemia
3. Cbl-C	increase MMA	responsive to B$_{12}$	+ megaloblastic anemia
4. Cbl-D	increase MMA	responsive to B$_{12}$	unknown if megaloblastic anemia is present
5. Cbl-E (methionine synthase reductase deficiency)	increase Hcy	responsive to B$_{12}$	+ megaloblastic anemia

6. Cbl-F	increase MMA	responsive to B$_{12}$	no megaloblastic anemia
7. Cbl-G (methionine synthase deficiency)	increase Hcy	responsive to B$_{12}$	+ megaloblastic anemia
8. Complete mutase deficiency of enzyme methylmalonyl CoA mutase	increase MMA	no response to B$_{12}$	no megaloblastic anemia
9. Partial mutase increase deficiency of enzyme methyl malo-nyl CoA mutase	increase MMA	no response to B$_{12}$	no megaloblastic anemia

HOMOCYSTINURIA IS ALSO CAUSED BY:

cystathionine β-synthase (CBS) deficiency	increase Hcy	not respon-sive to B$_{12}$	no megaloblastic anemia
Methylene-tetrahy-drofolate reductase (MTHFR) deficiency	increase Hcy	not respon-sive to B$_{12}$ (treatment: betaine, folate, and methionine)	no megaloblastic anemia

pediatrician did—that "nobody gets a B$_{12}$ deficiency." Instead, all doctors must realize that B$_{12}$ testing and treatment are powerful tools in the fight against autism and other childhood developmental disabilities. If you are a physician who treats children, please remember the ABCs—*Autism B$_{12}$ Connection*—because a quick diagnosis can save a child and that child's family from a lifetime of tragedy.

INBORN ERRORS OF B$_{12}$ METABOLISM AND TRANSPORT

Physicians caring for developmentally disabled children should be-come well-versed regarding the following inborn errors of B$_{12}$ metabo-lism, which can cause mental retardation or autistic behavior. There is growing evidence that some children labeled as autistic have functional

B$_{12}$ deficiency. It may be possible to cure a significant number of these children, but only if they are diagnosed early.

In our opinion, all children diagnosed with developmental delay or autism need to be evaluated for inborn errors of B$_{12}$ metabolism. There are ten different inherited defects that are known to disrupt the pathway of B$_{12}$; three are involved in B$_{12}$ transport and seven are involved in B$_{12}$ metabolism. Some are not responsive to B$_{12}$ therapy. Thus, determining which defect is present is critical to designing an appropriate treatment plan.

Cbl-A, Cbl-B, Cbl-F Methylmalonyl coenzyme A mutase deficiency (mut) disorders:

- Defect in conversion of methylmalonyl coenzyme A to succinyl coenzyme A
- Complete and partial mutase deficiencies: typically occur at one to four weeks of age.
- Cbl-A and Cbl-B: typically occur between one and twelve months of age.
- Signs and symptoms: failure to thrive, vomiting, dehydration, metabolic acidosis, muscular hypotonia; may experience retarded development, hepatomegaly, hypoglycemia, coma.
- 50 percent of patients present with anemia, leukopenia, thrombocytopenia
- increased MMA
- Treatment: restriction of dietary amino acids that are MMA precursors (methionine, threonine, valine, and isoleucine). Complete and partial deficiencies of enzyme methylmalonyl CoA mutase are not responsive to B$_{12}$ therapy.

Cbl-C, Cbl-D:

- Impaired synthesis of both succinyl coenzyme A and methionine, resulting in elevated MMA and Hcy.
- Differentiated by genetic complementation analysis.

- Cbl-C: thought to begin during the first few months of life, but a documented case was found at age four, and another at age fourteen.

- Signs and symptoms: failure to thrive, poor feeding, lethargy, developmental retardation, megaloblastic anemia. Some have thrombocytopenia, and some have visual disturbance caused by perimacular degeneration.

- increased MMA and Hcy

- Treatment: hydroxocobalamin 1,000 mcg daily, protein restriction, oral antibiotics, betaine supplements.

CBL-E, CBL-G:

- Synthesis of homocysteine to methionine is impaired, resulting in homocystinuria and homocystinemia.

- Typically patient becomes ill in the first two years of life. A delay in diagnosis may result in irreversible neurologic or developmental abnormalities.

- Signs and symptoms: poor feeding, vomiting, lethargy, developmental delay, megaloblastic anemia, pancytopenia, muscular hypotonia, nystagmus, visual defects, seizures, cerebral atrophy. Documented patient became symptomatic in adulthood and was diagnosed with multiple sclerosis.

- Large doses of vitamin B_{12} (hydroxocobalamin), 1,000 mcg daily, need to be administered.

ABNORMAL VITAMIN B_{12} TRANSPORT:

The transport protein for vitamin B_{12} is transcobalamin II (TC II). This protein must be present for the cells to accept and use vitamin B_{12}. The gene responsible for this protein is on chromosome 22. There can be an absence of TC II or abnormal TC II molecules.

- TC II deficiency is a potentially deadly disease. It is typically detected within the first six to twenty weeks of life.

- Signs and symptoms: weakness, diarrhea, failure to thrive, pancytopenia, megaloblastic anemia, hypogammaglobulinemia, and mucosal ulcers. Neurologic disease may present at onset or may occur later. If

diagnosed late, these neurologic abnormalities may become permanent and disabling.

- Serum vitamin B$_{12}$ levels are often normal because in plasma the majority of the vitamin is bound to TC I or TC III. Some low B$_{12}$ levels
have been found in patients with other abnormalities of B$_{12}$-binding
proteins and in the properties of TC I. Occasionally an elevated
MMA or Hcy has been found.

- Diagnosis is made by using chromatography or radioimmunoassay
demonstrating a lack of TC II.

- Treatment: Large doses of injectable hydroxocobalamin (1,000 mcg
three times weekly). One child was treated orally with 2,000 mcg
daily.

- Some patients may have functionally abnormal TC II molecules.
There appears to be a faulty protein unable to bind to B$_{12}$. Yet other
patients were able to bind B$_{12}$ but could not deliver it to their cells.

- Betaine is a methyl group donor that works in the normal metabolic
cycle of methionine and is used to treat patients with inborn errors of
methionine metabolism, because it decreases plasma homocysteine
levels in the disorder homocystinuria.

Betaine is used to treat homocystinuria. It is used in the management
of cystathionine b-synthase (CBS) deficiency, 5-10-methylenetetrahy-
drofolate reductase (MTHFR) deficiency, and certain cobalamin cofactor
metabolism defects. Betaine corrects elevated plasma homocysteine but
does not correct the underlying basic genetic disorder. Early detection of
homocystinuria in infancy and initiation of betaine therapy are essential
in improving the long-term prognosis of the patient. Betaine can increase
plasma concentrations of methionine and S-adenosylmethionine (SAM)
in patients with homocystinuria secondary to MTHFR deficiency or
cobalamin defect.

CHAPTER 12 ADDITIONAL READING:

- Rasmussen, S. A., Fernhoff, P.M., Scanlon, K.S. Vitamin B$_{12}$ deficiency in children and adolescents. *The Journal of Pediatrics*,2001, Vol.
138(1):10–17.

- Casella, E. B., et al. Vitamin B$_{12}$ deficiency in infancy as a cause of developmental regression. *Brain and Development*, 2005,Vol. 27(8):592–594.

- Erol, I., Alehan, F., Gumus, A. West syndrome in an infant with vitamin B$_{12}$ deficiency in the absence of macrocytic anaemia. *Dev Med Child Neurol*, 2007 Oct;49(10):774–6.

- Lucke, T., et al. Maternal vitamin B$_{12}$ deficiency: cause for neurological symptoms in infancy. *A Geburtshilfe Neonatol*, 2007 Aug;211(4):157–61 (article in German—abstract in English).

- Monagle, P.T., Tauro, G.P. Infantile megaloblastosis secondary to maternal vitamin B$_{12}$ deficiency. *Clin Lab Hematol*, 1997 April, Vol. 19(3):23–25.

- Grattan-Smith, P.J., et al. The neurological syndrome of infantile cobalamin deficiency: developmental regression and involuntary movements. *Mov Disord* 1997;12:39–46.

- von Schenck, U., et al. Persistence of neurological damage induced by dietary vitamin B$_{12}$ deficiency in infancy. *Arch Dis Child* 1997;77:137–139.

- Avci, Z., et al. Involuntary movements and magnetic resonance imaging findings in infantile cobalamin (vitamin B$_{12}$) deficiency. *Pediatrics*, Sept 1, 2003;112(3):684–686.

- Wagnon, J., et al. Breastfeeding and vegan diet. *J Gynecol Obstet Biol Reprod*, 2005 Oct;34(6):610–2.

- Mathey, C., et al. Failure to thrive and psychomotor regression revealing vitamin B$_{12}$ deficiency in 3 infants. *Arch Pediatr* 2007 May;14(5):467–471.

- Benbir, G., et al. Seizures during treatment of vitamin B$_{12}$ deficiency. *Seizure* 2007 Jan;16(1):69–73.

- Katar, S., et al. Nutritional megaloblastic anemia in young Turkish children is associated with vitamin B$_{12}$ deficiency and psychomotor retardation. *J Pediatr Hematol Oncol.* 2006 Sep;28(9):559–62.

- Baatenburg de Jong, et al. Developmental delay in breastfed children due to inadequate diet of the mother. *Ned Tijdschr Geneeskd.* 2006 Mar 4;150(9):465–9. Dutch.

- Korenke, G. C., et al. Severe encephalopathy with epilepsy in an infant caused by subclinical maternal pernicious anaemia: case report and review of the literature. *European Journal of Pediatrics*, 2004 Apr 163(4–5):196–201.

- Smolka, V., et al. Metabolic complications and neurologic manifestations of vitamin B$_{12}$ deficiency in children of vegetarian mothers. *Cas Lek Cesk*. 2001 Nov 22;140(23):732–5 (article in Czechoslovakian).

- Graham, S.M., et al. Long-term neurologic consequences of nutritional vitamin B$_{12}$ deficiency in infants. *J Pediatr* Nov 1992, Number 5, Part 1,710–14.

- Ramakrishna, T. Vitamins and brain development. *Physiol Res.* 1999;48(3):175–87.

- Wighton, M.C., et al. Brain damage in infancy and dietary vitamin B$_{12}$ deficiency. *Med J Aust*, 1979,2:1–3.

- Murphy, M.M., et al. Longitudinal study of the effect of pregnancy on maternal and fetal cobalamin status in healthy women and their offspring. *J Nutr* 137: 1863–1867, 2007.

- Suarez, L., et al. Maternal serum B$_{12}$ levels and risk for neural tube defects in a Texas-Mexico border population. *Ann Epidemiol.* 2003;13:81–8.

- Specker, B. L., Miller, D., Norman, E. J., Hayes, K. C. Increased urinary methylmalonic acid excretion in breast-fed infants of vegetarian mothers and identification of an acceptable dietary source of vitamin B$_{12}$. *Am J Clin Nutr* 1988;47:89–92.

- Rasmussen, S. A., et al. Vitamin B$_{12}$ deficiency in children and adolescents. *J Pediatr* 2001;138:10–17.

- Jadhav, M., et al. Vitamin B$_{12}$ deficiency in Indian infants: a clinical syndrome. *Lancet* 1962;2:903–7.

- Garewal, G., et al. Infantile tremor syndrome: a vitamin B$_{12}$ deficiency syndrome in infants. *J Trop Pediatr* 1988;34:178–8.

- Higginbottom, M. C., et al. A syndrome of methylmalonic aciduria, homocystinuria, megaloblastic anemia and neurologic abnormalities in a vitamin B$_{12}$-deficient breast-fed infant of a strict vegetarian. *N Engl J Med* 1978;299:317–23.

- Allen, L. H., et al. Cognitive and neuromotor performance of Guatemalan schoolers with deficient, marginal, and normal plasma vitamin B$_{12}$. *FASEB J* 1999;13:A544.

- Bjorke Monsen, A. L., Ueland PM. Homocysteine and methylmalonic acid in diagnosis and risk assessment from infancy to adolescence. *Am. J. Clinical Nutrition*, July 1, 2003;78(1):7–21.

- Monsen, A. L., et al. Determinants of cobalamin status in newborns. *Pediatrics* 2001;108(3):624–30.

- Rosenblatt, D. S., Whitehead, V. M. Cobalamin and folate deficiency: acquired and hereditary disorders in children. *Semin Hematol* 1999;36:19–34.

- Casterline, J. E., Allen, L. H., Ruel, M.T. Vitamin B$_{12}$ deficiency is very prevalent in lactating Guatemalan women and their infants at three month postpartum. *J Nutr* 1997;127:1966–72.

- Shinwell, E. D., Gorodisher, R. Totally vegetarian diets and infant nutrition. *Pediatrics* 1982;70:582–6.

- Specker, B. L., Black, A., Allen, L., Morrow, F. Vitamin B$_{12}$: low milk concentrations are related to low serum concentrations in vegetarian women and to methylmalonic aciduria in their infants. *Am J Clin Nutr* 1990;52:1073–6.

- Dagnelie, P. C., et al. Increased risk of vitamin B$_{12}$ and iron deficiency in infants on macrobiotic diets. *Am J Clin Nutr* 1989;50:818–24.

- Saraya, A.K., et al. Nutritional macrocytic anemia of infancy and childhood. *Am J Clin Nutr* 1970;23:1378–84.

- Rogers, L. M., et al. High prevalence of cobalamin deficiency in Guatemalan schoolchildren: associations with low plasma holotranscobalamin II and elevated serum methylmalonic acid and plasma homocysteine concentrations. *Am J Clin Nutr* 2003;77:433–40.

- Davis, J. R., Goldenring, J., and Lurin, B. H. Nutritional vitamin B$_{12}$ deficiency in infants. *American Journal of Diseases of Children*, 1981, 135:566–567.

- Hermann, W., Geisel, J. Vegetarian lifestyle and monitoring vitamin B$_{12}$ status. *Clin Chim Acta* 2002;326:47–59.

- McNicholl, B., Egan, B. Congenital pernicious anemia: effects on growth, brain, and absorption of B$_{12}$. *Pediatrics*, Vol 42, No1 1, July 1968:149–156.

- Pearson, H. A., et al. Pernicious anemia with neurologic involvement in childhood. *J. Pediat*, 65:334,1964.

- Lee, G.R. Inherited and drug-induce megaloblastic anemia. In G. R. Lee (10th Ed.), *Wintrobe's Clinical Hematology*, 1999, 973–8. Baltimore: Williams & Wilkins.

- VanTiggelen, C. J. M., et al. Vitamin B$_{12}$ levels of cerebrospinal fluid in patients with organic mental disorder. *Journal of Orthomolecular Psychiatry* 12: 305–11, 1983.

- VanTiggelen, C. J. M., Perperkamp, J. P. C., TerToolen, J. F. W. Assessment of vitamin-B$_{12}$ status in CSF. *American Journal of Psychiatry* 141, 1: 136–7, 1984.

CHAPTER 12 NOTES:

1. Lee, G. R. Inherited and drug-induced megaloblastic anemia. In G. R. Lee (10th Ed.), *Wintrobe's Clinical Hematology*, 1999, 973–8. Baltimore: Williams & Wilkins.

13

The Cost Effectiveness of Early Screening and Treatment for B$_{12}$ Deficiency

What is the cost of failing to diagnose vitamin B$_{12}$ deficiency early? The answer may stun you: billions of dollars. Not only are insurance companies and the government (through Medicare and Medicaid) paying out enormous amounts of money, but so are taxpayers and society.

Why? People who are injured as a result of B$_{12}$ deficiency often become disabled. These people are out of the workforce, unable to provide for their families, and collect disability payments provided by the government or private insurers. Many dip into their life savings, becoming bankrupt or even homeless.

When you consider the results of undiagnosed or untreated B$_{12}$ deficiency, it is clear why this problem is contributing to the bankrupting of America's health care system. The consequences of this invisible epidemic include:

- Fall-related trauma
- Frequent emergency department visits
- Frequent medical office visits
- Repeated hospitalizations
- Cognitive decline (dementia)
- Nursing home placements
- Unnecessary prescriptions
- Blood transfusions and/or erythropoietin use
- Psychiatric care (office visits and admissions)
- Unnecessary radiologic and invasive testing

> **People who are injured as a result of B$_{12}$ deficiency often become disabled.**

- Malpractice settlements and payouts
- Need for mobility devices (wheelchairs, scooters, walking devices)
- Rehabilitation (in-patient and out-patient)
- Physical therapy
- Occupational therapy
- Loss of income due to disability
- Social Security payments or disability insurance
- Family stress, as relatives become caretakers of disabled individuals

So why aren't we screening patients? Is B_{12} screening or treatment expensive? The answer to this question is a very clear "no." Table 1 compares B_{12} screening to other diagnostic tests.

Table 1: Costs of B_{12} tests and other lab and diagnostic tests

Lab tests for B_{12} deficiency	Cost
Vitamin B_{12}	$90
Urinary MMA	$150
Serum MMA	$246
Holo TC (Active B_{12})	$228
Homocysteine	$176
Other commonly ordered medical tests	
Complete blood count (CBC w/diff)	$48
Serum iron	$36
Ferritin, TIBC, iron sat (panel)	$144
TSH	$93
T-4 (free)	$109
BNP	$230
Lipid profile	$120
Vitamin D, 25-hydrox	$215
CT brain w/o contrast	$1,255
Hip x-ray (2 view)	$189
Femur x-ray	$230

There is a misconception that B_{12} screening is not cost-effective compared to other screening tests. This is simply not true. The 25-hydroxy-vitamin D test costs $215, yet physicians don't bat an eye at ordering it. Ruling out iron deficiency costs around $180, and screening for hypothyroidism costs $202. Routine cholesterol testing is $120, and physicians often order the B-type natriuretic peptide (BNP) test, which costs $230, to diagnose, manage, and treat heart failure. By comparison, a serum B_{12} test costs an average of $90, and the urinary MMA, when needed, costs $150.

Moreover, a failure to treat B_{12} deficiency creates massive costs in other areas, including hospital and rehabilitation care for patients whose symptoms continue to worsen. Table 2 shows the cost of room rates for hospitalization. This table does not include physician fees, treatment fees, equipment, supplies, or medications used.

Table 2. Cost of hospitalization (2009)

Type of hospitalization	Cost per day
Emergency room visit (level 4)	$450
Room and board, semi-private bed	$841
Room and board, telemetry bed	$1,283
Room and board for ICU medical or ICU surgical bed	$2,720
Room and board, rehabilitation facility bed	$248
Room and board, psychiatric facility	$1,076 to $1,368

To analyze the costs of this hidden epidemic from a different perspective, let's explore six main areas of expense related to untreated B_{12} deficiency.

1. Fall-related trauma:

In 2005, more than $19 billion was spent treating injuries from falls. As we've noted, a significant percentage of such falls are related to B_{12} deficiency.

The average hospitalization for a fall costs around $17,500. By 2020, the annual cost for fall-related injuries is expected to reach $54.9 billion.

In 2009, the average hospital bill for a four-day admission to a general medical floor following a fall resulting in a hip fracture without complications was greater than $30,000. An average fourteen-day rehabilitation room charge is $12,400, and it costs an additional $7,200 for services and supplies. The average physician's fee for fourteen days is $1,600, and nineteen home physical therapy sessions cost on average $2,200. This equates to more than $23,000 worth of additional expenses. Thus, the total cost for the average hip fracture exceeds $50,000.

2. Mental Illness:

In any given year, more than 57.7 million U.S. adults (26.2%) are diagnosed with a mental disorder. Depression, in particular, is epidemic; in fact, major depressive disorders are the leading cause of disability for people between the ages of fifteen and forty-four.

As we discussed in Chapter 4, undiagnosed B$_{12}$ deficiency can cause depression as well as a wide range of other mental symptoms ranging from paranoia to hallucinations. Doctors often fail to screen patients with these symptoms for B$_{12}$ deficiency, opting instead to prescribe antidepressants and other psychotropic drugs. In doing this, they condemn many B$_{12}$-deficient patients to a lifetime of mental illness—and they waste millions of healthcare dollars as well.

For example, one man whose case we discussed earlier in this book was placed in a psychiatric facility for eight days. His stay cost nearly $11,000 and was covered by his insurance company. He was also placed on Cymbalta for over a year, without his doctors investigating B$_{12}$ deficiency as a cause of his depression. Although this man's health began to rapidly decline, it took more than two years for his doctors (primary care doctor, psychiatrist, and two neurologists) to diagnose his severe B$_{12}$ deficiency, which almost cost him the use of his legs as well as his sanity and his life.

> Undiagnosed B$_{12}$ deficiency can cause depression as well as a wide range of other mental symptoms ranging from paranoia to hallucinations.

While the cost of such mistakes in human terms is incalculable, we can determine some of the financial costs. For example, Table 3 lists the costs of some commonly prescribed anti-depressant and psychiatric medications, as well as the annual cost of self-administered hydroxocobalamin (B$_{12}$) shots.

Table 3: Costs of Antidepressant and Psychiatric Medications (2010)

Medication	Dose/quantity	Cost per month	Cost per year
Lexapro	10mg daily	$92	$1,104
Celexa	10mg daily	$99	$1,188
Cymbalta	30mg daily	$135	$1,620
Zoloft	50mg daily	$101	$1,212
Risperdal	2mg daily	$246	$2,952
Abilify	2mg daily	$492	$5,904
Prozac	10mg daily	$163	$1,956
Hydroxocobalamin injectable (30 ml vial)	1,000 mcg IM bi-monthly or 500mcg SC weekly (this also includes the loading dose of 6 initial daily injections)	$3	$36

Health care leaders must do the math. Clearly, prescribing psychiatric medications to B_{12}-deficient patients isn't just dangerous and negligent—it strains our over-burdened healthcare system as well.

3. Dementia:

As we explained in Chapter 2, prolonged B_{12} deficiency often leads to permanent dementia. Thus, B_{12} deficiency must be ruled out in all patients with beginning cognitive changes, forgetfulness, or dementia, as well as in patients with a diagnosis of Alzheimer's disease, Pick's disease, or cortical basal ganglionic degeneration (CBGD). There is a critical window of opportunity to treat B_{12} deficiency before permanent cognitive changes or injury result. If medical providers miss that window, there is no way to repair the damage—and that damage is costly in both human and financial terms.

Tables 4 through 7 review the costs of different drugs used to treat dementia, as well as the costs associated with caring for someone with dementia:

Table 4: Cost of dementia or Alzheimer's medications (2010)

Medication	Dose/quantity	Cost per month	Cost per year
Aricept	5mg daily	$232	$2,784
Namenda	5mg daily	$107	$1,284
Cognex	10mg daily	$94	$1,128
Exelon	1.5mg BID	$270	$3,240

Table 5: Cost of assisted living memory care for dementia patient—non-skilled nursing (2010)

Level of care	Cost per day	Cost per month	Cost per year	Cost for 2 years	Cost for 5 years
Semi-private room (base rate)	$136	$4,080	$49,640	$99,280	$248,200
Meds—memory care	$ 136 + $43	$5, 370	$65,335	$130,670	$326,675
Meds, memory care + dressing + showering	$136 + $64	$6,000	$73,000	$146,000	$365,000

Table 6: Cost of nursing home care 2010 (dementia, post hip fracture, chronic disease, multiple sclerosis, etc.)

Level of care	Cost per day	Cost per month	Cost per year	Cost for 2 years	Cost for 5 years
Room charge semi-private (Base rate)	$172	$5,160	$62,780	$125,560	$313,900
Dressing, hygiene, dining, toileting Semi-private room	$211	$6,330	$75,960	$151.920	$379,800
Same as above (private room)	$271	$8,130	$98,915	$197,830	$494,575
Wander guard and flight risk	+ $10	+ $300	+ $3,650	+$ 7,300	+$18,250
Catheter care	+$4	+ $120	+ $1,460	+$2,920	+$ 7,300

Table 7: Cost of rehabilitation care 2010 (transfer from hospital)

Level of care	Cost per day	First 20 days Medicare pays 100%	Remaining 80 days per calendar year, patient responsible for partial payment
Daily Base Rate	$248	$4,950	$19,840
Dressing, hygiene, dining, toileting, semi-private room	$287	$5,740	$28,700
Wander guard and flight risk	+$10	+$200	+$1,000
Catheter care	+$4	+$80	+$80

4. Neurologic diseases: multiple sclerosis [MS], transverse myelitis, ALS, neuropathy, Guillain Barré, chronic inflammatory demyelinating polyneuropathy [CIDP], Parkinson's disease

What is the cost of diagnosing a patient with multiple sclerosis or another neurologic disorder when that person actually has a vitamin B_{12} deficiency? For patients, the toll is high: devastating and permanent neurologic injury and disability. And the economic cost is extraordinary as well; Table 8 shows the cost of MS drugs and intravenous immunoglobulin (IVIG) compared to injectable hydroxocobalamin and methylcobalamin (two forms of B_{12}).

Table 8: Cost of MS drugs vs. injectable vitamin B$_{12}$

Medication	Dose/quantity	Cost per month	Cost per year
MS Drugs			
Avonex	30 mcg SC weekly	$2,775	$33,299
Betaseron	0.3mg SC every other day	$2,765	$33,165
Copaxone	20mcg SC daily	$3,075	$36,904
Intravenous immunoglobulin (IVIG)	1 gram/kg IV every 3 weeks (70 kg patient)	$4,550 (every 3 weeks)	$77,350 (does not include fee for administration)
Injectable Vitamin B$_{12}$			
Hydroxocobalamin	1,000 mcg SC every day x 6; then 500 mcg SC every week	$3	$36
Methylcobalamin	1,000 mcg SC every day	$25.15	$302
Methylcobalamin	5,000 mcg SC every other day	$29.50	$354

In 2007, 400,000 Americans were diagnosed with MS. If 4.2 percent of them actually suffered from vitamin B$_{12}$ deficiency—the lowest estimate we can find in the medical literature, and almost certainly an underestimate—this would equate to 16,800 misdiagnosed people. If these 16,800 people were placed on the cheapest MS drug (Betaseron), the total cost would be $557 million each year. If these 16,800 misdiagnosed patients eventually required nursing home care, it would cost more than $1.3 billion per year to care for them. By contrast, if these 16,800 people were actually diagnosed correctly, it would cost $604,800 yearly for treatment with hydroxocobalamin, including the initial series of shots and then weekly injections. The savings would be over 1.299 billion dollars!

This is not mere speculation. We have personally heard from patients who were suspected to have or were actually diagnosed with other neurologic disorders (MS, ALS, Guillain Barre), but who actually had a misdiagnosed B$_{12}$ deficiency. We found it odd that their neurologists had performed an array of tests but had not included serum B$_{12}$ or other B$_{12}$

markers. These doctors had no problem ordering CT scans and MRIs of the brain and spinal cord and conducting EMG and NCV tests. They also had no problem prescribing medications for neuropathy without ruling out B_{12} deficiency. The financial toll of this error becomes clear when you compare the cost of diagnosing and treating B_{12} deficiency (which averages $300) with the costs of neurology office visits, diagnostic testing, and medications—see Table 9 below.

Table 9. Cost of neurology visits, tests, and medications

Office visit or test	Cost
New patient neurology office visit initial exam	$160–$398
Follow-up neurology office visit	$60–$215
CT brain w/o contrast	$1,255
MRI brain w/o contrast	$1,300
MRI c-spine, T-spine, LS-spine	$1,300 (each)
MRI brain or c-spine w/contrast	$ 1,950 (each)
MRI t-spine or LS-spine w/contrast	$1,950 (each)
EMG/NCV	($400–$800 per limb) All limbs ($1,600–$3,200)
EEG	$118
Myasthenia gravis panel 1	$478
Myasthenia gravis panel 2	$750
Myasthenia gravis panel 3	$1,033
Lyme disease panel	$386

Medication	Dose/quantity	Cost per month	Cost per year
Lyrica	50mg daily	$75	$903
Neurontin	300mg TID	$180	$2,160
Ativan	1mg daily	$95	$1,140
Lorazepam (generic for Ativan)	1 mg daily	$18	$216
Cymbalta	30 mg daily	$135	$1,620

Research also needs to be done to determine if bi-weekly methyl-B$_{12}$ injections would reduce the need for (or even replace) expensive intravenous immunoglobulin (IVIG) therapy used to treat CIDP, Guillain Barre, and other neuromuscular disorders. IVIG therapy costs a patient or insurance company more than \$75,000 per year for the drug, and thousands more for it to be infused by a nurse. Thus, the cost of misdiagnosing patients with CIDP who actually have a vitamin B$_{12}$ deficiency is enormous. IVIG is in phase III testing in the U.S. (as of December 2008) for the treatment of Alzheimer's disease, yet our country fails to screen for B$_{12}$ deficiency, fails to treat symptomatic patients in the gray zone, and fails to do trials of methyl-B$_{12}$ injections in dementia and other neurologic disorders.

5. Anemia:

In the emergency department, we commonly see anemic patients. Anemia can stem from blood loss due to GI bleeding, nutritional deficiency (iron, B$_{12}$, and folic acid), chronic disease (renal failure), cancer (chemotherapy agents), or a combination of these. When we diagnose B$_{12}$ deficiency and go back and review patients' charts, we commonly see these patients being worked up for iron deficiency anemia or GI bleeding. What we fail to see are physicians ruling out B$_{12}$ deficiency as the cause of anemia.

We have seen many patients whose anemia became so severe as a result of B$_{12}$ deficiency that they required blood transfusions. Many elderly patients with undiagnosed B$_{12}$ deficiency have endoscopies and colonoscopies performed because their doctors are searching for bleeding to explain their severe anemia. These procedures and transfusions are costly; in 2010, the average cost of a colonoscopy was \$2,750 and an upper endoscopy was \$2,440. Moreover, they are not without risk, exposing patients to anesthesia as well as the possibility of accidental perforation or exposure to blood-borne diseases.

> We have seen many patients whose anemia became so severe as a result of B$_{12}$ deficiency that they required blood transfusions.

We also see elderly patients with undiagnosed B$_{12}$ deficiency who are admitted, receive blood transfusions, and undergo workups for GI bleeding and a battery of other diagnostic tests. When no cause for the anemia is found, these patients are sent home, only to return months later to repeat the process, all because B_{12} deficiency was not contemplated or ruled out.

Some patients who are chronically anemic due to chronic renal failure, cancer, or HIV receive erythropoietin (Procrit, Epogen) to improve their anemia. In these cases as well, physicians routinely screen for iron deficiency but typically do not screen for B_{12} deficiency. Is it cost-effective to place a patient on Procrit, which costs $4,240 for eight weeks of treatment, without ruling out B_{12} deficiency?

One woman we saw in the emergency department had lung cancer and was on Procrit because of chronic anemia. She had lost her job because of her illness and was paying out of pocket for her Procrit. A review of her medical records and lab reports for the past few years showed that not a single physician checked her B_{12} status. She had many signs and symptoms of B_{12} deficiency, but they were blamed on her cancer. We tested her, and she was severely deficient.

In a similar case recently, a 36-year-old with a history of colon cancer came to the emergency department. She was on chemotherapy and was experiencing chronic pain and depression. She had undergone surgery on her ileum years before. She had never received B_{12} treatment, but she should have because of the ileal surgery. We tested her and she was found to be grossly B_{12} deficient at 126pg/ml. She had received multiple blood transfusions in the past for her "anemia of chronic disease."

How costly are such oversights? Table 10 shows the cost of blood products and their administration. Table 11 reviews the cost of erythropoietin compared to vitamin B_{12}.

Table 10: Cost of transfusing two units of packed red blood cells

Description	Cost
Leukopoor blood (2 units)	$736
Blood Administration	$312
Inj IV Push, Init/Sngl	$126
Furosemide 100 mg injectable	$47
0.9% NaCl 250 ml	$34
TOTAL	**$1,255**

Table 11: Cost of erythropoietin (Procrit, Epogen) versus B₁₂

Description	Cost
Procrit 50–100 units/kg (starting dose) 100 units x 70 kg = 7,000 units Starting dose: Chronic renal failure: 50–100units/kg Cancer patients:　　　150units/kg (3 x weekly) HIV patients:　　　100units/kg (3 x weekly) Ordering dose: 7,000 units (3 times per week) x (8 weeks)	($176.67) x (3) = $530/week ($530) x (8 weeks) = $4,240 for 8 weeks of treatment
Hydroxocobalamin 1,000 mcg/ml 1 ml IM q day x 6; then 1ml every wk x 2; then 1 ml every 2 weeks for next 11 months; or 0.5 ml every week for next 11 months	$36.00 for entire year or **10 cents per day**

Sometimes patients even undergo a bone marrow biopsy to determine the reason for their anemia, which verifies that simple vitamin B_{12} deficiency was the cause. The cost of a bone marrow biopsy can run up to $840, not including the costs for individual pathology tests and pathologists' fees for examining and interpreting the slides.

To us, these cases raise an important question: Why aren't all cancer patients being tested for B_{12} deficiency? In addition, we wonder if weekly B_{12} therapy could improve anemia even in cancer patients who are not B_{12}-deficient (an effect much like that of Procrit), saving billions of dollars for patients, insurance companies, and the government.

Our personal experience in this area has been positive. A close friend of ours, age 60, has stage IV colon cancer. She had been in remission for 18 months when the cancer returned with metastasis to her liver and lungs. After her bi-monthly chemotherapy treatments, she receives an intravenous multi-vitamin infusion with high doses of folic acid, but only 6mcg of B_{12}—not enough to keep optimal B_{12} stores when undergoing chemotherapy, and certainly not enough to treat a B_{12} deficiency. With the permission of her oncologist, we began giving her weekly hydroxocobalamin injections. Nineteen months later, she has not needed a transfusion of blood or platelets. Her oncologist admits that she is one of very few patients with good blood counts. Not only does B_{12} treatment prevent anemia, but it reduces her fatigue and improves her energy and overall mental wellbeing. More research in this area is needed to determine the potential for substantial savings and improved quality of life.

6: *Autism vs. B₁₂ Deficiency Acquired Brain Injury (BABI)*

The U.S. Centers for Disease Control and Prevention reports that one in 110 children have autism. As we discussed in Chapter 12, B_{12} deficiency in infants and children can easily be mistaken for autism. It is unknown how many children labeled as autistic have B_{12} Deficiency Acquired Brain Injury (BABI), but our guess is that the number is high.

Identifying such children *before* they suffer brain injury would prevent many tragedies, and it would do so while creating a huge savings in healthcare dollars. Michael Ganz, Assistant Professor of Society, Human Development, and Health at Harvard School of Public Health, puts the lifetime cost of caring for an autistic child at around $3.2 million. But Ganz believes this is likely an underestimate because this consists only of medical costs, such as visits to doctors' offices, medications, and therapies, and non-medical costs, such as adult care, childcare, and special education, and does not include costs due to lost parental income and income for people with autism.

Thus, it is critical that all children with developmental delay or a diagnosis on the autism spectrum have B_{12} deficiency ruled out. The cost of life-long care for a patient with BABI is similar to that of an individual with autism. Table 12 highlights the costs of occupational and speech therapy, as well as a typical autism program.

Table 12: Therapies/programs for children with autism in 2010

Therapy	Initial Evaluation	Cost per session	Cost per week	Cost per month	Cost per year
Speech	$300–$600	$67	$201 (3x/wk)	$804	$10,452
Occupational	$225–$400	$132	$264 (2x/wk)	$1,056	$13,728
Autism Program (2.5 hours per day, 5 days per week)				$4,000 for 19 sessions in a 4-week period	$48,000 (Less than 10% of all medical insurances cover any part of this cost.)

Table 13 outlines medications used to treat children on the autism spectrum. The prices reflect the usual starting doses of these medications, which are then adjusted on an individual basis.

Table 13: Medications commonly prescribed for autistic children

Medication	Approved age (in years)	Cost per month	Cost per year
Mellaril	2 and older	$16.77	$201
Haldol	3 and older	$12.74	$153
Adderall XR (extended release)	6 and older	$226.43	$2,717
Concerta	6 and older	$170.65	$2,048
methylphenidate (generic for Ritalin)	6 and older	$37.76	$453
Strattera	6 and older	$172.00	$2,064
Sinequan	12 and older	$24.14	$290
Wellbutrin	18 and older	$114.00	$1,368
Zyprexa	18 and older	$244.30	$2,932
Risperdal	18 and older	$246	$2,952
Seroquel	18 and older	$ 82.50	$990

Autism is largely considered an incurable disorder. B$_{12}$ deficiency, in contrast, is simple to diagnose and correct. In human terms, identifying B$_{12}$ deficiency in a child can mean the difference between a healthy, independent life and a lifetime of disability and dependence. Viewed from a financial perspective, early diagnosis of pediatric B$_{12}$ deficiency can save society millions of dollars. That's a huge return on an investment of only a few hundred dollars' worth of lab tests.

OTHER COSTLY CONCERNS

Two other costly areas of medical care deserve examination in this chapter, because both, as we have detailed, are linked to B$_{12}$ deficiency. These are the wide prescription of proton pump inhibitors, and the use of gastric bypass surgery as a treatment for obesity.

Chronic proton-pump inhibitor use:

Proton-pump inhibitors (PPIs) have been available for more than 20 years. Doctors prescribe these drugs for patients who have gastric or duodenal ulcers, for patients hoping to prevent stress ulcers, and also for patients who have gastroesophageal reflux disease (GERD), laryngopharyngeal reflux, Barrett's esophagus, gastrinomas, and Zollinger-Ellison syndrome.

Initially, proton-pump inhibitors were only intended for short-term use. However, most patients now remain on these drugs indefinitely. The majority are taking them to control symptoms of GERD. Doctors are complacent about prescribing these drugs, perceiving them to be very safe.

This is a misconception, because doctors are failing to remember the stomach's role in the absorption of vitamin B_{12}. Proton-pump inhibitors reduce stomach acid, which is needed to separate B_{12} from proteins—the first step in absorption. As a result, patients who take these medications chronically can easily become B_{12} deficient, especially if they have low B_{12} stores to begin with.

In 2008, $25.6 billion dollars were spent worldwide on proton-pump inhibitors. In 2001, General Motors Corporation spent $55 million just to buy Prilosec for its employees and retirees. Proton-pump inhibitors do have their uses, but we question why older adults are frequently placed on them, given that 30 percent of seniors suffer from inadequate stomach acid and gastric atrophy. Proton-pump inhibitors offer no value to these patients. Instead, these drugs reduce their existing B_{12} absorption as well as depleting their pocket books.

Gastroenterologists who perform endoscopies should always measure the stomach pH as part of the procedure. Many patients may have hypochlorhydria or achlorhydria. These patients may improve their symptoms by taking apple cider vinegar with meals, eating smaller and more frequent meals, and avoiding lying down after meals. Some patients may also have H. pylori and need an accurate diagnosis and treatment.

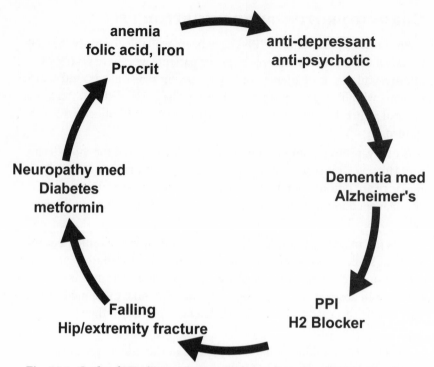

anemia
folic acid, iron
Procrit

anti-depressant
anti-psychotic

Neuropathy med
Diabetes
metformin

Dementia med
Alzheimer's

Falling
Hip/extremity fracture

PPI
H2 Blocker

Fig. 13.1. Cycle of Misdiagnosis: symptoms and medication history that
raise suspicion for B$_{12}$ deficiency.

GASTRIC BYPASS:

In 2010, gastric bypass surgery (GBS) cost on average between $20,000
and $36,000. In 2008, it was estimated that about 220,000 people in the
U.S. had weight loss surgery. Insurance providers, including Medicare and
in some states Medicaid, are paying all or part of the cost.

Physicians often recommend GBS for obese patients because they
believe it will prevent death or disability. Often, however, it does the
opposite. Why? Because clinicians fail to understand the role vitamin
B$_{12}$ plays in GBS (see Chapter 11). Most doctors do not screen for B$_{12}$
deficiency before surgery and, worse yet, many fail to prophylactically
place their patients on B$_{12}$ therapy or monitor their status. We have seen
countless GBS patients come to the emergency department with severe
anemia, fall-related trauma, or mental status changes because their health

care providers failed to understand that gastric bypass surgery will cause severe B_{12} deficiency over time.

For example, one patient was admitted due to mental status changes and to rule out a transient ischemic attack (mini-stroke), even though her symptoms were bilateral. She proved to have severe B_{12} deficiency and had undergone GBS four years earlier. Her hospital admission and array of diagnostic tests to rule out TIA and other B_{12}-related symptoms cost more than $18,000. This patient did not have a TIA, but proven B_{12} deficiency.

A more high-profile case involves Joanne Pearson, a 40-year-old woman who was crowned Miss Wheelchair Alabama in 2009. Joanne is in a wheelchair because her GBS led to severe B_{12} deficiency that destroyed her myelin, causing subacute combined degeneration of the spinal cord. By the time her deficiency was diagnosed, it was too late to reverse the damage. As a result, Joanne has no use of her legs and has only 60 percent use of her arms. Prior to developing B_{12} deficiency, Joanne had a high-paying job as a financial analyst for a Detroit radio station. She is now unemployed and on disability.

THE 10-CENT SECRET

As you can see from the numbers in this chapter, undiagnosed B_{12} deficiency costs society billions of dollars annually. Now, let's look at the other side of the coin: How much would it cost to prevent this tragedy? The answer, astonishingly, is less than ten cents per person per day.

If you're curious, here's the math. A 30ml vial of injectable B_{12} (hydroxocobalamin 1,000 mcg/ml) costs on average $36.00. Thirty-six dollars divided by 365 days equals $0.098, or 10 cents. This cost includes the initial series of injections followed by maintenance therapy. A 30ml vial of B_{12} contains enough for a patient to receive six initial injections (1,000 mcg) every day or every other day for six days, leaving a sufficient amount for bi-monthly 1,000-mcg injections over the next 12 months. Methyl-B_{12} lozenges (2,000 mcg daily) are slightly more expensive,

> Treating B_{12} deficiency costs as little as 10 cents per day.

costing around 13 cents per day. That's still quite a bargain, although as we've noted, more research needs to be done on the efficacy of oral B_{12} treatment.

Tables 14 and 15 list the monthly and yearly costs of different prescription and non-prescription forms of B_{12}.

Table 14: Monthly and yearly costs of different forms of B₁₂.

Prescription (Rx) B₁₂ and Non-prescription B₁₂	Cost per month	Cost per year
Folgard (cyanocobalamin 115 mcg, folic acid 800 mcg, vitamin B₆ 10mg)	$18.85	$226.20
Folgard RX (Rx) (cyanocobalamin 1,000 mcg, folic acid 2.2 mg, vitamin B6 25mg)	$25.68	$308.16
Metanx (Rx) (methyl-B₁₂ 2mg, L-methyl-folate 3 mg, vitamin B₆ 35 mg)	$35.92	$431.04
Cerefolin(Rx) (methylcobalamin 2 mg, L-methylfolate 5.6 mg, N-acetylcysteine 600mg)	$61.42	$737.04
Nascobal nasal spray (Rx) 500mcg/spray (2.3ml container) 8 doses in each container (given weekly)= $245.88/2months	$122.94	$1,475.28
Methyl-B₁₂ lozenges 2,000 mcg daily (Non-Rx) OTC	$4.04	$48.50
B₁₂ transdermal patch 1,000 mcg (4 patches) applied once weekly	$24.50	$294.00

Table 15: Monthly and yearly cost of injectable B₁₂

Medication	Qty	Dispensed	Cost per month	Cost per year
Cyanocobalamin (injectable) 1,000 mcg/ml = 1mg/ml IM or SC monthly	1ml	1 vial = 1ml 1 injection	$8.78	$105.36
Cyanocobalamin (injectable) 1mg/ml IM or SC bi-monthly	1ml	2 vials = 2ml 2 injections	$14.86	$178.32
Hydroxocobalamin (injectable) 1mg/ml IM or SC bi-monthly + initial 6 injections or 0.5mg SC every week + initial 6 injections (1mg = 1,000 mcg)	30ml	30ml multi-dose vial 30 injections	$3.00	$36.00
Methylcobalamin (injectable) Costs more because made up by compounding pharmacy. Used in patients with neuro-logical disorders (demyelinating diseases, CIDP, autism, MS, B₁₂ deficiency injury)	(varies) 7.2 ml	3 month supply 2.5mg/0.2ml SC 3 times/week 36 doses/ 3 months	$82.00 cost for 3 months	$328.00

THE BOTTOM LINE: SAVING LIVES AND SAVING MONEY

The statistics in this chapter paint a clear picture. The medical community's rampant failure to diagnose B_{12} deficiency is costing society billions of dollars annually for medical tests and treatments, nursing home or residential care, and disability payments. By comparison, the solution to this problem—testing for B_{12} and providing effective treatment for those who need it—costs next to nothing. The necessary tests add up to only a few hundred dollars, and we can provide treatment for about a dime a day.

> As you can see from the numbers in this chapter, undiagnosed B_{12} deficiency costs society billions of dollars annually.

So why does B_{12} deficiency continue to destroy so many lives and cost society so many billions of dollars? The answer is simple: ignorance. To combat this misunderstood and costly epidemic, we must educate medical professionals, the public, and government officials about the need for B_{12}-deficiency testing and treatment. In the next chapter, we lay out an effective plan for accomplishing this crucial goal.

14

A Call for a United Effort

In this book, we have exposed a major breakdown in America's medical system. An epidemic is raging, invisible to the public and virtually undetected by medical professionals. A safe, simple, and inexpensive cure exists, but only a minority of sufferers ever receives this treatment, or even an accurate diagnosis. As a result, hundreds of thousands of people suffer from this crippling disorder, or even lose their lives.

Clearly, action is needed to combat this invisible epidemic. On a national scale, all of us involved in the health-care system must combat B_{12} deficiency by standing up for the patients who count on us. This includes not only physicians, nurses, and other direct-care providers, but all others in a position to take positive action. For example:

- Nursing home and assisted living administrators must demand B_{12} testing for all of their patients, treat symptomatic patients in the gray zone, and use the urinary MMA test when indicated.

- Federal, state, and local agencies that provide medical screenings and other health-care services for the elderly need to make B_{12} screening part of their routine services.

> Each of us must play our part in stopping the B_{12} deficiency epidemic.

- Mental health professionals and psychiatric facilities must insist on B_{12} screening as part of their basic workup for all patients, including those with postpartum depression or postpartum psychosis.

- Professionals treating children with developmental disabilities must understand the role that B_{12} deficiency or impaired B_{12} metabolism can play in these disorders, and they must insist on B_{12} screening for all developmentally delayed or disabled children.

WHAT CAN WE DO TO STOP THIS EPIDEMIC IN ITS TRACKS?

✓ Raise the current lower limit of normal serum B_{12} from 200 pg/ml to 450 pg/ml.

✓ Raise the current daily recommended intake (DRI) to 1,000 mcg for adults and children (including during preconception, throughout pregnancy, and during breast-feeding).

✓ Raise awareness among medical professionals and consumers.

✓ Identify victims early.

✓ Test symptomatic and at-risk patients.

✓ Screen all adults age sixty or older.

✓ Include B_{12} screening in fall-prevention programs.

✓ Screen all people entering assisted living residences and nursing homes.

✓ Screen all patients diagnosed with mental illnesses.

✓ Screen all children with developmental delay or symptoms of autism.

✓ Develop state-of-the-art protocols for identifying and treating B_{12} deficiency.

✓ Use the active coenzyme form (methyl-B_{12}) rather than cyanocobalamin in tablets and lozenges.

✓ Pass legislation that recognizes an annual B_{12} Awareness Month.

✓ Enlist help from the media and governmental agencies to educate medical care providers and the public about the billions of health care dollars spent unnecessarily to treat serious medical disorders that could be prevented if patients with B_{12} deficiency were diagnosed early.

✓ Work with other countries to create a Worldwide B_{12} Awareness Day.

- Medical insurers must promote B_{12} awareness as a means of dramatically reducing health care expenses.

- Nurse case managers and clinical social workers must become aware of the problem of B_{12} deficiency and the role it plays in causing injury, reduced independence, disability and crowding of our long-term care facilities.

- Government agencies responsible for promoting public health must put the problem of B_{12} deficiency on their agendas, particularly with the huge Baby Boomer generation aging into the high-risk senior years.

- Consumers, too, must accept the responsibility for protecting their own health. To do this, they must insist on proper diagnosis and treatment if they are at risk for B_{12} deficiency (see Chapter 1). In addition, they must protect their loved ones—especially their children and their aging parents or grandparents—by serving as their advocates, if those in their care are in need of testing or treatment.

- Medical researchers need to study the absorption and neurologic efficacy of different forms of oral and injectable B_{12} in large patient populations.

Each of us must play our part in stopping the B_{12} epidemic—but to be truly effective, this effort must reach the highest levels. Thus, we call on the Surgeon General of the United States to implement an immediate "Call for Action" to combat B_{12} deficiency. This easily-diagnosed condition can be treated effectively for a few dollars per month per patient (literally ten cents per day!). Left undiagnosed, it costs our country's health-care system billions of dollars each year. We can think of no more crucial issue for the Surgeon General to address.

Education, awareness, prevention, and screening are desperately needed to combat this epidemic. A new protocol and standard of care change must be implemented in the medical community in the U.S. and around the world.

Whether you are a medical consumer or a medical professional, we hope you will join us in this battle to save millions of lives, save billions of healthcare dollars, and prevent untold numbers of tragedies. Together, we can stop this epidemic in its tracks. This is one of the most preventable and most curable of all medical scourges—*but only if we choose to act.*

Appendices

APPENDIX A: CAUSES OF VITAMIN B12 DEFICIENCY

- decreased stomach acid
- atrophic gastritis
- autoimmune pernicious anemia
- helicobacter pylori
- gastrectomy (partial or complete)
- gastric bypass surgery (weight loss)
- intestinal resection
- partial or complete ileectomy
- gastrointestinal neoplasms
- malnutrition
- inadequate diet
- vegetarianism
- eating disorders
- malabsorption syndromes
- alcoholism
- celiac disease (gluten enteropathy)
- Crohn's disease
- diphyllobothrium infection
- blind loop syndrome
- diverticulosis
- inflammatory bowel disease
- small bowel overgrowth
- tropical sprue
- gastric irradiation
- ileal irradiation (bladder, cervix, uterus, prostate)
- inborn errors of B_{12} metabolism

- transcobalamin II deficiency
- pancreatic exocrine insufficiency
- Imerslund-Gräesbeck syndrome
- Zollinger-Ellison syndrome
- advanced liver disease

DRUG INDUCED

- antacids
- colchicine
- H2-blockers (Zantac, Tagamet, Pepcid)
- metformin (Glucophage)
- proton pump inhibitors (omeprazole, Nexium, Prevacid, Protonix)
- nitrous oxide anesthesia
- nitrous oxide abuse (Whippets)
- mycifradin sulfate (Neomycin)
- phenytoin (Dilantin)
- para-aminosalicylates
- potassium chloride (K-Dur)
- cholestyramine (Questran)

INCREASED DEMANDS

- chronic hemolytic anemia
- hyperthyroidism
- multiple myeloma
- myeloproliferative disorders
- neoplasms
- pregnancy

APPENDIX B: SYSTEMS AFFECTED BY B12 DEFICIENCY

System	Pathology	Outcome
Neurologic	demyelination of CNS: posterior column disease, lateral column disease, spinothalamic tract, brain atrophy	paresthesia, ataxia, extremity weakness, paralysis, confusion dementia, depression, psychosis, incontinence, visual disturbances
Hematologic	bone marrow hypercellular, megaloblastosis, hemolysis, large metamyelocytes, pancytopenia	fatigue, weakness, anemia, hepatomegaly, splenomegaly, blood transfusions
Immunologic	impaired DNA synthesis, leukopenia, hypersegmented neutrophils	poor wound healing, increased susceptibility to infections, poor response to vaccines
Vascular	hyperhomocystinemia, enlarged heart, decreased left ventricular ejection fraction	occlusive vascular disorders (PE, CAD, DVT, CVA, TIA, MI) chest pain, exertional dyspnea, tachycardia, palpitations, CHF
Gastrointestinal	atrophic gastritis: increased goblet cells, parietal and chief cell atrophy gastric cytology: atypical cells, hepatomegaly, splenomegaly	indigestion, malabsorption, abdominal pain, weight loss, constipation, gastric stasis increased risk of gastric cancer
Musculoskeletal	proliferation of bone marrow, stromal osteoprogenitors and osteoblastic cells suppressed activity of osteoblasts	osteoporosis, poor bone density pathological fractures
Genitourinary	cervical dysplasia (atypical cells), neurogenic bladder	repeated Pap smears and GYN procedures (D&C, LEEP), hysterectomy, recurrent cystitis, incontinence, impotence, infertility

APPENDIX C: NEUROLOGICAL SIGNS AND SYMPTOMS OF B12 DEFICIENCY

- paresthesia (numbness, tingling, burning)
- weakness of legs, arms, trunk
- balance problems
- difficulty ambulating
- unsteady or abnormal gait—falls
- dizziness
- visual disturbances
- confusion/disorientation
- forgetfulness, memory loss, dementia
- disturbances in taste/smell
- tremor
- restless legs
- nocturnal cramping in arms and legs
- impaired pain perception
- diminished vibration sense
- impaired position
- impaired fine motor coordination
- muscular spasticity
- abnormal reflexes
- paralysis
- bladder or bowel incontinence
- impotence
- depression

APPENDIX D: PSYCHIATRIC MANIFESTATIONS OF VITAMIN B12 DEFICIENCY

- apathy
- irritability
- paranoia
- mania
- delusions
- violent behavior
- hallucinations
- psychosis
- personality changes
- post-partum depression/psychosis

APPENDIX E: HEMATALOGIC MANIFESTATIONS OF VITAMIN B12 DEFICIENCY

- anemia
- leukopenia
- ovalocytes
- macrocytosis (need not be present)
- thrombocytopenia
- low or normal reticulocyte count
- hypersegmented neutrophils
- anisocytosis
- poikilocytosis
- pancytopenia
- Howell-Jolly bodies

APPENDIX F: OTHER SIGNS AND SYMPTOMS OF VITAMIN B12 DEFICIENCY

- fatigue
- generalized weakness
- lack of energy
- pallor
- weight loss
- lightheadedness
- orthostatic hypotension
- syncope
- falls
- tinnitus
- shortness of breath
- exertional dyspnea
- tachycardia
- hepatomegaly
- splenomegaly
- loss of appetite
- anorexia
- sore tongue/glossitis
- constipation
- diarrhea
- premature graying of hair

APPENDIX G: SIGNS AND SYMPTOMS OF B12 DEFICIENCY IN INFANTS AND CHILDREN

- developmental delay
- developmental regression
- apathy
- irritability
- hypotonia
- weakness
- tremor
- involuntary movements
- seizures
- ataxia
- anorexia
- failure to thrive
- poor weight gain
- poor head growth
- poor socialization
- poor motor skills
- language delay
- speech problems
- lower IQ
- mental retardation
- anemia
- macrocytosis (need not be present)

APPENDIX H: WHO TO TEST AND WHO IS AT RISK FOR B12 DEFICIENCY?

- neurologic or motor symptoms
- mental status changes
- dementia or diagnosis of Alzheimer's
- psychiatric disorders (including depression)
- gastrointestinal disorders
- gastrointestinal surgeries
- gastric bypass patients
- anemia
- macrocytosis
- age 60 and over
- vegans, vegetarians, macrobiotic diets
- autoimmune disorders*
- family history of pernicious anemia
- proton pump inhibitor use
- metformin use
- anticonvulsant use
- diabetics
- cancer patients—chemotherapy and radiation
- hemodialysis patients
- nitrous oxide use or abuse
- eating disorders
- malnutrition
- occlusive vascular disorders (PE, DVT, CVA, MI)
- pregnant and nursing mothers
- breast fed infants of symptomatic or at risk mothers
- developmental delay in infants and children
- autism spectrum

APPENDIX I: DISORDERS WITH POSSIBLE UNDERLYING VITAMIN B12 DEFICIENCY

- dementia—Alzheimer's disease
- depression
- post-partum depression/psychosis
- multiple sclerosis
- peripheral neuropathies (e.g. diabetic, CIDP)
- vertigo
- anemia
- congestive heart failure
- autism
- AIDS dementia complex
- restless leg syndrome
- radiculopathy
- chronic pain disorder
- chronic fatigue syndrome
- fibromyalgia
- essential tremor
- Parkinson's disease
- erectile dysfunction
- infertility
- psychiatric disorders
- neurological disorders
- occlusive vascular disorders

*Hashimoto's thyroiditis, Graves' disease, Addison's disease, Type 1 diabetes, premature ovarian failure, hypoparathyroidism, hypogammaglobulinemia, agammaglobulinemia, vitiligo, idiopathic adrenocortical insufficiency.

APPENDIX J: REASONS THE ELDERLY ARE AT HIGH RISK FOR VITAMIN B12 DEFICIENCY

- poor stomach acid
- atrophic gastritis
- small bowel overgrowth
- preexisting diseases
- comorbid conditions
- low socioeconomic status
- antacid use
- prescribed PPI or H2 blockers
- metformin use
- elder discrimination
- depression/isolation
- alcoholism
- minimizing symptoms
- difficulty explaining symptoms
- increased incidence of thyroid disorders
- confusion—dementia
- poor appetites
- ill-fitting dentures/poor dentition
- sore tongue/mouth
- increased incidence of gastrointestinal disorders/surgeries
- increased number of gastrointestinal surgeries
- nitrous oxide administration

APPENDIX K: SIGNS AND SYMPTOMS OF VITAMIN B12 DEFICIENCY BLAMED ON AGING OR OTHER FACTORS

- fatigue
- depression
- neuropathy
- exertional dyspnea
- weakness
- anemia
- visual disturbances
- altered mental status
- confusion
- dementia
- dizziness
- syncope
- gait or balance disorder
- falls or fall-related trauma
- orthostatic hypotension
- increased susceptibility to infections
- tremor
- incontinence
- hyperhomocystinemia
- poor wound healing
- poor immune response to vaccinations
- another disorder diagnosed, therefore B$_{12}$ deficiency not considered

APPENDIX L: LABORATORY TESTS TO AID IN THE DIAGNOSIS OF VITAMIN B12 DEFICIENCY

- serum B$_{12}$
- urinary methylmalonic acid (uMMA)
- holotranscobalamin II (HoloTC)
- homocysteine
- serum MMA
- gastrin
- intrinsic factor antibody
- parietal cell antibody
- gastric secretion analysis (pH)
- peripheral blood smear

Note: The Schilling test I, II, and III are no longer readily available.

APPENDIX M: COBALAMIN DEFICIENCY CRITERIA LIST (CDCL) COBALAMIN DEFICIENCY RISK (CDR) SCORE

I. NEUROLOGICAL MANIFESTATIONS (+2 EACH)
- Numbness, tingling (including Dx of neuropathy)
- Weakness of legs, arms, or trunk
- Unsteady, abnormal gait or balance problems, including difficulty ambulating or near falls
- Dizziness or light-headedness
- Tremor (including Dx of Parkinson's)
- Restless legs or Dx of restless leg syndrome
- Visual disturbances
- Poor concentration or foggy thinking
- Forgetfulness, memory loss or (Hx of dementia/Alzheimer's)
- Mental status changes
- Impotence, erectile dysfunction
- Urinary or fecal incontinence
- Impaired vibration, position sense
- Abnormal reflexes
- Developmental delay (including Dx of autism)

II. PSYCHIATRIC MANIFESTATIONS (+2 EACH)
- Depression, suicidal ideations, post-partum depression, Rx of antidepressants or other psychiatric meds, Hx of any other psychiatric illness
- Irritability, anxiety
- Paranoia
- Mania
- Hallucinations
- Psychosis
- Violent behavior
- Personality changes

III. GASTROINTESTINAL RISK (+2 EACH)
- Decreased stomach acid or atrophic gastritis
- Gastric stasis or gastroparesis
- Helicobacter pylori
- GERD or ulcer disease
- Gastrectomy (partial or complete)
- Ileal resection (partial or complete)
- Gastric bypass or bariatric surgery
- Malabsorption syndromes
- Crohn's disease, IBD, IBS, celiac disease (gluten enteropathy)
- Chronic pancreatitis, pancreatic exocrine insufficiency
- Bacterial overgrowth (small bowel)
- Fish tapeworm
- Alcoholism
- Malnutrition or eating disorders
- (bulimia, anorexia)
- Advanced liver disease
- Zollinger-Ellison syndrome

IV. HEMATOLOGIC MANIFESTATIONS (+2 EACH)
- Anemia
- Macrocytosis
- Microcytosis
- Hypersegmented neutrophils
- Anisocytosis (elevated RDW)
- Leukopenia
- Thrombocytopenia

V. OTHER SIGNS / SYMPTOMS (+1 EACH)
- Generalized weakness or fatigue
- Apathy
- Shortness of breath, chest pain, or exertional dyspnea
- Pallor
- Orthostatic hypotension
- Hepatomegaly or splenomegaly
- Loss of appetite/weight loss
- Poor wound healing/ulcer/decubitus
- Cervical dysplasia
- Tinnitus
- Vitiligo
- Glossitis

VI. POPULATION AT RISK (+1 EACH)
- Age 60 and over
- Fall or fall-related injury in the past year
- Vegans, vegetarians, macrobiotic diets
- Autoimmune disorders including IDDM and/or thyroid disorders
- Family history of pernicious anemia
- Proton pump inhibitor or H2-blocker use
- Metformin use
- Nitrous oxide administration or abuse
- Multiple sclerosis patients
- Cancer patients
- Chemotherapy or radiation
- Occlusive vascular disorders (MI, CVA, DVT, PE)
- On folic acid therapy
- Pregnancy
- Breast-feeding
- Iron deficiency
- Infertility
- AIDS patients
- Fibromyalgia or chronic fatigue syndrome patients
- Chronic renal failure (hemodialysis patients)
- Neck/back surgery, or history of spinal stenosis

COBALAMIN DEFICIENCY RISK (CDR SCORE)

Low risk:	0–1
Moderate risk:	2–5
High risk:	6 or greater

APPENDIX N: LABORATORY DATA OF 12 PATIENTS PRESENTING TO A COMMUNITY ED WITH SYMPTOMS OF VITAMIN B12 DEFICIENCY

norms		211–911 pg/ml	4.5–11 s1000/mm3	11.7–15.7 gm/dl	34.9–46.9%	80.5–99.7 fl	11.5–14.5%		
Case #	age/sex	B$_{12}$	WBC	HgB	HCT	MCV	RDW	chief complaint	CDR score
1.*	44 F	185	8.4	10.7	31.8	80.7	15.6	syncope/trauma	12
2.*	51 F	211	6.5	6.8	20.3	97.9	16.2	dyspnea/weakness	11
3.	77 F	168	7.9	12.9	37.9	88.0	14.2	chest pain	10
4.	82 F	210	20.2	10.9	32.9	88.6	17.6	weakness (R side)	11
5.	89 F	156	4.4	12.2	35.5	102.5	12.3	fall - Fx wrist	9
6.*	52 F	146	4.6	11.4	33.5	109.8	15.5	abd. & back pain	18
7.	69 F	165	11.3	10.1	15.2	65.8	15.2	chest pain	11
8.	77 F	170	7.4	10.4	32.2	85.0	18.0	chest pain	16
9.*	57 F	186	3.1	14.3	41.1	92.1	12.8	left arm tremor	8
10.	59 F	172	3.9	12.9	40.6	87.6	14.4	fatigue/weakness	11
11.	51 F		2.9	6.3	19.0	136.3	32.2	severe fatigue	12
12.	19 F	240	7.52	14.6	43.9	102.2	15.4	elevated MCV	5

IBlank boxes: data not available
(*): Patient has history of thyroid disorder.

The first eight patients were from a 50-patient study from the Hospital A emergency department. Each had a Cobalamin Deficiency Risk (CDR) Score of three or more. Patients 9, 10, and 11 were not tallied in the percentages of the 50-patient study, for they presented after the 50-patient sample was collected. Patient 11 had a family history of pernicious anemia, and was treated with B$_{12}$ injections intermittently by her family doctor. Her MMA was 1.19 μmol/L (normal less than 0.4), Hcy 17 μmol/L (normal less than 15). Patient 12 presented before the 50-patient sample was started. Patient 12 was worked up and diagnosed with autoimmune pernicious anemia by a hematologist.

RESULTS:

1. 8/50 (16%) were found to have subnormal serum vitamin B$_{12}$ levels.
2. 10/50 (20%) were found to have serum B$_{12}$ levels from 212 to 350pg/ml.
3. 18/50 (36%) were found to have serum B$_{12}$ levels below 350pg/ml which warranted further workup.

DEFICIENT PATIENTS IN FIFTY-PATIENT STUDY:

- 8/8 (100%) were female
- 5/8 (62.5%) were anemic
- 2/8 (25%) were macrocytic
- 5/8 (62.5%) had elevated RDW
- 5/8 (62.5%) were over age sixty

- 3/8 (38%) had thyroid disorders
- 6/8 (75%) had decreased HCT
- 1/8 (12.5%) was microcytic
- 1/8 (12.5%) was anemic and macrocytic

APPENDIX O: LABORATORY DATA FROM HOSPITAL Z (SERUM VITAMIN B12<180 PG/ML); FORTY PATIENTS PRESENTING TO A COMMUNITY ED USING CDCL AND CDR SCORE

norms		180–914 pg/ml	M: 4.3–5.5 F: 3.7–5.3	M: 12.3–16.9 F: 11.4–15.9 gm/dl	M: 40–50 F: 34.8–46%	80–100 fl	11.9–15.1%		
Case #	age/sex	B₁₂	RBC	HGB	HCT	MCV	RDW	chief complaint	CDR score
1.*	42 F	134	4.46	13.3	38.3	85.9	12.1	chest pain	4
2.	46 F	177	4.83	13.7	41.8	86.5	17.1	chest pain	10
3.	54 F	131	1.37	5.5	15.2	111.2	21.1	unresponsive/fall	19
4,	59 M	157	5.94	16.0	48.0	80.9	14.4	seizure	5
5.	61 M	136	4.71	15.6	46.4	98.5	15.3	chest pain	6
6.	62 F	164	4.67	13.7	40.5	86.6	13.5	chronic back pain with radiculopathy	15
7.	69 M	143	4.59	15.7	45.7	99.5	11.8	dizziness/headache	10
8.*	74 F	107	5.05	14.9	44.5	88.0	14.5	syncope, (?) seizure	13
9.	74 F	151	3.99	10.7	32.5	81.4	13.8	chest pain	5
10.	78 M	167	3.44	10.4	31.6	91.7	13.6	weakness/TIA	7
11.*	79 F	90	3.19	11.7	34.7	108.5	19.0	dizziness/fall	10
12.*	80 M	84	4.33	14.2	41.9	96.5	13.6	right arm weakness with numbness	10
13.*	80 M	137	4.13	12.7	36.7	88.9	12.9	syncope	8
14.	81 F	99	4.46	11.5	34.4	77.0	16.5	TIA/fall/weakness	10
15.	81 F	161	4.44	14.2	42.3	95.0	13.9	weakness	14
16.*	82 F	147	2.82	8.6	25.2	89.2	14.0	light-headedness	13
17.	82 F	93	3.39	10.3	30.1	88.6	13.0	dizziness, fall	13
18.	83 F	166	3.91	12.2	36.2	92.4	14.3	cellulitis lower extremity	7
19.	86 M	131	4.26	12.9	37.4	87.7	13.6	fall	6
20.*	86 M	89	3.95	11.6	34.3	86.8	13.5	weakness/fall	12
21.	87 M	159	2.31	7.5	22.4	97.0	14.0	fall, left hip Fx	16
22.*	87 F	180	3.48	10.8	31.4	90.0	13.5	dyspnea, weakness	14
23.	89 F	179	4.50	13.4	40.5	90.1	13.1	unresponsive	8
24.*	92 F	132	3.59	11.3	32.8	91.2	12.1	fall, rib Fx	11

LABORATORY DATA FROM HOSPITAL Z (SERUM VITAMIN B12 181–211 PG/ML)

norms		180–914 pg/ml	M: 4.3-5.5 F: 3.7–5.3	M: 12.3–16.9 F: 11.4–15.9 gm/dl	M: 40-50 F: 34.8-46%	80-100 fl	11.9-15.1%		
Case #	age/ sex	B$_{12}$	RBC	HGB	HCT	MCV	RDW	chief complaint	CDR score
25.	35 F	192	4.34	9.7	30.3	69.8	15.5	chest pain	5
26.	39 M	208	4.22	14.8	43.0	101.8	12.1	headache	3
27.	44 F	200	3.35	11.5	33.6	100.1	12.6	abdominal pain	2
29.*	66 F	208	3.74	10.3	30.8	82.1	12.4	DVT/cellulitis	10
30.	66 M	208	4.83	15.6	46.1	95.3	13.1	abdominal pain, constipation	5
31.	69 F	205	3.62	10.3	31.4	86.7	15.2	fall/right hip Fx	15
32.*	70 F	194	4.73	13.9	40.7	85.9	14.1	mental status change	16
33.	73 M	210	4.67	15.0	43.7	93.6	13.1	syncopal episode	9
34.	74 F	198	4.36	13.5	39.3	90.2	11.8	abdominal pain	7
35.	77 F	190	4.26	13.2	39.0	91.4	13.4	dizziness, fall x 2	13
36.	79 F	199	4.13	11.8	35.2	85.2	14.2	cellulitis right foot	7
37.	82 F	203	4.80	14.8	43.9	91.6	13.6	syncope, confusion, gait disorder	11
38.	82 M	207	4.47	9.1	28.8	64.3	18.6	dyspnea, new onset of atrial fibrillation	7
39.	88 M	187	4.47	14.2	42.4	94.8	13.6	weakness, fell six months ago - Fx L5	12
40.	90 F	205	4.01	12.8	38.2	95.4	13.3	right-sided weakness	9

- 15/40 (37.5%) male
- 25/40 (62.5%) female
- 5/40 (12.5%) macrocytic
- 1/40 (.03%) macrocytic anemia
- 3/40 (.05%) microcytic
- 1/40 (.03%) microcytic anemia
- 13/40 (32.5%) anemic
- 24/40 (60%) decreased hematocrit
- 10/40 (25%) elevated RDW
- 8/40 (21%) under 60 years

- 6/40 (15%) chest pain
- 10/40 (25%) CHF
- 10/40 (25%) thyroid disease (designated with *symbol)
- 8/40 (21%) dementia
- 9/40 (23%) psychiatric disorder
- 24/40 (60%) neurologic manifestation
- 18/40 (45%) TIA/CVA
- 15/40 (38%) fell within the past year
- 15/40 (38%) H2-blocker/anti-secretory proton pump inhibitor

APPENDIX P: REASONS PHYSICIANS DO NOT SCREEN FOR OR TREAT VITAMIN B12 DEFICIENCY

- Knowledge deficit
- Not up-to-date with current literature
- Past prejudices
- Fear of poor reimbursement with treatment
- Do not believe it is their specialty's job or responsibility to screen for it
- Resistance to change
- Do not believe it is cost effective or needed
- Not familiar with reimbursement codes
- Believe too much effort in following up with patient's results (contacting family physician or patient)
- Ego
- Apathy
- Overworked, uninterested in adding another disease process to rule out
- Fear of increased liability to follow up with tests ordered (ED)

APPENDIX Q: EXAMPLES OF SUBSTANDARD CARE

- Telling patients they do not require parenteral B12 therapy when they have been receiving injections for years
- Obtaining a serum B12 level to disprove a patient's need, months or years after the patient has started receiving injections or B12 therapy
- Assuming a patient cannot have B12 deficiency because he or she is not anemic or macrocytic
- Not working up a patient for B12 deficiency when anemia or macrocytosis is present
- Not inquiring about a patient's B12 status when neurologic or psychiatric manifestations are present
- Prescribing other medications for B12 signs and symptoms
- Giving B12 treatment before testing for B12 deficiency
- Giving occasional B12 injections
- Withholding treatment
- Not screening the elderly
- Not screening symptomatic or at-risk patients
- Making the diagnosis of dementia/Alzheimer's without ruling out B12 deficiency
- Prescribing anti-depressants and anti-psychotics without ruling out B12 deficiency
- Medically clearing a psychiatric patient and sending to psychiatric facility before ruling out B12 deficiency
- Diagnosing B12 deficiency late when severe anemia has developed, requiring blood transfusions
- Improper, inconsistent, or miserly treatment
- Not giving a series of injections to rebuild a patient's B12 stores when found to be deficient
- Giving patients standard RDA doses of oral B12 supplements instead of high-dose (1,000 mcg or more) oral therapy or injectable therapy
- Placing patients on PPIs or H2-blockers and not periodically screening patients or placing them on B12 therapy for prevention
- Not giving injectable B12 to patients who have a diseased ileum or partial/total ileectomy
- Not placing gastric bypass patients on high-dose B12 or B12 injections prophylactically
- Not ruling out B12 deficiency in elderly patients who have sustained fall-related trauma

Appendix R: Why Is B12 deficiency an epidemic?

- Knowledge deficit among physicians and other health care providers
- Poor or absent screening in symptomatic and at-risk patients
- Current range for "normal" serum B$_{12}$ extends far too low
- Clinicians ignoring the neurologic manifestations of B$_{12}$ deficiency
- Clinicians not treating symptomatic patients whose serum B$_{12}$ levels are in the gray zone (200–450 pg/ml)
- Clinicians wait for enlarged red blood cells or macrocytic anemia to be present before testing or treating patients
- Elderly are frequently misdiagnosed due to increased incidence of preexisting diseases and comorbid conditions
- B$_{12}$ screening not included in older adults who fall or are at risk for falling
- B$_{12}$ screening not included in older adults with cognitive changes or dementia

Appendix S: Diagnostic ICD-9 Reimbursement Codes for B12 Deficiency

Anemia
281.0 pernicious anemia
281.1 vitamin B$_{12}$ deficiency anemia
281.9 megaloblastic anemia
285.9 unspecified anemia

Neurologic
355.9 neuropathy (unspecified site)
356.9 peripheral neuropathy
331.7 cerebral degeneration
336.2 subacute combined degeneration of spinal cord
780.97 altered mental status
781.9 neurological deficit

Other Symptoms
780.7 weakness/lethargy
781.2 gait disturbance
781.3 ataxia and lack of coordination
780.4 dizziness
780.2 syncope
783.2 weight loss

Malabsorption Etiologies
555.2 ileocolitis
555.9 enterocolitis (unspecified site)
579.3 gastrointestinal surgery
579.9 malabsorption not otherwise specified

Dementia
290.0 senile dementia, uncomplicated
290.1 presenile dementia
290.2 senile dementia with depression
294.1 dementia
297.1 paranoid psychosis, chronic
297.9 paranoid state, unspecified
300.9 mental status change
331.0 Alzheimer's disease/dementia

Psychiatric
296.2 depression
296.3 major depression
296.80 bipolar disorder, unspecified deficiency
266.2 vitamin B$_{12}$ or folate deficiency
266.9 unspecified vitamin B-complex deficiency

APPENDIX T: RECOMMENDED TREATMENT PROTOCOL FOR B12 DEFICIENCY

1. Serum B_{12} < 200 pg/ml: Severe B_{12} deficiency
    Serum B_{12} 200–350pg/ml: Moderate B_{12} deficiency
    Serum B_{12} 351–450pg/ml: Beginning B_{12} deficiency

2. If the patient is symptomatic and serum B_{12} levels are less than 450 pg/ml, treat the patient. Urinary MMA, holoTC, and homocysteine tests are optional regardless of stage. We advise treating all patients who are symptomatic regardless of metabolite markers or holoTC results.

3. If the patient is symptomatic and the serum B_{12} level is greater than 450 pg/ml

    A) Inquire if patient recently began self-treating with high-dose B_{12}

    B) Inquire if another clinician administered B_{12} shot in the past 12 months, patient received TPN or MVI intravenously

    C) Consider therapeutic trial of B_{12} and monitor response

4. If the patient has neurologic manifestations, consider a therapeutic trial of B_{12} injections. We recommend methyl-B_{12} or hydroxo-B_{12} (initial series; then weekly for 3 months) regardless of test results. Monitor response.

APPENDIX U: TREATMENT COST FOR INJECTABLE B12

Vitamin B_{12} (hydroxocobalamin) 1,000 mcg/ml (30ml) vial costs approximately $36.00 per year for treatment

1,000 MCG = 1MG = 1ML INJECTED = $1.20

- Initial 7 injections daily or every other day then;

- Maintenance: 1 ml IM or SC every 2 weeks = 24 ml per year or 0.5 ml SC every week = 24 ml per year

- Syringes with needles (quantity 30): 1 ml syringe with 25 gauge needle costs 29 cents each or $8.70 per year (we recommend using 27 gauge needle) or insulin syringe with needle

- 1 box of 100 insulin syringes with needles costs $28.56 and lasts over three years

- Injectable hydroxocobalamin (1,000mcg/ml) is manufactured by Abraxis BioScience, Phoenix, AZ 85043, USA, and distributed by Watson Pharma, Inc. Corona, CA 92880 USA. Prescription only: NDC 0591-2888-30 (30ml sterile multiple dose vial).

APPENDIX V: COUNTRIES AND TERRITORIES IN WHICH B12 DEFICIENCY HAS BEEN DESCRIBED IN MEDICAL JOURNALS

- Australia
- Belgium
- Brazil
- Canada
- China
- Costa Rica
- Cuba
- Denmark
- Dominican Republic
- Finland
- France
- Germany
- Guatemala
- Hong Kong
- India
- Indonesia
- Ireland
- Israel
- Italy
- Japan
- Korea
- Kuwait
- Mexico
- Netherlands
- New Zealand
- Norway
- Poland
- Portugal
- Russia
- Saudi Arabia
- South Africa
- Spain
- Sweden
- Switzerland
- Taiwan
- Thailand
- Turkey
- Ukraine
- United Kingdom
- United States

APPENDIX W: HISTORY OF VITAMIN B12*

- 1824: Combe describes the first case of pernicious anemia and its possible relation to the GI system.
- 1855: Combe and Addison identify clinical signs and symptoms of pernicious anemia.
- 1925: Whipple and Robscheit-Robbins discover factor in liver reverses anemia in anemic dogs.
- 1926: Minot and Murphy discover feeding large amounts of raw liver to patients with PA reverses their anemia. Study is underway for the active component in liver reversing anemia ("antipernicious anemia factor").
- 1929: Castle theorizes that an "extrinsic factor" in food and an "intrinsic factor" in normal stomach secretions are involved in the development of pernicious anemia. Administering both of these factors alleviates pernicious anemia.
- 1934: Whipple, Murphy, and Minot share the Nobel Prize in Physiology or Medicine for their life-saving discovery found in liver.
- 1948: Isolation of a crystalline red pigment is undertaken by Rickes (USA) and Smith and Parker (England). Substance is named vitamin B$_{12}$.
- 1948: Injections of B$_{12}$ shown to dramatically benefit pernicious anemia patients, demonstrated by West.
- 1949: Pierce and coworkers isolate and identify two crystalline forms of B$_{12}$, (cyanocobalamin and hydroxocobalamin), both effective in the treatment of pernicious anemia.
- 1955: Dorothy Crowfoot Hodgkin and colleagues discover the molecular structure of cyanocobalamin and its coenzyme forms using X-ray crystallography.
- 1955: Robert Burns Woodward and colleagues (USA) and Eschenmoser and coworkers (Switzerland) synthesize vitamin B$_{12}$ from cultures of specific bacteria and fungi.
- 1973: The entire chemical synthesis of vitamin B$_{12}$ is documented by Woodward and colleagues.

---

* http://www.vitamin-basics.com/index.php?id=57

Appendix X: Facts Regarding B12 Deficiency in Children

1. Inadequate B_{12} during pregnancy has been associated with adverse outcomes including neural tube defects, preterm birth, intrauterine growth-retardation, and recurrent miscarriage.

2. The most common cause of B_{12} deficiency in young children is maternal dietary deficiency, which typically manifests in breastfed infants at four to eight months of age.

3. Vitamin B_{12} is necessary for the normal growth and development of infants and children.

4. Cerebral and spinal cord lesions resulting from B_{12} deficiency are well-documented.

5. B_{12} deficiency can cause neurologic damage if untreated, and diagnosis must be made early to prevent permanent neurologic injury. Infants are more vulnerable to permanent damage.

6. B_{12} deficiency identified late in the infant or child causes lower IQ.

7. B_{12} deficiency is capable of causing mental retardation.

8. B_{12} deficiency can rapidly lead to failure to thrive, and if not promptly treated can lead to coma or death.

9. High-dose folic acid supplementation masks the traditional signs of B_{12} deficiency in the blood count (anemia and/or macrocytosis). High-dose folic acid is prescribed to all pregnant women in prenatal vitamins.

10. Many women of child-bearing age have undiagnosed celiac disease, autoimmune pernicious anemia, or B_{12} deficiency stemming from other causes (primarily dietary). These women's children are at high risk for B_{12} deficiency. Their risk of brain injury is increased if the mother breastfeeds.

11. Children who were found to be B_{12} deficient and then treated have lower IQs, "which suggests that at some stage minor cerebral damage may have occurred: this may have been in the latter part of their first years when they showed regression or slowing in motor development, or during their long periods without B_{12}." (McNicholl and Egan, *Pediatrics*, 1968, 42(1):149–156). As reported in a study of children of vegetarians, reduced IQ is common in children who have B_{12} deficits during early development, even if these children receive adequate amounts of B_{12} later in life.)

12. There is an increased use of proton-pump inhibitor (PPI) drugs in infants and young children due to gastroesophageal reflux disease (GERD). These drugs cause B_{12} deficiency with chronic use.

APPENDIX Y: KEY POINTS FOR DIAGNOSTICIANS

B$_{12}$ deficiency in infants that goes undiagnosed will lead to irreversible neurological damage. B$_{12}$ deficiency is progressive, and variable damage occurs to the brain, spinal cord, and peripheral nerves, depending on the duration of misdiagnosis. Early diagnosis and treatment may prevent significant long-term sequelae.

Vitamin B$_{12}$ deficiency in infants and young children may produce the following neurologic and hematologic signs:

- developmental delay
- developmental regression
- irritability
- weakness
- hypotonia
- ataxia
- apathy
- tremor
- myoclonus of the head, limbs, and tongue
- involuntary movements
- seizures
- anorexia
- failure to thrive
- poor weight gain
- poor head growth (microcephaly)
- poor socialization

- poor motor skills
- language delay
- speech problems
- lower IQ
- mental retardation
- hematologic abnormalities (but not a requirement)
- macrocytosis
- anemia
- thrombocytopenia
- pancyotpenia

Common Diagnostic Findings

- abnormal brain CT: cerebral brain atrophy, enlarged ventricles
- abnormal brain MRI: cerebral brain atrophy, enlarged ventricles
- abnormal EEG: generalized slow activity

APPENDIX Z: B12 AWARENESS

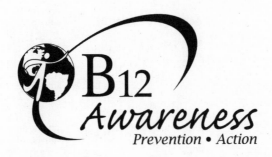

MISSION STATEMENT: UNMASKING THE EPIDEMIC OF UNDIAGNOSED VITAMIN B$_{12}$ DEFICIENCY THROUGH EDUCATION AND ADVOCACY.

B$_{12}$ AWARENESS GOALS:

1. Raise awareness of the dangers of B$_{12}$ deficiency by reeducating the medical community and educating the public

2. Promote early diagnosis and treatment to prevent neurologic injury, disability, poor outcomes, and premature death

3. Educate society on the role B$_{12}$ deficiency plays in overall health, cognitive decline and fall-related trauma

4. Enlist help from the media, Congress, and governmental agencies to expose and eliminate billions of wasted health care dollars

5. Protect the public and save lives

6. Promote further research

7. Pass legislation in the U.S. that recognizes September as B$_{12}$ Awareness Month

8. Work with other countries to create Worldwide B$_{12}$ Awareness Day

VISIT US AT: WWW.B12AWARENESS.ORG

OTHER INFORMATIVE B$_{12}$ WEBSITES:

www.B12D.org

www.B12.com

www.Pernicious-Anaemia-Society.org

Index

About the Authors

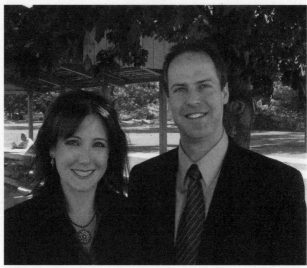

Sally Pacholok, R.N., B.S.N., an emergency room nurse with twenty-four years of experience, received her bachelor's degree in nursing from Wayne State University. Prior to entering the field of nursing, she received an Associate's Degree of Applied Science with magna cum laude honors. She was also an Advanced Emergency Medical Technician (A-EMT), and worked as a paramedic prior to and during nursing school. She has worked in health care for a total of thirty-two years, and has cared for thousands of patients. In addition, she is an Advanced Cardiac Life Support (ACLS) provider, and has assisted instructors at a local community college in training paramedics in ACLS. She is a Trauma Nursing Core Course (TNCC) Provider, an Emergency Nurse Pediatric Course (ENPC) Provider, and a member of the Emergency Nurses Association (ENA).

In 1985, Pacholok diagnosed herself with vitamin B_{12} deficiency, after her doctors had failed to identify her condition. As a result, she is passionate about the need to educate the public about the dangerous consequences of this hidden and all-too-common disease.

Jeffrey J. Stuart, D.O., a physician who has practiced emergency medicine for eighteen years, is board certified in this field. He is also certified in Advanced Trauma Life Support, Advanced Cardiac Life Support (ACLS), Advanced Pediatric Life Support, and Neonatal Resuscitation. Stuart received his Doctor of Osteopathy degree from the Chicago College of Osteopathic Medicine. His training includes field amputation and hazardous materials decontamination, and he has also participated in training sessions with the Detroit Metropolitan Airport SWAT team. Dr. Stuart participated in visual brain research at the National Institute of Mental Health in Bethesda, Maryland, in 1987, and was involved in cholesterol metabolism research at the Rockefeller University Hospital in New York City in 1985. He is a member of the American Osteopathic Association, the American College of Osteopathic Emergency Physicians, the Macomb County Osteopathic Medical Association, and the Michigan Osteopathic Association.